Probability and its Applications

Editors: J. Gani, C.C. Heyde, T.G. Kurtz

Springer
New York
Berlin
Heidelberg
Barcelona
Hong Kong
London
Milan
Paris
Singapore
Tokyo

Probability and its Applications

Rick Durrett

Probability Models for DNA Sequence Evolution

With 62 Illustrations

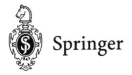 Springer

Rick Durrett
Department of Mathematics
Cornell University
Ithaca, NY 14853
USA

Series Editors

J. Gani
Stochastic Analysis
  Group, CMA
Australian National
  University
Canberra, ACT 0200
Australia

C.C. Heyde
Stochastic Analysis
  Group, CMA
Australian National
  University
Canberra, ACT 0200
Australia

T.G. Kurtz
Department of
  Mathematics
University of Wisconsin
480 Lincoln Drive
Madison, WI 53706
USA

Library of Congress Cataloging-in-Publication Data
Durrett, Richard, 1951–
    Probability models for DNA sequence evolution / Rick Durrett.
      p. cm. — (Probability and its applications)
    Includes bibliographical references and index.
    ISBN 0-387-95435-X (alk. paper)
      1. Genetics—Statistical methods.   2. Nucleotide sequence—Statistical methods.
    3. Probabilities.   4. Evolutionary genetics—Statistical methods.   5. Variation
    (Biology)—Statistical methods.   I. Title.   II. Series.
    QH438.4.S73 D87 2002
    572.8′38′0727—dc21   2002016001

Printed on acid-free paper.

Manufacturing supervised by Jacqui Ashri.
Photocomposed pages prepared by the author.
Printed and bound by Edwards Brothers Inc., Ann Arbor, MI.
Printed in the United States of America.

9 8 7 6 5 4 3 2 1

ISBN 0-387-95435-X   SPIN 10864650

Springer-Verlag   New York Berlin Heidelberg
A member of BertelsmannSpringer Science+Business Media GmbH

Preface

The generic question we address here is: Given a collection of DNA sequences, what underlying forces are responsible for the observed patterns of variability? Our tools are a variety of probability models. We begin in Chapter 1 with the simplest of these: the Wright-Fisher model, the coalescent, the infinite alleles model, and the infinite sites model. In Chapter 2, we confront the complications that come from nonconstant population size, recombination, and population subdivision in the form of the island (metapopulation) model or the spatially explicit stepping stone model. Chapter 3 considers the consequences of three forms of natural selection: directional selection, balancing selection, and background selection.

Chapters 2 and 3, which describe the footprints of various departures from neutral evolution in a homogeneously mixing population, prepare for Chapter 4, where we introduce four statistical tests that have been used to detect departures from this null model. The first four chapters are concerned primarily with the evolution of DNA sequences by small-scale processes: nucleotide substitutions, and insertions and deletions. In Chapter 5, we tackle the newer and less well-developed study of the evolution of whole genomes by chromosomal inversions, reciprocal translocations, and genome duplication. Throughout the book, the theory is developed in close connection with more than 50 examples from the biology literature that illustrate the use of these results.

This book is written for mathematicians and for biologists alike. With the first group in mind we assume no knowledge of concepts from biology. Section 1.1 gives a rapid introduction to the terminology. Other explanations are given as concepts arise. The only formal prerequisite for reading this book is a one-semester undergraduate course in probability, but some familiarity with Markov chains and Poisson processes will be very useful. My book *Essentials of Stochastic Processes*, also published by Springer-Verlag, provides all that you need to know in its Chapters 1, 3, and the first few sections of Chapter 4.

One of my motivations for writing this book was to help further my education about a subject that I find extremely interesting. I have worked in probability theory for twenty-five years but only for about five years in genetics. A number of the insights in this book are new, and quite likely some of those are wrong. However, I think that new readers will find this a generally reliable introduction to an exciting new area, and I think that experienced readers will find some new ideas as well.

Family Update. This is my sixth book and each has contained a family snapshot. My two children, David and Greg, are now teenagers (15 and 13). In the three years since the previous book, they played the online role-playing game *Everquest* for fifteen months and have played a number of computer games. Some of these games have been wholesome entertainment (*Civilization, Age of Empires, The Sims*) but most have involved killing things from a first- or third-person perspective. PC Gamer magazine with its demo disks has been extremely useful in allowing them to indulge their fascination in games for very little cost.

Everquest introduced David and Greg to the Internet, and they have taken to it like ducks to water, finding online games and a wide variety of comic strips. Sometimes they even use it as a resource for school projects, or they help their computer-challenged mother paddleboard around the Internet or cope with the high-tech chore of attaching a file to an email. Susan's lack of computer skills probably comes from the fact that she spends a lot of her energy dealing with her kid's braces, clarinet lessons, high school newspaper story writing, tutoring, homework, and social life. It is for this reason that we were all thankful that she had a good rest on our most recent summer vacation – having an appendectomy and spending five days in the hospital during our trip to visit her parents in California.

At this point, experienced readers probably expect a list of hard rock tunes that served as the background music while this book was being written. Unfortunately, my favorite alternative rock station, WNRV from Rochester, was bought by a corporation and now appeals to the type of person who drinks beer and plays Sega Dreamcast at 10 in the morning on Sunday, calling up every hour to request Ozzy Osborne's "Crazy Train." It remains to be seen whether my new Ithaca based Lite Rock stations will make the book better or worse. As usual, I look forward to learning from your feedback. Send your comments to *rtd1@cornell.edu* and watch *www.math.cornell/~durrett* for typos and other updates.

Rick Durrett   Ithaca, NY

Contents

1
Basic Models

1.1 The ATGCs of Life

Before we can discuss modeling the evolution of DNA sequences, the reader needs a basic knowledge of the object being modeled. Biologists should skip this very rapid introduction, the purpose of which is to introduce some of the terminology used in later discussions. Mathematicians should concentrate here on the description of the genetic code and the notion of recombination. An important subliminal message is that DNA sequences are not long words randomly chosen from a four-letter alphabet; chemistry plays an important role as well.

The hereditary information of most living organisms is carried by deoxyribonucleic acid (DNA) molecules. DNA usually consists of two complementary chains twisted around each other to form a double helix. Each chain is a linear sequence of four nucleotides adenine (A), guanine (G), cytosine (C), and thymine (T). Adenine pairs with thymine by means of two hydrogen bonds, while cytosine pairs with guanine by means of three hydrogen bonds. The $A = T$ bond is weaker than the $C \equiv G$ one and separates more easily.

The backbone of the DNA molecule consists of sugars (deoxyribose, dR) and phosphates (P) and is oriented. There is a phosphoryl radical (P) on one end (the 5' end) and a hydroxyl (OH) on the other (3' end). By convention, DNA sequences are written in the order in which they are transcribed from the 5' to the 3' end. Schematically we have

$$5' \qquad P-dR-P-dR-P-dR-P-dR-OH \qquad 3'$$

$$
\begin{array}{cccc}
| & | & | & | \\
A & C & C & T \\
\cdot\cdot & \cdots & \cdots & \cdot\cdot \\
T & G & G & A \\
| & | & | & |
\end{array}
$$

$$3' \qquad HO-dR-P-dR-P-dR-P-dR-P \qquad 5'$$

The structure of DNA guarantees that the overall frequencies of A and T are equal and the frequencies of C and G are equal. Indeed this observation was one of the clues to the structure of DNA. If DNA sequences were constructed by rolling a four-sided die, then all four nucleotides would have a frequency near 1/4, but they do not. If one examines the 12 million nucleotide sequence of the yeast genome, which consists of the sequence of one strand of each of its 16 chromosomes, then the frequencies of the four nucleotides are

$$A = 0.3090 \quad T = 0.3078 \qquad C = 0.1917 \quad G = 0.1913$$

Watson and Crick (1953a), in their first report on the structure of DNA, wrote: "It has not escaped our attention that the specific [nucleotide base] pairing we have postulated immediately suggests a possible copying mechanism of the genetic material." Later that year at a Cold Spring Harbor meeting, Watson and Crick (1953b) continued: "We should like to propose ... that the specificity of DNA replication is accomplished without recourse to specific protein synthesis and that each of our complimentary DNA chains serves as a template or mould for the formation onto itself of a new companion chain." This picture turned out to be correct. When DNA is ready to multiply, its two strands pull apart, along each one a new strand forms in the only possible way, and we wind up with two copies of the original. The precise details of the replication process are somewhat complicated but are not important for our study.

Much of the sequence of 3 billion nucleotides that make up the human genome apparently serves no function, but embedded in this long string are about 60,000 protein-coding genes. These genes are *transcribed* into ribonucleic acid (RNA), so-called messenger RNA (mRNA), which subsequently is *translated* into proteins. RNA is usually a single stranded molecule and differs from DNA by having ribose as its backbone sugar and by using the nucleotide uracil (U) in place of thymine (T).

Amino acids are the basic structural units of proteins. All proteins in all organisms, from bacteria to humans, are constructed from 20 amino acids. The next table lists them along with their three-letter and one-letter abbreviations.

Ala	A	Alanine	Leu	L	Leucine
Arg	R	Arginine	Lys	K	Lysine
Asn	N	Asparagine	Met	M	Methionine
Asp	D	Aspartic acid	Phe	F	Phenylalanine
Cys	C	Cysteine	Pro	P	Proline
Gly	G	Glycine	Ser	S	Serine
Glu	E	Glutamic acid	Thr	T	Threonine
Gln	Q	Glutamine	Trp	W	Tryptophan
His	H	Histidine	Tyr	Y	Tyrosine
Ile	I	Isoleucine	Val	V	Valine

Amino acids are coded by triplets of adjacent nucleotides called codons. Of the 64 possible triplets, 61 code for amino acids, while 3 are stop codons, which terminate transcription. The correspondence between triplets of RNA nucleotides and amino acids is given by the following table. The first letter of the codon is given on the left edge, the second on the top and the third on the right. For example, CAU codes for Histidine.

	U	C	A	G	
	Phe	Ser	Tyr	Cys	U
U	”	”	”	”	C
	Leu	”	Stop	Stop	A
	”	”	”	Trp	G
	Leu	Pro	His	Arg	U
C	”	”	”	”	C
	”	”	Gln	”	A
	”	”	”	”	G
	Ile	Thr	Asn	Ser	U
A	”	”	”	”	C
	”	”	Lys	Arg	A
	Met	”	”	”	G
	Val	Ala	Asp	Gly	U
G	”	”	”	”	C
	”	”	Glu	”	A
	”	”	”	”	G

Note that in 8 of 16 cases the first two nucleotides determine amino acid, so a mutation that changes the third base does not change the amino acid that is coded for. Such mutations are called *synonymous substitutions*; the others are *nonsynonymous*. For example, a change at second position always changes the amino acid coded for, except for $UAA \to UGA$, which are both stop codons.

In DNA, adenine and guanine are *purines* while cytosine and thymine are *pyrimidines*. A substitution that preserves the type is called a *transition*; the others are called *transversions*. As we will see in the discussion of Example 3.1 later in this chapter, transitions occur 10–20 times more frequently than transversions. One reason for this can be seen in the genetic code. At the third position, only the transition $UGA \rightarrow UGG$ (or vice versa) changes the meaning of the triplet but roughly half of the transversions do.

Roughly speaking, a gene is a collection of nucleotides that specify the amino acid sequence of a protein. The rules that govern genes are considerably more complicated than the genetic code. Genes in bacteria are typically one continuous piece of DNA. However, in higher organisms, genes typically consist of regions that are transcribed (called *exons*) separated by others (called *introns*) that are not. Some genes have only a few exons. In contrast, the *Dmd* gene discussed in Example 1.2 of Chapter 4 has 79 exons spread over 2.4 megabases of DNA that code for a 3685 amino acid protein.

The nontranscribed parts of the DNA upstream and downstream of the gene are called the 5′ and 3′ flanking sequences respectively. The 5′ flanking sequence contains several specific sequences that determine the point of initiation of the transcription process. The 3′ region contains signals for the termination of the transcription, and the introns have signals that guarantee they are spliced out of the mRNA. The details of these signals are not important for what follows, but we must remember that some mutations in introns or in the flanking sequence may not be harmless.

Most of the genes in our bodies reside on DNA in the nucleus of our cells and are organized into chromosomes. Lower organisms such as bacteria are *haploid*: they have one copy of their genetic material. Most higher organisms are *diploid* (i.e., have two copies). However, some plants are *tetraploid* (4 copies), *hexaploid* (6 copies, e.g., wheat), or *polyploid* (many copies, e.g., sorghum, which has more than 100 chromosomes of 8 basic types). Sex chromosomes in diploids are an exception to the two-copy rule. In humans, females have two X chromosomes, while males have one X and one Y. In birds, males have two Z chromosomes, while females have one Z and one W.

When haploid individuals reproduce, there is one parent that passes copies of its genetic material to its offspring. When diploid individuals reproduce, there are two parents, each of which contributes one of each of its pairs of chromosomes. Actually one parent's contribution may be a combination of its two chromosomes, since *homologous* pairs (e.g., the two copies of human chromosome 14) undergo recombination, a reciprocal exchange of genetic material that may be diagrammed as follows

$$aaaaaaaaaaaaaaa \qquad aaaaavvvvvvvvvv$$
$$\rightarrow$$
$$vvvvvvvvvvvvvvv \qquad vvvvvaaaaaaaaaa$$

Recombination will greatly complicate our analysis, so it is natural to want to ignore it. We will take our first steps studying the Y chromosome (which except for a small region near the tip does not recombine) and the mitochondria, about 16,000 nucleotides of DNA that exist in multiple identical copies outside the nucleus and are inherited from the maternal parent. However, recombination is important for limiting the effect of deleterious mutations and for determining the order of genes on chromosomes so we must eventually come to grips with it.

These definitions should be enough to get the reader started. We will give more explanations as the need arises. Readers who find our explanations of the background insufficient should read the *Cartoon Guide to Genetics* by Gonick and Wheelis (1991) or the first chapter of Wen-Hsiung Li's (1997) *Molecular Evolution.*

1.2 Wright-Fisher Model and the Coalescent

We will begin by considering a genetic locus with two alleles A and a that have the same fitness in a diploid population of constant size N with nonoverlapping generations that undergoes random mating. To explain the terms

A *genetic locus* is just a location in the genome of an organism. A common example is the sequence of nucleotides that makes up a gene.

The *two alleles, A and a,* could be the "wrinkled" and "round" types of peas in Mendel's experiments. More abstractly, alleles are just different versions of the genetic information encoded at the locus.

The *fitness* of an individual is a measure of the individual's ability to survive and to produce offspring. Here we consider the case of *neutral evolution* in which the mutation changes the DNA sequence but this does not change the fitness.

Diploid individuals have two copies of their genetic material in each cell. In general, we will treat the N individuals as $2N$ copies of the locus and not bother to pair the copies to make individuals. Note: It may tempting to set $M = 2N$ and reduce to the case of M haploid individuals but that makes it harder to compare with formulas in the literature.

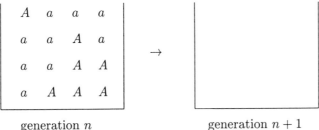

generation n $\qquad\qquad\qquad$ generation $n+1$

To explain the terms *nonoverlapping generations* and *random mating*, we use the picture on the previous page. In words, we can represent the state of the population in generation n by an "urn" that contains $2N$ balls: i with A's on them and $2N - i$ with a's. Then, to build up the $(n + 1)$th generation, we choose at random from the urn $2N$ times with replacement.

Remembering the definition of the binomial distribution, it is easy to see that the probability there are j A's at time $n + 1$ when there are i A's in the urn at time n is

$$(2.1) \qquad p(i,j) = \binom{2N}{j} p_i^j (1 - p_i)^{2N-j}$$

where $p_i = i/2N$ is the probability of drawing an A on one trial when there are i in the urn and

$$\binom{2N}{j} = \frac{(2N)!}{j!(2N - j)!}$$

is the number of ways of choosing j things out of $2N$ and $j! = 1 \cdot 2 \cdots j$ is "j factorial."

The long-time behavior of the Wright-Fisher model is not very exciting. Eventually, the number of A's in the population, X_n, will become 0, indicating the loss of the A allele, or $2N$, indicating the loss of a. Once one allele is lost from the population, it never returns, so the states 0 and $2N$ are *absorbing states* for X_n. That is, once the chain enters one of these states, it can never leave. Let

$$\tau = \min\{n : X_n = 0 \text{ or } X_n = 2N\}$$

be the *fixation time*; that is, the first time that the population consists of all a's or all A's. Since the number of individuals is finite, and it is always possible to draw either all A's or all a's, fixation will eventually occur. To compute the probability of fixation in the all A's state, let X_n be the number of A's at time n. Since the mean of the binomial in (2.1) is $2Np$ it follows that

$$(2.2) \qquad E(X_{n+1}|X_n = i) = 2N \cdot \left(\frac{i}{2N}\right) = i = X_n$$

In words, the average value of X_n stays constant in time. From this it follows easily that

$$(2.3) \qquad P_i(X_\tau = 2N) = \frac{i}{2N}$$

Why is this true? In the jargon of probability, X_n is a *martingale*, a process that can be thought of as a gambler's winnings in a fair game. Intuitively, if the game is fair then, on the average, the amount of money the gambler has at the end is the amount he had at the beginning. Thus, if we use P_i to denote the probability distribution of the process X_n starting from $X_0 = i$, and E_i to denote expected value with respect to P_i, then

$$(2.4) \qquad\qquad E_i X_\tau = E_i X_0 = i$$

Since X_τ is either 0 or $2N$, we have $i = E_i X_\tau = 2N P_i(X_\tau = 2N)$ and the desired result follows. $\qquad\square$

Proof of (2.3). It suffices to show (2.4). To do this, we note that (2.2) and induction implies that for any n, $E_i X_n = E_i X_0 = i$. Since $X_n = X_\tau$ when $n > \tau$,

$$E_i X_n = E_i(X_\tau; \tau \le n) + E_i(X_n; \tau > n)$$

where $E(X; A)$ is short for the expected value of X over the set A. Now let $n \to \infty$ and use the fact that $|X_n| \le 2N$ to conclude that the first term converges to $E_i X_\tau$ and the second to 0. $\qquad\square$

Remark. Throughout the book we will often derive formulas first by informal reasoning, as we have done here, and then follow up with a formal proof. Biologists (and even mathematicians) should feel free to skip the latter.

To get an idea how long fixation takes to occur, we will examine the *heterozygosity*, which we define here to be the probability that two copies of the locus chosen (without replacement) at time n are different:

$$H_n^o = \frac{2X_n(2N - X_n)}{2N(2N - 1)}$$

Let $h(n) = E H_n^o$ be the average value of the heterozygosity at time n. As we will now show,

$$(2.5) \qquad\qquad h(n) = \left(1 - \frac{1}{2N}\right)^n \cdot h(0)$$

Proof. It is convenient to number the $2N$ copies of the locus $1, 2, \ldots 2N$ and refer to them as individuals. Suppose we pick two individuals numbered $x_1(0)$ and $x_2(0)$ at time t. Individuals $i = 1, 2$ are each a descendent of some individual $x_i(1)$ at time $t-1$, who is a descendent of $x_i(2)$ at time $t-2$, etc. When $x_1(m) \ne x_2(m)$ the two choices of parents are made independently. Of course, if $x_1(m) = x_2(m)$, then we will have $x_1(\ell) = x_2(\ell)$ for $m < \ell \le n$.

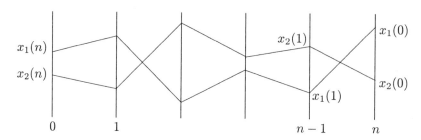

In the jargon of probability, $x_1(m)$ and $x_2(m)$ are *discrete time coalescing random walks*. In that model, $1, 2, \ldots 2N$ are thought of as spatial locations and are referred to as sites, while the moving objects are referred to as particles. When particles are on different sites, they jump independently, but when they land on the same site, they coalesce to become one. In order for the two chosen particles to be distinct at time n, the coalescing random walk paths must avoid each other at all times $1 \le m \le n$. Since, on each try, the second particle will land on the same site as the first one with probability $\frac{1}{2N}$, this event has probability $(1 - \frac{1}{2N})^n$. When the two paths avoid each other, $x_1(t)$ and $x_2(t)$ are two individuals chosen at random from the population at time 0, so the probability that they are different is $H_0 = h(0)$.   □

A Minor Detail. If we choose with replacement above then the statistic is

$$H_n = \frac{2X_n(2N - X_n)}{(2N)^2} = \frac{2N - 1}{2N} H_n^o$$

and we again have $EH_n = \left(1 - \frac{1}{2N}\right)^n \cdot H_0$. This version of the statistic is more commonly used but is not very nice for the proof given above.

When x is small we have $(1 - x) \approx e^{-x}$. Thus, when N is large, (2.5) can be written as $h(n) \approx e^{-n/(2N)} h(0)$, so the heterozygosity decays to zero exponentially fast as $n/(2N) \to \infty$. If we look at k individuals, then the probability of a collision when they all pick their parents from the previous generation is

$$\approx \frac{k(k - 1)}{2} \cdot \frac{1}{2N}$$

where the first factor gives the number of ways of picking two of the k individuals to be the ones to collide and the second the probability they will choose the same parent. Here we are ignoring the probability that two different pairs collide on one step or that three individuals will all choose the same parent, events of probability of order $1/N^2$.

By the reasoning used above, the probability of no collision in the first n generation is (when the population size N is large)

$$\approx \left(1 - \frac{k(k-1)}{2} \cdot \frac{1}{2N}\right)^n \approx \exp\left(-\frac{k(k-1)}{2} \cdot \frac{n}{2N}\right)$$

Recalling that the exponential distribution with parameter λ is defined by

$$P(T > t) = e^{-\lambda t}$$

and has mean $1/\lambda$, we see that if we let the population size $N \to \infty$ and express time in terms of $2N$ generations, that is, we let $t = n/(2N)$, then the time to the first collision has an exponential distribution with mean $2/k(k-1)$. Using terminology from the theory of continuous time Markov chains, k particles coalesce to $k-1$ at rate $k(k-1)/2$.

Here is a picture of the coalescent. For simplicity, we do not depict how the particles move around in the set before they collide but only indicate when the collisions occur.

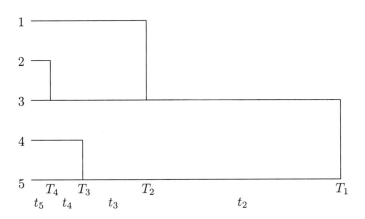

Let T_j be the first time that there are j lineages and let t_j be the amount of time that there are exactly j lineages. By the reasoning above,

(2.6) *When measured in units of $2N$ generation, the amount of time during which there are j lineages, t_j, has approximately an exponential distribution with mean $2/j(j-1)$.*

If we start with a sample of size k from the population, then the total time T_1 needed to reduce the sample through coalescence to a single lineage has

$T_1 = t_k + \cdots + t_2$ so the mean

$$(2.7) \qquad ET_1 = \sum_{j=2}^{k} \frac{2}{j(j-1)} = 2 \sum_{j=2}^{k} \left(\frac{1}{j-1} - \frac{1}{j} \right) = 2 \cdot \left(1 - \frac{1}{k} \right)$$

The reader should note that this quantity converges to 2 as the sample size $k \to \infty$, but the time, t_2, at which there are only two lineages has $Et_2 = 1$, so the amount of time spent waiting for the last collision is always at least half of the total coalescence time (in expected value).

In addition to keeping track of the number of lineages, we would like to record the genetic relationship between the individuals. To do this we will number the individuals in the sample as $1, \ldots, k$. The genetic state of the population at any time can then be represented as a *partition*, $A_1, \ldots A_m$, of $\{1, 2, \ldots k\}$. That is, $\cup_{i=1}^{m} A_i = \{1, 2, \ldots k\}$, and if $i \neq j$ the sets A_i and A_j are disjoint. In words, each A_i consists of one subset of particles that have coalesced and hence are identical by descent. To explain this notion, we will use the previous example. In this case, as we work backwards in time, the partitions are

$$
\begin{array}{llllll}
time & 0 & \{1\} & \{2\} & \{3\} & \{4\} & \{5\} \\
& T_4 & \{1\} & \{2,3\} & \{4\} & \{5\} \\
& T_3 & \{1\} & \{2,3\} & \{4,5\} \\
& T_2 & \{1,2,3\} & \{4,5\} \\
& T_1 & \{1,2,3,4,5\}
\end{array}
$$

Initially the partition consists of five singletons since there has been no coalescence. After 2 and 3 coalesce at time T_4, they appear in the same set. Then 2 and 3 coalesce at time T_3, etc. Finally, at time T_1 we end up with all the labels in one set.

Let $\mathcal{E}_k$ be the collection of partitions of $\{1, 2, \ldots k\}$. If $\xi \in \mathcal{E}_k$, let $|\xi|$ be the number of sets that make up ξ, i.e., the number of lineages that remain in the coalescent. If, for example, $\xi = \{\{1\}, \{2,3\}, \{4,5\}\}$, then $|\xi| = 3$. Let ξ_i^k, $i = k, k-1, \ldots 1$ be the partition of $\{1, 2, \ldots k\}$ at time T_i, the first time there are i lineages. Kingman (1982a) has shown

(2.8) *If ξ is a partition of $\{1, 2, \ldots k\}$ with $|\xi| = i$, then*

$$P(\xi_i^k = \xi) = c_{k,i} \, w(\xi)$$

Here the weight $w(\xi) = \lambda_1! \cdots \lambda_i!$, where $\lambda_1, \ldots \lambda_i$ are the sizes of the i sets in the partition and the constant

$$c_{k,i} = \frac{(k-i)! \, i! \, (i-1)!}{k! \, (k-1)!}$$

is chosen to make the sum of the probabilities equal to one.

The reader should note that the weight favors partitions that are uneven. For example if $k = 9$ and $i = 3$, a 3-3-3 split has weight $(3!)^3 = 216$ while a 7-1-1 split has weight $7! = 5040$.

Proof of (2.8). We proceed by induction working backwards from $i = k$. When $i = k$, the partition is always $\{1\}, \ldots \{k\}$, all the $\lambda_i = 1$, and $c_{k,k} = 1$ (by definition $0! = 1$). To begin the induction step now write $\xi < \eta$ if $|\xi| = |\eta| + 1$ and η is obtained by combining two of the sets in ξ. For example, we might have

$$\xi = \{1\}, \{2,3\}, \{4,5\} \quad \text{and} \quad \eta = \{1,2,3\}, \{4,5\}$$

When $\xi < \eta$, there is exactly one coalescence event that will turn ξ into η so

$$P(\xi^k_{i-1} = \eta | \xi^k_i = \xi) = \begin{cases} \frac{2}{i(i-1)} & \text{if } \xi < \eta \\ 0 & \text{otherwise} \end{cases}$$

and we have

$$(\star) \qquad P(\xi^k_{i-1} = \eta) = \frac{2}{i(i-1)} \sum_{\xi < \eta} P(\xi^k_i = \xi)$$

If $\lambda_1, \ldots \lambda_{i-1}$ are the sizes of the sets in η, then for some ℓ with $1 \le \ell \le i-1$ and some ν with $1 \le \nu < \lambda_\ell$, the sets in ξ have sizes

$$\lambda_1, \ldots \lambda_{\ell-1}, \nu, \lambda_\ell - \nu, \lambda_{\ell+1}, \ldots \lambda_{i-1}$$

Using the induction hypothesis, the right-hand side of $(\star)$ is

$$= \frac{2}{i(i-1)} \sum_{\ell=1}^{i-1} \sum_{\nu=1}^{\lambda_\ell - 1} c_{k,i} \, w_{\ell,\nu} \binom{\lambda_\ell}{\nu} \cdot \frac{1}{2}$$

where the weight

$$w_{\ell,\nu} = \lambda_1! \cdots \lambda_{\ell-1}! \, \nu! \, (\lambda_\ell - \nu)! \, \lambda_{\ell+1}! \cdots \lambda_{i-1}!$$

and $\binom{\lambda_\ell}{\nu} \cdot \frac{1}{2}$ gives the number of ways of picking $\xi > \eta$ with the ℓth set in η subdivided into two pieces of size ν and $\lambda_\ell - \nu$. (We pick ν of the elements to form a new set but realize that we will generate the same choice again when we pick the $\lambda_\ell - \nu$ members of the complement.)

It is easy to see that $w_{\ell,\nu} \binom{\lambda_\ell}{\nu} = w(\eta)$ so the sum above is

$$= w(\eta) \frac{c_{k,i}}{i(i-1)} \sum_{\ell=1}^{i-1} \sum_{\nu=1}^{\lambda_\ell - 1} 1$$

The double sum $= \sum_{\ell=1}^{i-1} (\lambda_\ell - 1) = k - (i-1)$. The last detail to check is that

$$\frac{c_{k,i}}{i(i-1)} \cdot (k - i + 1) = c_{k,i-1}$$

but this is clear from the definition.   □

In (2.8), the first and last partitions are trivial. $\xi_k^k = \{\{1\}, \ldots \{k\}\}$ is the finest possible partition. $\xi_1^k = \{1, 2, \ldots k\}$ is the coarsest. Given any partition $\xi = \{A_1, \ldots A_j\}$, we let

$$\text{size}\,(\xi) = \{\lambda_1, \ldots \lambda_j\}$$

where λ_i is the number of points in A_i and the set braces are there to indicate that the order in which the sizes are written is not important. The second coarsest partition ξ_2^k consists of two sets. Using our new notation, $\text{size}\,(\xi_2^k) = \{i, k-i\}$ for some $i \in [1, k-1]$. (Note that if $i = k-i$ we regard this as a set with two identical elements.) Using (2.8) and supposing for the moment that $i \neq (k-i)$, we have

$$P(\text{size}\,(\xi_2^k) = \{i, k-i\}) = c_{k,2}\, i!(k-i)! \binom{k}{i}$$

where the third term gives the number of ξ with size $(\xi_2^k) = \{i, k-i\}$. It follows that if $i \neq k-i$

$$(2.9a) \qquad P(\text{size}\,(\xi_2^k) = \{i, k-i\}) = c_{k,2}\, k! = \frac{(k-2)!\,2!\,1!}{(k-1)!} = \frac{2}{k-1}$$

In the case $i = k-i$, the third term changes and the result is

$$(2.9b) \qquad P(\text{size}\,(\xi_2^k) = \{i, k-i\}) = c_{k,2}\, i!(k-i)! \binom{k}{i} \cdot \frac{1}{2} = \frac{1}{k-1}$$

To illustrate the use of these formulas, consider the special case $k = 6$. In this case, the probabilities for the various partitions are

$$1/5 : \frac{2}{5} \qquad 2/4 : \frac{2}{5} \qquad 3/3 : \frac{1}{5}$$

Note that if we randomly assign the label "left" to one half of the partition then the left half has size 1, 2, 3, 4, or 5 with probability 1/5 each. The last observation generalizes easily to a sample of size k. If we randomly label the two sets then the left one has a size that is uniformly distributed on $1, 2, \ldots k-1$. This result is due to Tajima (1983).

We leave it to the reader to use (2.8) to compute the distribution of size(ξ_3^k). In the proof of (3.14) we will see that if the three sets in the partition are randomly labeled 1, 2, 3 and λ_i is the size of the ith set, then $(\lambda_1, \lambda_2, \lambda_3)$ is uniformly distributed over the set of all triples of positive integers that add up to k.

We turn now to a result of Cannings (1974) that is remarkable because it gives ALL of the eigenvalues of the transition matrix for a collection of models that generalize the Wright-Fisher model. To explain the generalization we need some definitions. Let y_i be the number of children of the ith individual and suppose that $(y_1, \ldots y_{2N})$ is *exchangeable*, i.e., the joint distribution is not changed if we permute the labels. This is true for the Wright-Fisher model since in that case the y_i have a symmetric multinomial distribution. However, one can also consider conditioned branching processes in which the family sizes are independent and identically distributed random variables conditioned to have their sum equal to $2N$.

(2.10) Let X_n denote the number of A alleles in generation n and define the transition probability $p_{ij} = P(X_{n+1} = j | X_n = i)$. The eigenvalues of p_{ij} are $\lambda_0 = 1$ and

$$\lambda_j = E(y_1 y_2 \ldots y_j) \quad \text{for } 1 \leq j \leq 2N$$

Proof. Suppose a nonsingular matrix Z and an upper triangular matrix A can be found so that $PZ = ZA$. Since this implies $P = ZAZ^{-1}$, the eigenvalues of P are the same as those of A. Since A is upper triangular, its eigenvalues are its diagonal elements. To check this matrix fact, note that $A - a_{ii}I$ is not invertible since a linear combination of rows numbered i and higher will be 0.

Let $Z_{kj} = k^j$ with the convention that $0^0 = 1$. With this choice of Z,

$$(PZ)_{ij} = \sum_k p_{ik} k^j = E(X_{n+1}^j | X_n = i)$$

To prove the result now, we want to show that there is an upper triangular matrix A so that

$$E(X_{n+1}^j | X_n = i) = (ZA)_{ij} = \sum_{k=0}^{j} i^k a_{kj}$$

The result is trivial for $j = 0$ since $a_{00} = 1$. When $j = 1$ we have $a_{11} = 1 = Ey_1$ since $E(y_1 + \cdots + y_{2N}) = 2N$. To verify the result for $j = 2$ we note that exchangeability implies

$$\begin{aligned} E(X_{n+1}^2 | X_n = i) &= E(y_1 + \cdots + y_i)^2 = i(i-1)E(y_1 y_2) + iE(y_1^2) \\ &= i^2 E(y_1 y_2) + i[E(y_1^2) - E(y_1 y_2)] = a_{22} i^2 + a_{12} i \end{aligned}$$

Careful readers will note that the second equality implicitly assumes $i \geq 2$ but also holds for $i = 1$. When $j = 3$ we have

$$E(X_{n+1}^3 | X_n = i) = i(i-1)(i-2)E(y_1 y_2 y_3) + 3i(i-1)E(y_1^2 y_2) + iE(y_1^3)$$

a result that remains valid for $i < 3$. Rearranging the right-hand side gives an expression of the form $a_{33} i^3 + a_{23} i^2 + a_{13} i$ with $a_{33} = E(y_1 y_2 y_3)$. There are more terms on the right-hand side when $j > 3$, but the same pattern continues. The highest-order term in i is i^j and has coefficient $a_{jj} = E(y_1 y_2 \cdots y_j)$. Since the diagonal entries of a are the eigenvalues of P, the proof is complete. $\square$

The eigenvalues $\lambda_0 = 1$ and $\lambda_1 = 1$ correspond to the eigenvectors $(1, 0, \ldots, 0)$ and $(0, \ldots, 0, 1)$. The first nontrivial eigenvalue is

$$\lambda_2 = E(y_1 y_2)$$

To compute this we note that $y_1 + \cdots + y_{2N} = 2N$ and $Ey_i = 1$ so

$$0 = \text{var}(y_1 + \cdots + y_{2N}) = 2N \text{ var}(y_1) + 2N(2N - 1)\{E(y_1 y_2) - 1\}$$

From this we see that if $\text{var}(y_1) = \sigma^2$ then

$$E(y_1 y_2) = 1 - \frac{\sigma^2}{2N - 1}$$

In the Wright-Fisher model, y_1 is binomial$(2N, 1/2N)$, so $\text{var}(y_1) = 1 - 1/2N$ and $\lambda_2 = 1 - 1/2N$. Comparing this with the rate of decay of the homozygosity given in (2.5), we conclude that the corresponding eigenvector has components $v_i = i(2N - i)$.

Mutations

Suppose now that after you sample from the urn at time n, and before you drop the result in the urn at time $n + 1$, an a turns to A with probability u and an A turns into an a with probability v. Again, the probability there are j A's at time $n + 1$ when there are i at time n is given by the formula in (2.1)

$$(2.11a) \qquad p(i, j) = \binom{2N}{j} p_i^j (1 - p_i)^{2N-j}$$

but now the probability p_i of drawing an A when the number of A's in the urn is i becomes:

$$(2.11b) \qquad p_i = \frac{i}{2N} \cdot (1 - v) + \frac{2N - i}{2N} \cdot u$$

In words, either we draw an A and it doesn't change or we draw an a and it does. The transition probability for the model with mutation has $p(i, j) > 0$ for all i, j. Since the number of possible states of our system is finite, it follows that as the number of generations $n \to \infty$, $P(X_n = i)$ converges to a limit $\pi(i)$, which is the unique *stationary distribution* for the Markov chain, that is, the unique solution of

$$\sum_i \pi(i) p(i, j) = \pi(j)$$

with $\pi(i) \geq 0$ and $\sum_i \pi(i) = 1$.

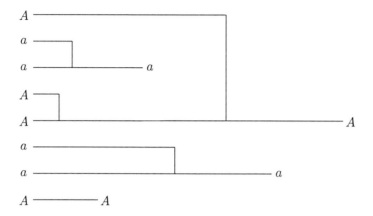

The stationary distribution can be calculated from the last formula but it is easier to understand when it is described in terms of a modification of the coalescent in which particles are killed and labeled with A with probability u, killed and labeled with a with probability v, or jump to a randomly chosen point with probability $1-u-v$. (Again we assume u and v are small and ignore two mutations on one time step.) Killing a particle determines its state and that of all of its descendents. If all of the particles are killed before we work our way back to the initial condition, then the state at time n does not depend on the initial configuration and the process is in equilibrium. Therefore, the random configuration determined by running this process to completion gives the stationary distribution for the Wright-Fisher model with mutation and X_n converges to this distribution as $n \to \infty$. The figure above shows a possible realization of the construction.

To gain some insight into the properties of the limiting distribution $X_\infty = \lim_{n\to\infty} X_n$, we will now compute its moments

(2.12) $$EX_\infty = 2N\rho = 2N \cdot \frac{u}{u+v}$$

If one thinks in terms of the coalescent with killing, the last conclusion is obvious. Each of the $2N$ lineages will eventually encounter an A or an a. The probability that an A will be encountered first is $\rho = u/(u+v)$.

Proof of (2.12). We first look at the behavior of the mean $\mu(n) = EX_n$. From (2.11) it follows that

(a) $$EX_{n+1} = (1-v) \cdot EX_n + (2N - EX_n) \cdot u$$

Setting $x = EX_n = EX_{n+1}$ gives

(b) $$x = (1-v)x + (2N - x)u$$

Solving, we have $(v + u)x = 2Nu$ or $x = 2Nu/(u + v)$. To see that EX_n will converge to this limit, we note that setting $x = 2N\rho$ in (b) gives

$$2N\rho = 2N(1 - v)\rho + 2N(1 - \rho)u$$

and subtracting this from (a) we have

$$E(X_{n+1} - 2N\rho) = (1 - u - v)E(X_n - 2N\rho)$$

so if $0 < u + v < 2$ we have $EX_n \to 2N\rho$ as $n \to \infty$.   □

Notation. In this proof and the ones that follow we use letters to label formulas that are only of local importance. We will reuse the same letters in later proofs, see e.g., (2.14).

With a little more work one can compute the second moment of the equilibrium distribution. The first step in doing this is the following result that is of interest in its own right. We say that two individuals are *identical by descent* if their lineages coalesce before a mutation affects either lineage. In the current application $\mu = u + v$ but later it will be useful to have the formula for a general mutation rate μ.

(2.13) If μ is the probability of mutation in one generation, then the probability that two individuals are identical by descent is (when μ is small and N is large)

$$\approx \frac{1/2N}{2\mu + 1/2N} = \frac{1}{1 + 4N\mu}$$

Proof. On each step, we can have mutation occur to one of the lineages, an event of probability $p_1 = 2\mu$, or coalescence, an event of probability $p_2 = 1/2N$. By considering one cycle, we see that the probability, ρ, of mutation before coalescence satisfies

$$\rho = p_1 + (1 - p_1)(1 - p_2)\rho$$

since if neither event happens the game starts again. Ignoring the possibility that both mutation and coalescence occur on one step we can write the last equation as

$$\rho = p_1 + (1 - p_1 - p_2)\rho$$

and solve to find $\rho = p_1/(p_1 + p_2)$.   □

We are now ready to state the formula for the variance:

$$(2.14) \qquad \text{var}\,(X_\infty) = \left(2N + \frac{2N(2N - 1)}{1 + 4N(u + v)}\right)\frac{uv}{(u + v)^2}$$

Proof. To compute EX_∞^2 now, we begin by writing $X_\infty = \sum_{i=1}^{2N} \eta_i$, where $\eta_i = 1$ if the ith individual is A and 0 otherwise. In probability theory, the η_i

are called *indicator variables* since they indicate whether an event occurred or not. As the next calculation indicates, they are a useful bookkeeping device. Squaring the sum, we have

$$
(a) \qquad\qquad X_\infty^2 = \sum_{i=1}^{2N} \sum_{j=1}^{2N} \eta_i \eta_j
$$

Separating the $2N$ terms with $i = j$ from the $2N(2N-1)$ with $i \neq j$ gives

$$
(b) \qquad E(X_\infty^2) = 2NP(\eta_1 = 1) + 2N(2N-1)P(\eta_1 = 1, \eta_2 = 1)
$$

From (2.12), $P(\eta_1 = 1) = u/u + v$. Considering the possibilities of coalescence before mutation or not, and using (2.13) with $\mu = u + v$, it follows that

$$
(c) \qquad P(\eta_1 = 1, \eta_2 = 1) = \frac{1}{1 + 4N\mu} \frac{u}{u+v} + \frac{4N\mu}{1+4N\mu} \left(\frac{u}{u+v} \right)^2
$$

Writing

$$
(EX_\infty)^2 = \left(2N + 2N(2N-1) \left\{ \frac{1}{1+4N\mu} + \frac{4N\mu}{1+4N\mu} \right\} \right) \cdot \left(\frac{u}{u+v} \right)^2
$$

and using (a)–(c) gives the stated result.   □

With more work, one can compute higher moments $E(X_\infty^k)$. To simplify things, we will only consider $m_k = \lim_{N\to\infty} E(X_\infty/2N)^k$. One motivation for doing this is that if one knows all of the moments, then (in most cases) one can compute the underlying distribution. See (2.17).

(2.15) If $4Nu \to q$ and $4Nv \to r$ then

$$
m_k = \frac{(q+k-1)\cdots(q+1)q}{(q+r+k-1)\cdots(q+r+1)(q+r)}
$$

Proof. To begin, we recall that the generating function of a probability distribution p_m on the nonnegative integers is defined by $\sum_{m=0}^\infty p_m s^m$. The binomial$(n,p)$ distribution has generating function

$$
\sum_{m=0}^{n} \binom{n}{m} p^m (1-p)^{n-m} s^m = (ps + 1 - p)^n
$$

Differentiating k times with respect to s gives

$$
\sum_{m=0}^{n} \binom{n}{m} p^m (1-p)^{n-m} s^{m-k} m(m-1)\cdots(m-k+1)
$$
$$
= n(n-1)\cdots(n-k+1)(ps+1-p)^{n-k}p^k
$$

Setting $s = 1$, it follows that if $X = $ binomial(n,p), then

$$
E(X(X-1)\cdots(X-k+1)) = n(n-1)\cdots(n-k+1)p^k
$$

Using this with (2.11), it follows that

$$E(X_n(X_n - 1)\cdots(X_n - k + 1)|X_{n-1} = i) = 2N(2N - 1)\cdots(2N - k + 1)p_i^k$$

where $p_i = (\frac{i}{2N})(1 - u - v) + u$. A little algebra shows

$$(2N)^{-k}2N(2N - 1)\cdots(2N - k + 1) = 1 - \frac{1}{2N}\sum_{j=1}^{k-1} j + O(N^{-2})$$

$$= 1 - \frac{k(k - 1)}{4N} + O(N^{-2})$$

where $O(N^{-2})$ indicates that we have ignored terms of order $1/N^2$ or smaller. An almost identical computation shows

$$E((2N)^{-k}X_n(X_n - 1)\cdots(X_n - k + 1))$$

$$= E\left(\frac{X_n}{2N}\right)^k - \frac{k(k - 1)}{4N}E\left(\frac{X_n}{2N}\right)^{k-1} + O(N^{-2})$$

A similar computation shows that if $u = q/4N$ and $v = r/4N$, then

$$p_i^k = \left(\frac{i}{2N}\right)^k + k\left(\frac{i}{2N}\right)^{k-1}\left(\frac{q}{4N} - \frac{i}{2N}\frac{q + r}{4N}\right) + O(N^{-2})$$

Combining the last four equations, we have

$$E\left(\frac{X_n}{2N}\right)^k - \frac{k(k - 1)}{4N}E\left(\frac{X_n}{2N}\right)^{k-1} + O(N^{-2})$$

$$= E\left(\frac{X_{n-1}}{2N}\right)^k\left(1 - \frac{k(k - 1)}{4N}\right) + \frac{qk}{4N}E\left(\frac{X_{n-1}}{2N}\right)^{k-1}$$

$$- \frac{(q + r)k}{4N}E\left(\frac{X_{n-1}}{2N}\right)^k + O(N^{-2})$$

Letting $n \to \infty$, it follows that the stationary distribution has

$$\frac{k(q + r + k - 1)}{4N}E\left(\frac{X_\infty}{2N}\right)^k = \frac{k(q + k - 1)}{4N}E\left(\frac{X_\infty}{2N}\right)^{k-1} + O(N^{-1})$$

Letting $N \to \infty$ now, we have

$$m_k = \frac{q + k - 1}{q + r + k - 1}m_{k-1}$$

Since (2.11) implies $m_1 = u/(u + v) = q/(q + r)$, the result follows.   □

Moran model

The Wright-Fisher model considers nonoverlapping generations, as one has in annual plants and the deer herds of upstate New York. However, in many species, e.g., humans, the generations are not synchronized and it is convenient to use a model due to Moran (1958) in which only one individual changes at a time. In the Wright-Fisher model, the $2N$ copies of our locus could come either from N diploid individuals or $2N$ haploid individuals (who have one copy of their genetic material in each cell). As the reader will see, in our formulation of the *Moran model* we must think in terms of $2N$ haploid individuals. We use $2N$ rather than N to get rid of one factor of two that differentiates the Moran model from the Wright-Fisher model.

(i) Each individual is replaced at rate 1. That is, individual x lives for an exponentially distributed amount with mean 1 and then is "replaced."

(ii) To replace individual x, we choose at random from the set of individuals (including x itself).

(iii) An a that is chosen mutates to A with probability u. An A that is chosen mutates to a with probability v.

(iv) The new, possibly mutated, letter replaces the old one at x.

By (2.11) the probability that a choice results in an A when there are i in the population is

$$p_i = \frac{i}{2N} \cdot (1 - v) + \frac{2N - i}{2N} \cdot u$$

With this notation in hand, we can write the transition rates for the Moran model as

$$i \to i+1 \quad \text{at rate} \quad b_i = \frac{2N - i}{2N} \cdot p_i$$

$$i \to i-1 \quad \text{at rate} \quad d_i = \frac{i}{2N} \cdot (1 - p_i)$$

In words, we can only gain an A if a site with a is chosen to be replaced and we succeed in picking an A. If $\pi(i)$ is the probability of i in equilibrium, then by considering the rate at which jumps occur across a line drawn between $i - 1$ and i, we have

$$\pi(i)d_i = \pi(i - 1)b_{i-1}$$

Rearranging shows $\pi(i) = \pi(i - 1)b_{i-1}/d_i$. Iterating gives that if $k < i$

(2.16)
$$\pi(i) = \pi(k) \prod_{j=k+1}^{i} \frac{b_{j-1}}{d_j}$$

(2.16) shows that if we specify one probability $\pi(k)$ we can compute all of the others. This gives us one free parameter we can choose to make the probabilities sum to 1.

This formula in (2.16) is not very explicit but is easy to evaluate numerically. To see what the stationary distribution looks like in a concrete case we will consider a population of size $2N = 20$ (that is, $N = 10$ diploid individuals). If we choose mutation rates $u = 0.1$ and $v = 0.2$ so that $2Nu = 2$ and $2Nv = 4$, then the stationary distribution has the following shape

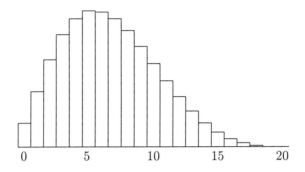

Increasing the population size to $2N = 200$ (that is, $N = 100$ diploid individuals) and dividing the mutation rates by ten, $u = 0.01$ and $v = 0.02$, so that we still have $2Nu = 2$ and $2Nv = 4$, the shape of the curve stays roughly the same.

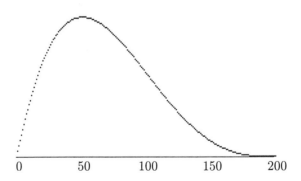

Keeping the population size as $2N = 200$ and reducing the mutation rates to $u = 0.0025$ and $v = 0.0035$, so that $2Nu = 0.5$ and $2Nv = 0.7$, the curve changes shape and is largest at the endpoints of the interval. As one might guess from the large masses at 0 and 200, coalescence of the entire sample often occurs before any mutation has occurred.

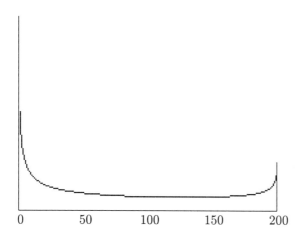

The exact solution in (2.16) is nice but must be evaluated numerically, so it is also useful to have a more easily computed approximation.

(2.17) Suppose the population size N is large and let $q = 2Nu$, $r = 2Nv$. Then the stationary distribution for the Moran model, when rescaled to lie on the unit interval $[0, 1]$, is close to a beta(q, r) distribution that has density

$$f(x) = c_{q,r} x^{q-1}(1-x)^{r-1}$$

and $c_{q,r}$ is a constant chosen to make $\int_0^1 f(x)\, dx = 1$.

From (2.17) we can see immediately that if $q < 1$ the density tends to ∞ at 0, while if $r < 1$ this will occur at 1. Note that in our third example $p = 0.5$ and $q = 0.7$ so it approaches ∞ at each end, but at a faster rate near 0 ($x^{-0.5}$ versus $(1-x)^{-0.3}$ at 1). Differentiating the density function we have

$$f'(x) = \frac{q-1}{x}f(x) - \frac{r-1}{1-x}f(x)$$

so $f'(x_0) = 0$ when $x_0 = (q-1)/(q+r-2)$. When $p, q > 1$, $f(x)$ vanishes at 0 and 1, so x_0 will be a maximum. Since this is the only place where $f'(x) = 0$, the distribution will be unimodal, i.e., have a single hump. This is the case in our first example where $q = 2$ and $r = 4$, so $x_0 = 1/4$.

Proof of (2.17). It is convenient to rewrite (2.16) as

(a)
$$\pi(i) = \pi(k) \cdot b_k \cdot \prod_{j=k+1}^{i-1} \frac{b_j}{d_j} \cdot \frac{1}{d_i}$$

Recalling that $u = p/2N$ and $v = q/2N$ and writing

$$p_i = \frac{i}{2N} + u - (u+v)\frac{i}{2N}$$

it is easy to see that if $i/2N \to x$ as $N \to \infty$ then

(b) $$d_i = \frac{i}{2N} \cdot (1 - p_i) \to x(1 - x)$$

This factor gives the $x^{-1}(1-x)^{-1}$ in the limiting density. To tackle the product, we note that it follows from the definition that

$$\frac{b_j}{d_j} = \frac{(2N-j)\left\{\frac{j}{2N} + u - (u+v)\frac{j}{2N}\right\}}{j\left\{\frac{2N-j}{2N} - u + (u+v)\frac{j}{2N}\right\}}$$

$$= \frac{(2N-j)\cdot\{j + 2Nu - (u+v)j\}}{j\cdot\{2N - j - 2Nu + (u+v)j\}}$$

$$= \left(1 + \frac{2Nu}{j} - (u+v)\right)\bigg/\left(1 - \frac{2Nu}{2N-j} + \frac{(u+v)j}{2N-j}\right)$$

When x and y are small, $(1+x)/(1-y) \approx 1 + x + y$ so the above

$$\approx 1 + 2nu\left(\frac{1}{j} + \frac{1}{2N-j}\right) - (u+v)\frac{2N-j}{2N-j} - (u+v)\frac{j}{2N-j}$$

$$= 1 + \frac{2Nu}{j} - \frac{2Nv}{2N-j}$$

Taking the logarithm of the formula in (a) we see that

$$\log\left(\frac{\pi(i)d_i}{\pi(k)b_k}\right) = \sum_{j=k+1}^{i-1} \log\left(1 + \frac{2Nu}{j} + \frac{2Nv}{2N-j}\right)$$

Using $\log(1+x) \approx x$ for small x, and plugging in $2Nu = q$ and $2Nv = r$ the above is

$$\sum_{j=k+1}^{i-1}\left\{\frac{q}{(j/2N)} - \frac{r}{1 - (j/2N)}\right\} \cdot \frac{1}{2N}$$

Recognizing the last quantity as a Riemann sum approximating the integral

$$\int_{k/2N}^{i/2N} \frac{q}{x} - \frac{r}{1-x}\, dx = q\log x + r\log(1-x)\big|_{k/2N}^{i/2N}$$

Taking $k = N$ as our reference point it follows that

$$\log\left(\frac{\pi(i)d_i}{\pi(N)b_N}\right) \approx \int_{1/2}^{i/2N} \frac{q}{x} - \frac{r}{1-x}\, dx = 2^{q+r}(i/2N)^q(1 - i/2N)^r$$

Now $b_N = (1/2)p_N \to 1/4$ as $N \to \infty$ so we have

(c) $$\pi(i) \approx \frac{\pi(N)}{d_i}2^{p+q+2}(i/2N)^p(1 - i/2N)^q$$

and the desired result follows from (a).   □

For a second proof of this result one can observe that the limiting moments given in (1.15) are those of beta(q,r) distribution.

When we looked at the Wright-Fisher model going backwards in time, the resulting genealogical process was a discrete time coalescing random walk. If we do this for the Moran model, the result is a *continuous time coalescing random walk*. In this process, when there are k lineages, each jumps at rate 1 and goes to a site chosen at random so collisions occur at rate $k \cdot (k-1)/2N$. If we speed up time by a factor of $2N$, then coalescence occurs at rate $k(k-1)$ compared with rate $k(k-1)/2$ in the large population limit of the genealogy of the Wright-Fisher model. This factor of 2 is easily explained. In the discrete time model, two particles jump at once, so two jumps give only one chance of a collision. In continuous time, each particle jumps separately, affording twice as many opportunities for collisions.

Apart from this factor of 2, the genealogy of the large population limit of the Moran model is the same as that of the Wright-Fisher model. This observation implies that if mutation rates in the Moran model are twice what they are in the Wright-Fisher model, then (in the limit $N \to \infty$) the stationary distributions are the same. This observation allows us to translate the approximation in (2.17) into a corresponding result for the Wright-Fisher model.

(2.18) *Suppose the population size N is large and let $q = 4Nu$, $r = 4Nv$. Then the stationary distribution for the Wright-Fisher model, when rescaled to lie on the unit interval $[0,1]$, is close to a beta(q,r) distribution that has density*

$$f(x) = c_{q,r} x^{q-1}(1-x)^{r-1}$$

and $c_{q,r}$ is a constant chosen to make $\int_0^1 f(x)\, dx = 1$.

1.3 Ewens Sampling Formula

In this section, we will give an explicit formula for the stationary distribution of the Wright-Fisher model under the *infinite alleles model*. As the name should suggest, there are so many alleles that each mutation is always to a new type never seen before. To explain the reason for this assumption, we use the reasoning of one of two inventors of this model, Kimura and Crow (1964). Kimura (1971) argued that if a gene consists of 500 nucleotides, the number of possible DNA sequences is

$$4^{500} = 10^{500 \ln 4 / \ln 10} = 10^{301}$$

For any of these, there are $3 \cdot 500 = 1500$ sequences that can be reached by single base changes, so the chance of returning where one began in two mutations is $1/1500$ (assuming an equal probability for all replacements). Thus the total number of possible alleles is essentially infinite.

As in the case of the two alleles, the genealogical process associated with the infinite alleles version of the Wright-Fisher model is the coalescent with killing. When there are k lineages, coalescence and mutation occur on each step with probabilities

$$\frac{k(k-1)}{2} \cdot \frac{1}{2N} \quad \text{and} \quad k\mu$$

respectively. Speeding up the system by running time at rate $2N$, the rates become $k(k-1)/2$ and $k\theta/2$, where $\theta = 4N\mu$.

Turning the coalescent with killing around backwards leads to *Hoppe's (1984) urn model*. This urn contains a black ball with mass θ and various colored balls with mass 1. At each time, a ball is selected at random with a probability proportional to its mass. If a colored ball is drawn, that ball and another of its color are returned to the urn. If the black ball is chosen, it is returned to the urn with a ball of a new color that has mass 1.

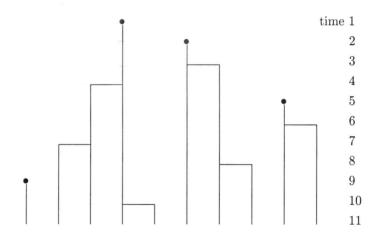

Clearly, the choice of the black ball corresponds to a new mutation and the choice of a colored ball corresponds to a coalescence event. The simulation above should help explain the definition. Here a black dot indicates that a new color was added at that time step.

As we go backwards from time $k+1$ to time k in Hoppe's urn we lose a particle with probability $\theta/(\theta+k)$ and have a coalescence with probability $k/(\theta+k)$. Since in the coalescent there are $k+1$ particles that are each exposed to mutations at rate $\theta/2 = 2N\mu$ and collisions occur at rate $(k+$

1)$k/2$, this is the correct ratio. Since by symmetry all of the coalescence events have equal probability, it follows that

(3.1) *The genealogical relationship between k particles in the coalescent can be simulated by running Hoppe's urn for k time steps.*

The observation in (3.1) is useful in computing properties of the stationary distribution. To illustrate this, let K_n be the random variable that counts the number of different alleles found in a sample of size n. Let $\eta_i = 1$ if the ith ball added to Hoppe's urn is a new type and 0 otherwise. It is clear from the definition of the urn scheme, that $K_n = \eta_1 + \cdots + \eta_n$ and

(3.2) $\eta_1, \ldots \eta_n$ *are independent with* $P(\eta_i = 1) = \theta/(\theta + i - 1)$.

Using (3.2) we can immediately compute the asymptotic behavior of the mean, variance, and distribution of K_n. The first step is the mundane detail.

(3.3) *Suppose* $P(\eta = 1) = p$ *and* $P(\eta = 0) = 1 - p$. *Then* $E\eta = p$ *and* $\mathrm{var}\,(\eta) = p(1 - p)$.

With this in hand, we can prove Watterson's (1975) result:

(3.4) *For fixed θ, as the sample size $n \to \infty$*

$$EK_n \sim \theta \ln n \quad \text{and} \quad \mathrm{var}\,(K_n) \sim \theta \ln n$$

where $a_n \sim b_n$ means that $a_n/b_n \to 1$ as $n \to \infty$. In addition, the central limit theorem holds. If χ has the standard normal distribution, then

$$P\left(\frac{K_n - EK_n}{\sqrt{\mathrm{var}\,(K_n)}} \le x \right) \to P(\chi \le x)$$

Proof. Since the η_i are independent, the final claim follows from the triangular array form of the central limit theorem. See, for example, (4.5) in Chapter 2 of Durrett (1995). To compute the asymptotic behavior of EK_n we note that (3.2) implies

$$EK_n = \sum_{i=1}^{n} \frac{\theta}{\theta + i - 1}$$

Viewing the right-hand side as a Riemann sum approximating an integral, it follows that

$$\sum_{i=1}^{n} \frac{1}{\theta + i - 1} \sim \int_{\theta}^{n+\theta} \frac{1}{x}\, dx = \ln(n + \theta) - \ln(\theta) \sim \ln n$$

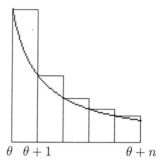

$$\theta \quad \theta + 1 \qquad\qquad\qquad \theta + n$$

From this, the first result follows. To prove the second, we note that (3.2) and (3.3) imply

$$\operatorname{var}(K_n) = \sum_{i=1}^{n} \operatorname{var}(\eta_i) = \sum_{i=2}^{n} \frac{\theta(i-1)}{(\theta+i-1)^2}$$

As $i \to \infty$, $(i-1)/(\theta+i-1) \to 1$, so

$$\operatorname{var}(K_n) \sim \sum_{i=1}^{n} \frac{\theta}{\theta+i-1} \sim \theta \ln n$$

by the reasoning for EK_n.   □

An immediate consequence of (3.4) is that $K_n / \ln n$ is an asymptotically normal estimator of the scaled mutation rate θ. However, the asymptotic standard deviation of $K_n / \ln n$ is quite large, namely of order $1/\sqrt{\ln n}$. Thus, if the true $\theta = 1$ and we want to estimate θ with a standard error of 0.1, a sample of size e^{100} is required. Given this depressingly slow rate of convergence, it is natural to ask if there is another way to estimate θ from the data. The answer is NO, however. As we will see below, K_n is a sufficient statistic. That is, it contains all the information in the sample that is useful for estimating θ.

The last result describes the asymptotic behavior of the number of alleles. The next one, due to Ewens (1972), deals with the entire distribution of the sample.

(3.5) *Ewens sampling formula.* Let a_i be the number of alleles present i times in the sample. When the scaled mutation rate is $\theta = 4N\mu$

$$P_\theta(a_1, \ldots a_n) = \frac{n!}{\theta_{(n)}} \prod_{j=1}^{n} \frac{(\theta/j)^{a_j}}{a_j!}$$

where $\theta_{(n)} = \theta(\theta+1)\cdots(\theta+n-1)$.

The formula may look strange at first but becomes more familiar if we rewrite it as

$$c_{\theta,n} \prod_{j=1}^{n} e^{-\theta/j} \frac{(\theta/j)^{a_j}}{a_j!}$$

where $c_{\theta,n}$ is a constant that depends on θ and n. In words, if we let $Y_1, \ldots Y_n$ be independent Poisson random variables with means θ/j the allelic partition $a_1, a_2, \ldots a_n$ has the same distribution as

$$\left(Y_1, Y_2, \ldots, Y_n \middle| \sum_m mY_m = n\right)$$

One explanation of this can be found in (3.17).

Proof of (3.5). In view of (3.1), it suffices to show that the distribution of the colors in Hoppe's urn at time n, Π_n, is given by the Ewens sampling formula. We proceed by induction. When $n = 1$, the partition $a_1 = 1$ has probability 1 so the result is true. Suppose that the state at time n is $(a_1, \ldots, a_n)$ and let $\bar{a}$ be the state at the previous time. There are two cases to consider

(i) $\bar{a}_1 = a_1 - 1$, i.e., a new color was just added. In this case, the transition probability for Hoppe's urn is

$$p(\bar{a}, a) = \frac{\theta}{\theta + n - 1}$$

and the ratio of the probabilities in the Ewens sampling formula is

$$\frac{P_\theta(a)}{P_\theta(\bar{a})} = \frac{n}{\theta + n - 1} \cdot \frac{\theta}{a_1}$$

(ii) For some $1 \le j < n$, we have $\bar{a}_j = a_j + 1$, $\bar{a}_{j+1} = a_{j+1} - 1$, i.e., an existing color with j representatives was chosen and increased to size $j+1$. In this case, the transition probability is

$$p(\bar{a}, a) = \frac{j\bar{a}_j}{\theta + n - 1}$$

and the ratio of the probabilities in the Ewens sampling formula is

$$\frac{P_\theta(a)}{P_\theta(\bar{a})} = \frac{n}{\theta + n - 1} \cdot \frac{j\bar{a}_j}{(j+1)a_{j+1}}$$

To complete the proof now we observe

$$\sum_{\bar{a}} \frac{P_\theta(\bar{a})}{P_\theta(a)} p(\bar{a}, a) = \frac{\theta}{\theta + n - 1} \cdot \frac{\theta + n - 1}{n} \cdot \frac{a_1}{\theta}$$

$$+ \sum_{j=1}^{n-1} \frac{j\bar{a}_j}{\theta+n-1} \cdot \frac{\theta+n-1}{n} \cdot \frac{(j+1)a_{j+1}}{j\bar{a}_j}$$

Canceling on the right-hand side, we have

$$= \frac{a_1}{n} + \sum_{j=1}^{n-1} \frac{(j+1)a_{j+1}}{n} = 1$$

since $\sum_k ka_k = n$. Rearranging, we have

$$\sum_{\bar{a}} P_\theta(\bar{a})p(\bar{a},a) = P_\theta(a)$$

Since the distribution of Hoppe's urn also satisfies this recursion with the same initial condition, the two must be equal. $\qquad\square$

As an example of the use of Ewens' sampling formula, we will answer

Q. *What is the conditional distribution of the number of individuals with the two alleles given that there was exactly one mutation?*

Consider first the situation in which one allele has m and the other $n-m > m$ representatives. Let $a^{m,n-m}$ be the allelic partition with $a_m^{m,n-m} = 1$ and $a_{n-m}^{m,n-m} = 1$. Writing $q(m, n-m)$ as shorthand for $P_\theta(a^{m,n-m})$, (3.5) gives

$$(3.6a) \quad q(m, n-m) = \frac{n!}{\theta_{(n)}} \cdot \frac{\theta}{m^1 \cdot 1!} \cdot \frac{\theta}{(n-m)^1 \cdot 1!} = \frac{n!\theta^2}{\theta_{(n)}} \cdot \frac{1}{m(n-m)}$$

In the exceptional case that $n-m = m$, the allelic partition has $a_m = 2$ so

$$(3.6b) \qquad\qquad q(m, m) = \frac{n!}{\theta_{(n)}} \cdot \frac{\theta^2}{m^2 \cdot 2!}$$

The asymmetry between the cases can be made to disappear if we arbitrarily designate one half of the partition as the left half, for then

(3.7) *the left half has size m with probability*

$$\frac{C_n}{m \cdot (n-m)} \qquad \text{for } 1 \le m \le n-1$$

where C_n is a constant chosen to make the sum equal to 1.

In the case of $n = 7$ individuals the probabilities are

$$1/6: \frac{2C_7}{1 \cdot 6} \qquad 2/5: \frac{2C_7}{2 \cdot 5} \qquad 3/4: \frac{2C_7}{3 \cdot 4}$$

A little arithmetic shows that $2C_7 = 60/21$, so the probabilities are

$$1/6: \frac{10}{21} = 0.476 \qquad 2/5: \frac{6}{21} = 0.286 \qquad 3/4: \frac{5}{21} = 0.238$$

Example 3.1. Our interest in the case $n = 7$ comes from a data set of Aquadro and Greenberg (1983) for mitochondrial DNA (mtDNA). The first column contains the position (base pair number) in the sequence. Small numbers are adjacent to large ones since mtDNA forms a loop. Here we have omitted positions numbered 315.1, 302.2, 302.1, and 16222 from their data set where insertions or deletions have changed the length of the sequence. The seven columns in the table give the mtDNA sequences from 7 individuals. To make it easier to spot the mutations, only the first sequence is given in full, while the others have dashes where they agree with sequence 1.

	1	2	3	4	5	6	7	partition
→ 456	G	A	-	-	-	-	-	
→ 444	T	C	-	-	-	-	-	
→ 316	C	-	-	T	-	-	-	
263	T	C	C	C	C	C	C	
247	C	-	T	T	-	-	-	2/5
236	A	-	G	-	-	-	-	
200	T	-	C	-	-	-	-	
195	A	-	-	-	-	G	-	
→ 189	T	-	C	G	-	-	-	**
186	G	-	-	G	-	-	-	
185	C	-	T	-	-	-	-	
182	G	-	-	A	-	-	-	
152	A	-	-	G	G	G	-	3/4
151	G	-	-	A	-	-	-	
150	G	-	-	-	-	A	-	
146	A	-	-	-	G	-	-	
73	T	-	-	C	C	C	C	3/4
9	C	-	T	-	-	-	-	
7	T	-	C	-	-	-	-	
16519	A	-	-	G	G	G	G	3/4
16424	A	-	-	G	-	-	-	
16362	A	-	G	-	-	-	-	
16360	G	-	-	A	-	-	-	
16356	A	-	-	-	-	G	-	
16320	G	-	A	-	-	-	-	
16311	A	-	G	G	G	-	-	3/4
16304	A	G	-	-	-	-	-	
16294	G	-	-	A	-	-	-	
16293	T	-	-	C	-	-	-	
16280	T	-	-	C	-	-	-	
16278	G	-	-	A	-	-	A	2/5
16243	A	-	-	-	-	G	-	
16242	G	-	-	-	-	A	-	

16230	T	-	C	-	-	-	-	
16224	A	-	-	-	G	-	-	
16223	G	-	A	A	-	-	-	2/5
16189	A	-	G	G	-	-	-	2/5
16188	G	-	C	-	-	-	-	
16187	G	-	A	A	-	-	-	2/5
16172	A	G	G	-	-	-	-	2/5
16167	G	-	A	-	-	-	-	
16163	T	-	-	C	-	-	-	
16148	G	-	A	-	-	-	-	
16134	G	-	-	-	-	A	-	
16129	C	-	T	-	-	-	-	

Ignoring position 189 marked with **, which has had two mutations, we find

partition	observed	expected
3/4	4	10.48
2/5	6	12.58
1/6	34	20.94

These data show an excess of 1/6 splits over what is expected, suggesting that they are not consistent with a neutral genealogy in a homogeneously mixing population of constant size. A little more thought reveals that if we assume that each site has only been hit by one mutation, it is not consistent with any genealogy at all. To explain this, we first observe that any mutation that affects only one individual is consistent with any genealogy, so these sites are not informative. Removing these sites from the list and replacing the entries in the first column by dashes, we have

	1	2	3	4	5	6	7
16172	-	G	G	-	-	-	-
247	-	-	T	T	-	-	-
16223	-	-	A	A	-	-	-
16189	-	-	G	G	-	-	-
16187	-	-	A	A	-	-	-
16311	-	-	G	G	G	-	-
152	-	-	-	G	G	G	-
73	-	-	-	C	C	C	C
16519	-	-	-	G	G	G	G
16278	-	-	-	A	-	-	A

To explain why this pattern is inconsistent with only one mutation on each site on a single tree, consider the following example genealogy. The sets of individuals affected by mutations A, B, and C are $S_A = \{1, 2\}$,

$S_B = \{5, 6\}$, $S_C = \{5, 6, 7\}$. Note that $S_B \subset S_C$ while S_C and S_A are disjoint. A little thought reveals that any two mutations on this tree must obey this pattern. Their sets of affected individuals must be nested (i.e., one a subset of the other) or disjoint. If we introduce lowercase letters a, b, c to indicate the absence of the corresponding capital letter mutations, then this can be reformulated as saying that if all loci share the same genealogy it is impossible to observe all four combinations AB, Ab, aB, and aa in one data set.

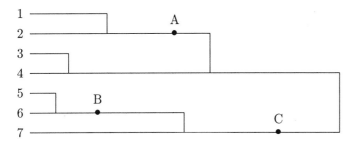

Loci 16172 and 247 show all four combinations, as do 16223 and 152, 16189 and 73, 16187 and 16519, and 16311 and 16278. Since there are five disjoint pairs of conflicting sites, at least five sites must have been hit by more than one mutation. The next figure shows a phylogenetic network with five double mutations. Only the informative sites are listed and are shown in the order given in the original data set. The five unnumbered sequences are hypothesized intermediates. Numbers along the edges indicate the positions at which mutations occur. There are 15 mutations, with sites 2, 3, 4, 6, and 10 hit twice.

Using methods of Fitch (1977), Aquadro and Greenberg (1983) showed that this is the only network with five double mutations and hence is the phylogenetic tree according to the maximum parsimony criterion. However, as they say on page 292, "since many different branching orders for the seven sequences differed from the most parsimonious network by only one or a few additional substitutions it would be unwise to ascribe very great significance to this most parsimonious tree as necessarily reflecting the true phylogenetic relationships among the seven human mtDNAs."

The network drawn on the next page is an unrooted tree. If we follow Aquadro and Greenberg and take the node between 3 and 4 as the ancestral sequence then the following substitutions have occurred.

	A	G	C	T
A	–	13	0	0
G	20	–	1	0
C	0	0	–	7

T   0   1   9   –

In words, G's have been substituted for A's 13 times, A's for G's 20 times, etc. To explain the departures from purely random substitution, we need some terminology. A's and G's are purines (mnemonic: AG's are pure) while C's and T's are pyrimidines. Substitutions of bases of the same type, called *transitions*, occurred 49 times, while those of the opposite type, called *transversions*, occurred only twice.

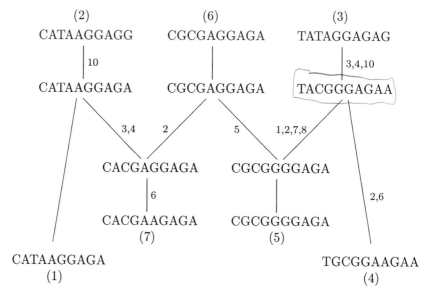

In the years since Aquadro and Greenberg (1983), there has been more investigation of the unexpectedly high ratio of transitions to transversions. Using 95 human sequences and comparing them to one chimpanzee sequence, Tamura and Nei (1993) observed the following substitution pattern. The entries in the table are the percentages of changes of the various types. The bold faced numbers are transitions and account for 93.3% of the changes.

	A	G	C	T	total
A	–	**14.1**	1.1	0.4	15.6
G	**20.0**	–	1.6	1.1	22.7
C	1.1	0.5	–	**25.8**	27.4
T	0.3	0.3	**33.4**	–	34.4
total	21.4	14.9	36.5	27.3	

Joyce and Tavaré (1987) enriched Hoppe's urn by adding bookkeeping to keep track of the relationship between particles as a permutation written in its cyclic decomposition. Numbering the balls according to the order that they enter the urn, the rules are simple: a new color starts a new cycle. If ball k's color was determined by choosing ball j it is inserted to the left of j. For an example consider the first eight events in the realization from the beginning of this section.

(1)	1 is always a new color
(1)(2)	2 is a new color
(1)(32)	3 is a child of 2
(41)(32)	4 is a child of 1
(41)(32)(5)	5 is a new color
(41)(32)(65)	6 is a child of 5
(741)(32)(65)	7 is a child of 4
(741)(832)(65)	8 is a child of 3

This scheme is also known as the "Chinese restaurant process", see Aldous (1985). In that formulation, one thinks of the numbers as successive arrivals to a restaurant and the groups as tables.

Let Π_n be the permutation when there are n individuals. An important property of this representation is that given a permutation, the path to it is unique. Indeed, one can compute the path by successively deleting the largest number that remains in the permutation. This property is the key to the following result.

(3.8) If π is a permutation with k cycles, then

$$P_\theta(\Pi_n = \pi) = \frac{\theta^k}{\theta_{(n)}}$$

When $\theta = 1$, the right-hand side is $1/n!$, i.e., all permutations are equally likely.

Proof. In our example $P^\theta(\Pi_8 = (741)(832)(65))$ is

$$\frac{\theta}{\theta} \cdot \frac{\theta}{\theta+1} \cdot \frac{1}{\theta+2} \cdot \frac{1}{\theta+3} \cdot \frac{\theta}{\theta+4} \cdot \frac{1}{\theta+5} \cdot \frac{1}{\theta+6} \cdot \frac{1}{\theta+7}$$

where the θ's in the numerators of the first, second, and fifth fractions are due to the new colors at those steps and the 1's in the other numerators come from the fact that each individual is the child of a specified parent. Generalizing from the example, we see that if a permutation of $\{1, 2, \ldots n\}$ has k cycles, then the numerator is always θ^k and the denominator is $\theta_{(n)}$. □

Comparing with the Ewens sampling formula in (3.5) and noting that $k = \sum a_j$ is the number of cycles, we see that the number of permutations of $\{1, 2, \ldots n\}$ with a_1 cycles of size 1, a_2 cycles of size 2, etc., is

$$\frac{n!}{\prod_{j=1}^{n}(j^{a_j} j!)}$$

Let $|S_n^k|$ be the number of permutations of $\{1, 2, \ldots n\}$ with exactly k cycles. Letting K_n be the number of alleles in a sample of size k, it follows from (3.8) that

(3.9) $$P_\theta(K_n = k) = \frac{\theta^k}{\theta_{(n)}} \cdot |S_n^k|$$

The $|S_n^k|$ are called the Stirling numbers of the second kind. In order to compute them, it is enough to know that they satisfy the relationship

(3.10) $$|S_n^k| = (n-1)|S_{n-1}^k| + |S_{n-1}^{k-1}|$$

In words, we can construct a $\pi \in S_n^k$ from a member of S_n^{k-1} by adding (n) as a new cycle, or from a $\sigma \in S_{n-1}^k$ by picking an integer $1 \leq j \leq n-1$ and setting $\pi(j) = n$, $\pi(n) = \sigma(j)$.

Combining (3.9) with (3.5), we see that

(3.11) $$P_\theta(a_1, \ldots, a_n | K_n = k) = \frac{n!}{|S_n^k|} \prod_{j=1}^{n} \left(\frac{1}{j}\right)^{a_j} \frac{1}{a_j!}$$

Since the conditional distribution of the allelic partition does not depend on θ, K_n is a sufficient statistic for estimating θ. To develop an estimate of θ based on K_n, we will use maximum-likelihood estimation. Let

$$L_n(\theta, k) = \frac{\theta^k}{\theta_{(n)}} \cdot |S_n^k|$$

be the likelihood of observing k when the true parameter is θ. The maximum-likelihood estimator finds the value of θ that maximizes the probability of the observed value of k. To find the maximum value we compute

$$\frac{\partial}{\partial \theta} L_n(\theta, k) = |S_n^k| \frac{k\theta^{k-1}\theta_{(n)} - \theta^k \theta'_{(n)}}{(\theta_{(n)})^2} = \frac{\theta^k |S_n^k|}{\theta_{(n)}} \cdot \left[\frac{k}{\theta} - \frac{\theta'_{(n)}}{\theta_{(n)}}\right]$$

Setting the right-hand side equal to 0 and solving for k yields

$$k = \theta \frac{\theta'_{(n)}}{\theta_{(n)}} = \theta \frac{d}{d\theta} \log \theta_{(n)}$$

Recalling $\theta_{(n)} = \theta(\theta + 1) \cdots (\theta + n - 1)$, we need to compute

$$\frac{d}{d\theta} \sum_{i=1}^{n} \log(\theta + i - 1) = \sum_{i=1}^{n} \frac{1}{\theta + i - 1}$$

and thus

$$k = \frac{\theta}{\theta} + \frac{\theta}{\theta + 1} + \cdots \frac{\theta}{\theta + n - 1} = EK_n$$

In words, the maximum-likelihood estimator is the θ that makes the mean number of alleles equal to the observed number.

The theory of maximum-likelihood estimation tells us that asymptotically $E\hat{\theta} = \theta$ and $\mathrm{var}(\hat{\theta}) = 1/I(\hat{\theta})$, where $I(\theta)$ is the Fisher information

$$I(\theta) = E\left(\frac{\partial}{\partial\theta} \log L_n(\theta, k)\right)^2$$

This is easy to compute here

$$\frac{\partial}{\partial\theta} \log L_n(\theta, k) = \frac{\partial}{\partial\theta} \log \frac{\theta^k |S_n^k|}{\theta_{(n)}} = \frac{k}{\theta} - \frac{\partial}{\partial\theta} \log \theta_{(n)}$$

$$= \frac{k}{\theta} - \sum_{i=1}^{n} \frac{1}{\theta + i - 1} = \frac{1}{\theta}\left(k - \sum_{i=1}^{n} \frac{\theta}{\theta + i - 1}\right)$$

Since $EK_n = \sum_{i=1}^{n} \frac{\theta}{\theta+i-1}$ it follows that

$$I(\theta) = \frac{1}{\theta^2} \mathrm{var}(K_n)$$

(3.4) implies that $\mathrm{var}(K_n) \sim \theta \log n$, so $\mathrm{var}(\hat{\theta}) \to 0$ but rather slowly.

Example 3.2. To illustrate the use of the theory just developed we will consider a study that Ward et al. (1991) made of an Amerindian tribe, the Nuu-Chah-Nulth of the Pacific Northwest. Sequencing of a 360 nucleotide segment of the mitochondrial control region for 63 individuals revealed the existence of 28 allelic types. The maximum likelihood estimate in this case is $\hat{\theta} = 19$. This estimate is much higher than the value $\hat{\theta} = 8.5$ that came from the study of 15 !Kung samples by Vigilant et al. (1989). Since $\theta = 2N_f\mu$, where N_f is the effective number of females, the population size could explain the difference. However, that goes in the wrong direction; the !Kung number some 10,000 individuals, while there are only 2000–2400 Nuu-Chah-Nulth. We will return to this example in the next section when we discuss the infinite sites model.

Since this distribution in (3.11) is independent of θ, one can use any function of the allele frequencies to test for departures from the infinite alleles model. Watterson (1977) suggested the use of the *sample homozygosity*

$$\hat{F} = \sum_{i=1}^{k} x_i^2$$

where x_i is the frequency of the ith allele. In words, $\hat{F}$ is the probability that two individuals chosen with replacement are the same. In terms of the allelic partition this statistic can be written as

$$\hat{F} = \sum_{j=1}^{n} a_j \left(\frac{j}{n}\right)^2$$

Example 3.3. Watterson (1978) used (3.11) to study data Coyne (1976) and Singh, Lewontin, and Felton (1976) obtained by performing electrophoresis under various conditions. Coyne (1976) found 23 alleles in 60 genes at the xanthine dehydrogenase locus of *Drosophila persimilis* that displayed the following pattern:

$$1^{18} 2^3 4^1 32^1$$

That is, there were 18 unique alleles, 3 alleles had 2 representatives, 1 had 4, and 1 had 32. Singh, Lewontin, and Felton (1976) found 27 alleles in 146 genes from the xanthine dehydrogenase locus of *D. pseudoobscura* with the following pattern

$$1^{20} 2^3 3^7 5^2 6^2 8^1 11^1 68^1$$

Using (3.11) on the Coyne data gives

$$\frac{60!}{2^3 \cdot 4 \cdot 32 \cdot 18! \cdot 3! \cdot |S_{60}^{23}|} = 5.952 \times 10^{-7}$$

Applied to the Singh, Lewontin, and Felton data, (3.11) gives

$$\frac{146!}{2^3 \, 3^7 \, 5^2 \, 6^2 \, 8^1 \, 11^1 \, 68^1 \, 20! \, 3! \, 7! \, 2! \, 2! \cdot |S_{146}^{27}|} = 2.326 \times 10^{-9}$$

The above calculations show that both sets of data are very unlikely to occur under the neutral allele distribution (3.11). It is not surprising that the samples have low probability since there are many possible samples. Therefore, to assess whether the data sets above afford evidence against neutrality, we need to consider the probability of getting data sets that are more extreme than this one. To decide what is extreme, we will again consider the homozygosity. For the Coyne data, $\hat{F} = 0.2972$. For that of Singh, Lewontin, and Felton, $\hat{F} = 0.2353$.

To assess the significance of the value for the Coyne data, Watterson (1978) generated 1000 samples of size 60 with 23 alleles. No sample had a value of $\hat{F}$ larger than 0.2972. For the Singh, Lewontin, and Felton data, 2000 samples of size 146 with 27 alleles produced only 8 values larger than 0.2353. We may thus conclude that both data sets depart significantly from the neutral alleles distribution in the direction of excess homozygosity.

In addition to introducing the bookkeeping described above, Joyce and Tavaré (1987) related Hoppe's urn to the *linear birth process with immigra-*

tion. In this process, immigrants enter the population at times of a Poisson process with rate θ, and each individual in the population follows the rules of the *binary branching process.* That is, they never die and they give birth to new individuals at rate 1. If we only look at the process when the number of particles increases, then we get a discrete time process in which a new type is added with probability $\theta/(k + \theta)$ and a new individual with a type randomly chosen from the urn is added with probability $k/(k + \theta)$. From this description, it should be clear that

(3.12) *If each immigrant is a new type and offspring are the same type as their parents, then the sequence of states the branching process with immigration moves through has the same distribution as those generated by Hoppe's urn.*

If we combine the last observation with the fact (see page 109 of Athreya and Ney 1972)

(3.13) *Starting from a single particle, the number of particles in a binary branching process at time t has a geometric distribution with success probability $p = e^{-t}$.*

we obtain the following:

(3.14) *Consider the coalescent starting with ℓ lineages. If we pick one of them at random when there are $k \leq \ell$ lineages, then the probability it will contain m of the ℓ starting lineages is*

$$s(k, m) = \binom{\ell - m - 1}{k - 2} \Big/ \binom{\ell - 1}{k - 1}$$

When $k = 2$, the numerator is $\binom{\ell-m-1}{0} = 1$ by definition and the denominator is $\binom{\ell-1}{1} = \ell - 1$, giving a new proof of (2.9).

Proof. Let Z_t^i, $1 \leq i \leq k$ be independent copies of the binary branching process. If $j_1, \ldots j_k$ are positive integers that add up to ℓ then

$$P(Z_t^1 = j_1, \ldots Z_t^k = j_k) = (1 - p)^{\ell - k} p^k$$

Since the right-hand side only depends on the sum ℓ and the number of terms k, all of the possible vectors have the same probability. To count the number of such vectors, note that a possible vector can be constructed by taking ℓ balls and using $k - 1$ pieces of cardboard to divide them into k groups. For example, if $\ell = 10$ and $k = 4$, then

$$O\,O\,O|O|O\,O\,O\,O|O\,O$$

yields $j_1 = 3, j_2 = 1, j_3 = 4, j_4 = 2$. Our $k - 1$ pieces of cardboard can go in any of the $\ell - 1$ spaces so there are $\binom{\ell-1}{k-1}$ possible vectors $(j_1, \ldots, j_k)$ of positive integers that add up to ℓ. From this it follows that

$$P\left(Z_t^1 = j_1, \ldots Z_t^k = j_k \middle| \sum_{j=1}^k Z_t^j = \ell\right) = 1 \middle/ \binom{\ell - 1}{k - 1}$$

that is, the conditional distribution is uniform over the set of possible vectors. Since the number of vectors $(j_2, \ldots, j_k)$ of positive integers that add up to $\ell - m$ is $\binom{\ell - m - 1}{k - 2}$

$$P\left(Z_t^1 = m \middle| \sum_{j=1}^k Z_t^j = \ell\right) = \binom{\ell - m - 1}{k - 2} \middle/ \binom{\ell - 1}{k - 1} \qquad \square$$

The passage from the discrete time urn model to the continuous time branching process with immigration is useful because it makes the growth of the various families independent. This leads to some nice results about the asymptotic behavior of the Ewens sampling distribution when n is large. The proofs are somewhat more sophisticated than the others in this section and we will not use the results for applications, so if the discussion becomes confusing, the reader should feel free to move on to the next section. Let $s_j(n)$ be the size of the jth family when there are n individuals. Donnelly and Tavaré (1986) have shown in their Theorem 6.1 that

(3.15) For $j = 1, 2, \ldots$, $\lim_{n \to \infty} s_j(n)/n = P_j$ with

$$P_j = Z_j \prod_{i=1}^{j-1}(1 - Z_i)$$

where the Z_i are independent and have a beta$(1, \theta)$ density: $\theta(1 - z)^{\theta - 1}$.

Note that when $\theta = 1$, the Z_i are uniform. In this case, (3.15) describes the "cycle structure" of a random permutation. To define the quantity in quotes, start with 1 and follow the successive iterates $\pi(1)$, $\pi(\pi(1))$ until you return to 1. This is the first cycle. Now pick the smallest number not in the first cycle and repeat the procedure to construct the second cycle, etc. As (3.8) shows, the cycle sizes in a random permutation have the same distribution as the family sizes when $\theta = 1$.

Sketch of Proof of (3.15). We content ourselves to explain the main ideas, referring the reader to Tavaré (1987) for details. Let $X(t)$ be the number of particles at time t in the binary branching process. It is well-known, see e.g., Athreya and Ney (1972), that as $t \to \infty$, $X(t)/e^t$ converges to a limit we will denote by $\mathcal{E}$. From (3.13) it follows that $\mathcal{E}$ has an exponential distribution. Let $X_i(t)$ be the number of individuals in the ith family at time t. From the previous result, it follows that

$$e^{-t}(X_1(t), X_2(t), \ldots) \to (e^{-T_1}\mathcal{E}_1, e^{-T_2}\mathcal{E}_2, \ldots)$$

where $T_1, T_2, \ldots$ are the arrival times of the rate θ Poisson process and $\mathcal{E}_1, \mathcal{E}_2, \ldots$ are independent mean 1 exponentials. Let $I(t) = X_1(t) + X_2(t) + \cdots$ be the total number of individuals at time t. Leaving the boring details of justifying the interchange of sum and limit to the reader, we have

$$e^{-t} I(t) \to \sum_{i=1}^{\infty} e^{-T_i} \mathcal{E}_i$$

A little calculation shows that the sum has a gamma(θ,1) distribution. From the last two results, it follows that

$$\frac{X_1(t)}{I(t)} \to \frac{e^{-T_1} \mathcal{E}_1}{\sum_{i=1}^{\infty} e^{-T_i} \mathcal{E}_i} = \frac{\mathcal{E}_1}{\mathcal{E}_1 + \sum_{i=2}^{\infty} e^{-(T_i - T_1)} \mathcal{E}_i} \equiv Z_1$$

where the last three-lined equality ($\equiv$) indicates we are making a definition. Writing $\stackrel{d}{=}$ to indicate that two things have the same distribution,

$$\sum_{i=2}^{\infty} e^{-(T_i - T_1)} \mathcal{E}_i \stackrel{d}{=} \sum_{i=1}^{\infty} e^{-T_i} \mathcal{E}_i$$

has a gamma(θ,1) distribution and is independent of $\mathcal{E}_1$, which has an exponential distribution, so the ratio has a beta($1, \theta$) distribution. To get the result for $i = 2$, we note that

$$\frac{X_2(t)}{I(t)} \to \frac{e^{-T_2} \mathcal{E}_2}{\sum_{i=1}^{\infty} e^{-T_i} \mathcal{E}_i}$$

$$= (1 - Z_1) \cdot \frac{e^{T_2} \mathcal{E}_2}{\sum_{i=2}^{\infty} e^{-T_i} \mathcal{E}_i} \equiv (1 - Z_1) Z_2$$

Similar algebra leads to the result for $i > 2$. □

As Donnelly, Kurtz, and Tavaré (1991) have shown, the ideas above can be used to prove a result of Hansen (1990) about

$$K_n(u) = \text{the number of parts of the partition of size } \le n^u$$

when the sample size is n.

(3.16) *As* $n \to \infty$

$$Y_n(u) = \frac{K_n(u) - \theta u \log n}{\sqrt{\theta \log n}}$$

converges to a normal distribution with mean 0 and variance u. Furthermore, the process $\{Y_n(u) : 0 \le u \le 1\}$ converges to Brownian motion.

Sketch of Proof. Let $\tau_n = \inf\{t : I(t) = n\}$. Since $I(t)$ grows like e^t, $\tau_n \approx \log n$. Applying the last reasoning to the $X_i(t)$ we see that most of the families founded since $(1-u)\log n$ will have size smaller than n^u at time τ_n, while most of those founded before $(1-u)\log n$ will have size larger than n^u. Thus $K_n(u, \pi)$ is like the number of families founded between $(1-u)\log n$ and $\log n$, and the result follows from the central limit theorem for the Poisson process. $\qquad\square$

(3.16) concerns the large parts of the partition. At the other end of the size spectrum, Arratia, Barbour, and Tavaré (1992) have studied $A_j(n)$, the number of parts of size j, and shown

(3.17) As $n \to \infty$, $(A_1(n), A_2(n), \ldots)$ converges to $(Y_1, Y_2, \ldots)$, where the Y_i are independent Poissons with mean θ/i.

Sketch of Proof. Let $T_{\ell,m} = (\ell + 1)Y_\ell + \cdots + mY_m$. By the remark after (3.5), if $z = y_1 + 2y_2 + \cdots + \ell y_\ell$, then

$$P(A_1(n) = y_1, \ldots A_\ell(n) = y_\ell) = \frac{P(Y_1 = y_1, \ldots Y_\ell = y_\ell)P(T_{\ell,n} = n - z)}{P(T_{0,n} = n)}$$

so it suffices to show that for each fixed z and ℓ,

$$P(T_{\ell,n} = n - a)/P(T_{0,n} = n) \to 1$$

When $\theta = 1$, this can be done using the local central limit theorem but for $\theta \neq 1$ this requires a simple large deviations estimate, see Arratia, Barbour, and Tavaré (1992) for details. $\qquad\square$

1.4   Infinite Sites Model

In the infinite alleles model, we say that two distinct sequences are different but we do not keep track of the number of differences between sequences, throwing away a lot of useful information. For example the entire Aquadro and Greenberg data set would be reduced to the statement that the seven individuals had different alleles. In this section we will introduce a model that keeps track of where in the sequence mutations occur. Thinking of the Aquadro and Greenberg data, suppose we are considering a genetic locus with 900 nucleotides with equal mutation probabilities. In this setting the first two dozen mutations are likely to occur at different sites.

   To explain the last claim we derive a result for the generalized birthday problem. Let $X_1, X_2, \ldots$ be independent and uniform on $\{1, 2, \ldots N\}$ and let $T_N = \min\{n : X_n = X_m \text{ for some } m < n\}$. When $N = 365$, T_N gives the number of people we have to ask before we find two with the same birthday.

(4.1) As $N \to \infty$, $P(T_N > xN^{1/2}) \to e^{-x^2/2}$

Proof. Since each X_m must miss the $m - 1$ previous values

$$P(T_N > n) = \prod_{m=2}^{n} \left(1 - \frac{m-1}{N}\right)$$

$$\approx \exp\left(-\sum_{k=1}^{n-1} \frac{k}{N}\right) = \exp\left(-\frac{n(n-1)}{2N}\right)$$

since $1 + 2 + \cdots + (n-1) = n(n-1)/2$. Letting $n = xN^{1/2}$ and $N \to \infty$ the desired result follows. □

Example 4.1. In the situation of Aquadro and Greenberg, $N = 900$ so $N^{1/2} = 30$. If we look at the data then there were 46 mutations with two at the same site. The 46 mutations correspond to $x = 1.5333$, so the limit is $e^{-0.32} = 0.308$, i.e., almost 70% of the time we expect two mutations at the same site. At first glance, the data agree well with (4.1). However, if one remembers that our analysis in Example 3.1 turned up five other sites where two mutations have occurred, then what we really had was 51 mutations with six nucleotides hit twice. There are $\binom{51}{2} = 1275$ pairs of mutations, each of which will hit the same site with probability $1/900$, so the expected number of double hits is only 1.41666. Since the events we are dealing with are almost independent, the number of double hits should have a Poisson distribution with mean 1.41666 and will be equal to 6 with probability

$$\approx e^{-1.41666} \frac{(1.41666)^6}{6!} = 0.00272$$

Taking the time to add the probabilities of 7, 8, 9, 10, etc., only increases the answer by about 25%, so if all sites mutate at the same rate this pattern is extremely unlikely.

Kocher and Wilson (1991) sequenced the control region in 13 humans and used a phylogeny to infer the number of changes. Their results are given in the next table.

hits	observed	Poisson	negative binomial
0	1044	1017	1046
1	52	100	54.2
2	21	4.9	14.2
3+	5	0.2	7.6

Note that the Poisson fits much worse than the negative binomial. The negative binomial is known to be generated when the Poisson parameter λ varies according to a gamma distribution (Johnson and Kotz 1973, pages 124–125). This provides support for the practice of supposing mutation rates have a gamma distribution in the reconstruction of phylogenies using maximum-likelihood methods. See e.g., Yang (1996). Here we will in general ignore rate variation in our modeling. For more on substitution rate variation in human mitochondrial DNA, see Wakeley (1993).

If we assume that the number of sites is infinite then mutations will always occur at distinct sites and we have the *infinite sites model* of Kimura (1969). In this section we will study several aspects of this model.

Pairwise differences

Given two DNA sequences of length L let Δ_2 be the number of pairwise differences. For example, the two sequences

$$AATCGCTTGATACC$$
$$A\underline{C}TCGC\underline{C}TGATA\underline{A}C$$

have three pairwise differences at positions 2, 7, and 13. To compute the distribution of Δ_2, let u be the mutation rate for the locus and note that (2.13) implies that the probability of coalescence before mutation is $1/(1 + 4Nu)$. If, however, mutation comes before coalescence, we have an equal chance of having another mutation before coalescence, so letting $\theta = 4Nu$ we have

$$(4.2) \qquad P(\Delta_2 = k) = \left(\frac{\theta}{\theta+1}\right)^k \frac{1}{\theta+1} \quad \text{for } k = 0, 1, 2, \ldots$$

To compute the mean and variance of Δ_2 now, we recall that the

(4.3) *shifted geometric distribution* $P(X = k) = (1-p)^k p$ for $k = 0, 1, 2, \ldots$ has mean $(1/p) - 1$ and variance $(1 - p)/p^2$.

Taking $p = 1/(\theta + 1)$, we find

$$(4.4) \qquad\qquad E\Delta_2 = \theta \qquad \text{var}(\Delta_2) = \theta(1 + \theta) = \theta + \theta^2$$

Given n DNA sequences, we can estimate the scaled mutation rate θ by Δ_n, the average number of pairwise differences between these sequences. To be precise, let Δ_{ij} be the number of pairwise differences between the ith and jth sequences, and let

$$\Delta_n = \binom{n}{2}^{-1} \sum_{\{i,j\}} \Delta_{ij}$$

where the sum is over all pairs $\{i, j\} \subset \{1, 2, \ldots n\}$. Since there are $\binom{n}{2}$ pairs, and $E\Delta_{ij} = E\Delta_2$, (4.2) implies

$$(4.5) \qquad\qquad\qquad E\Delta_n = \theta$$

In words, Δ_n is an *unbiased estimator* of θ. Tajima (1983) has shown that

$$(4.6) \qquad \text{var}(\Delta_n) = \frac{n+1}{3(n-1)}\theta + \frac{2(n^2+n+3)}{9n(n-1)}\theta^2$$

Note that the variance does not tend to 0 as the sample size n tends to infinity but

$$\text{var}(\Delta_n) \to \frac{\theta}{3} + \frac{2\theta^2}{9}$$

Before turning to the details of the proof, we will consider two examples.

Example 4.2. In the data of Aquadro and Greenberg (1983) from Section 1.3, the number of sequences is $n = 7$, and ignoring the locus that was hit twice we have:

partition	observed	differences
3/4	4	12/21
2/5	6	10/21
1/6	34	6/21

To explain the last column, we note that there are $(7 \cdot 6)/2 = 21$ ways of picking 2 of the 7 sequences. Doing all 21 choices will result in 12 pairwise differences when the partition is $3/4$, 10 when the partition is $2/5$, and 6 when the partition is $1/6$. Adding things up, we see that the average number of pairwise differences is

$$34 \cdot \frac{6}{21} + 6 \cdot \frac{10}{21} + 4 \cdot \frac{12}{21} = \frac{312}{21} = 14.86$$

Example 4.3. To further investigate the surprising value of θ found for the Nuu-Chah-Nulth, Ward et al. (1991) used Felsenstein's maximum-likelihood algorithm to construct a phylogeny for the 28 lineages. They found that the majority of lineages fell into four clusters. The average pairwise difference percentages between individuals in the four groups are given above the diagonal in the following table:

	I	II	III	IV
I	-	1.86	1.74	1.34
II	56,000	-	2.59	2.31
III	53,000	78,000	-	2.01
IV	41,000	70,000	61,000	-

Comparison of the amount of sequence divergence between humans and chimpanzees for the 360 nucleotide segment of the control region and using an estimate of 4 million years for the divergence of the two species which is at the lower end of accepted values, gives a maximum rate estimate of 33%

divergence per million years for this DNA segment. Using this with the observed divergences between the groups gives estimated divergence times that are in the lower part of the table. These estimates predate by a large margin the entrance of humans into the Americas about 15,000 years ago. For a more thorough study of the genealogy of this sample, see Griffiths and Tavaré (1994a) and Weiss and von Haeseler (1998).

Proof. The derivation of (4.6) is somewhat lengthy, so we won't blame the reader who skips it and goes to the next subsection on nucleotide diversity. To begin our calculation, we note that

$$\Delta_n^2 = \binom{n}{2}^{-2} \sum_{\{i_1,j_1\}} \sum_{\{i_2,j_2\}} \Delta_{i_1,j_1} \Delta_{i_2,j_2}$$

There are three types of terms:

(i) $|\{i_1, i_2, j_1, j_2\}| = 2$. That is, $i_1 = i_2$, $j_1 = j_2$. There are $\binom{n}{2}$ of these.

(ii) $|\{i_1, i_2, j_1, j_2\}| = 3$. There are $n \cdot n - 1 \cdot n - 2 = \binom{n}{2} 2(n-2)$ of these.

(iii) $\{i_1, j_1\} \cap \{i_2, j_2\} = \emptyset$. There are $\binom{n}{2}\binom{n-2}{2}$ of these.

To check the combinatorics, note that

$$1 + 2(n-2) + \frac{(n-2)(n-3)}{2} = \frac{2 + 4n - 8 + n^2 - 5n + 6}{2} = \frac{n^2 - n}{2} = \binom{n}{2}$$

Let i, j, k, ℓ be distinct indices and let

$$
\begin{aligned}
U_2 &= E(\Delta_{ij}^2) - \theta^2 \\
U_3 &= E(\Delta_{ij}\Delta_{ik}) - \theta^2 \\
U_4 &= E(\Delta_{ij}\Delta_{k\ell}) - \theta^2
\end{aligned}
$$

Using our new notation we can write

$$(\star) \qquad \mathrm{var}\,(\Delta_n) = \binom{n}{2}^{-1} \left(U_2 + 2(n-2)U_3 + \binom{n-2}{2} U_4 \right)$$

From (4.4) we have $U_2 = \theta + \theta^2$. Following Tajima (1983), we will compute U_3 and U_4 by computing $\mathrm{var}\,(\Delta_3)$ and $\mathrm{var}\,(\Delta_4)$, then using $(\star)$ to solve for U_3 and U_4. We begin with the case $n = 3$.

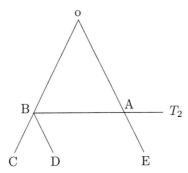

Writing $n_{AB} = n_{BA}$ as the number of mutations on the path AoB, $n_{BC} = n_{CB}$ the number on the edge CB, etc, we can write the three pairwise differences as

$$\begin{aligned}
\Delta_{CD} &= n_{CB} + n_{BD} \\
\Delta_{CE} &= n_{CB} + n_{BA} + n_{AE} \\
\Delta_{DE} &= n_{DB} + n_{BA} + n_{AE}
\end{aligned}$$

Adding these equations (and rearranging the subscripts) gives

(a) $$3\Delta_3 = 2n_{AB} + 2n_{BC} + 2n_{BD} + 2n_{AE}$$

From (4.4) it follows that

(b) $$En_{AB} = \theta \quad \text{and} \quad \text{var}(n_{AB}) = \theta + \theta^2$$

Note that n_{AB} is independent of n_{BC}, n_{BD}, and n_{AE}, and that the last three random variables have the same distribution since each is the number of mutations that hit a given lineage before the first coalescence at time T_2. The last observation implies

$$\text{cov}(n_{BC}, n_{BD}) = \text{cov}(n_{BD}, n_{AE}) = \text{cov}(n_{AE}, n_{BC})$$

so we have

(c) $$\frac{9}{4} \text{var}(\Delta_3) = \text{var}(n_{AB}) + 3 \text{var}(n_{BC}) + 6 \text{cov}(n_{BC}, n_{BD})$$

To compute the mean of n_{BC}, note that in units of $2N$ generations the time of the first coalescence T_2 has an exponential distribution with mean $1/\binom{3}{2} = 1/3$ and that mutations occur at rate $2N\mu = \theta/2$, so if we condition on the time T_2 then the number of mutations is Poisson with mean $T_2\theta/2$. $E(n_{BC}|T_2) = T_2\,\theta/2$ and hence

(d) $$En_{BC} = \frac{\theta}{2} ET_2 = \frac{\theta}{2} \cdot \frac{1}{3}$$

To compute the variance of n_{BC} we recall that if Z has a Poisson distribution with mean λ, then $EZ^2 = \lambda + \lambda^2$ so

$$E(n_{BC}^2|T_2) = T_2\,\theta/2 + (T_2\,\theta/2)^2$$

Recalling that if X has an exponential distribution with mean μ then $EX^2 = 2\mu^2$, we have

(e)
$$E(n_{BC}^2) = \frac{\theta}{6} + \frac{\theta^2}{4} \cdot \frac{2}{9}$$

and it follows that

(f)
$$\text{var}\,(n_{BC}) = E(n_{BC}^2) - (En_{BC})^2 = \frac{\theta}{6} + \frac{\theta^2}{36}$$

Since n_{BC} and n_{BD} are conditionally independent given T_2 we have

$$E(n_{BC}\, n_{BD}|T_2) = \left(\frac{T_2\,\theta}{2}\right)^2$$

and hence

(g)
$$E(n_{BC}\, n_{BD}) = \theta^2/18$$

From this it follows that

(h)
$$\text{cov}\,(n_{BC}, n_{BD}) = \frac{\theta^2}{18} - \left(\frac{\theta}{6}\right)^2 = \frac{\theta^2}{36}$$

Combining (b), (c), (f), and (h), we have

$$\text{var}\,(\Delta_3) = \frac{4}{9}\left(\theta + \theta^2 + 3\left[\frac{\theta}{6} + \frac{\theta^2}{36}\right] + 6 \cdot \frac{\theta^2}{36}\right)$$

Simplifying gives

(i)
$$\text{var}\,(\Delta_3) = \frac{2}{3}\theta + \frac{5}{9}\theta^2$$

which agrees with (4.6) in the case $n = 3$.

We turn now to the case $n = 4$, where there are two types of coalescence events to consider and a larger number of segments to consider.

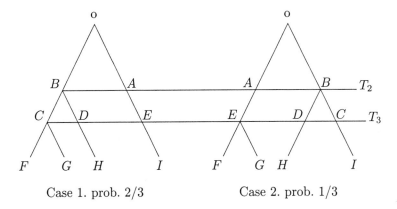

Case 1. prob. 2/3   Case 2. prob. 1/3

Our first step is to observe that if we use the notation of the computation for $n = 3$, then in Case 1

$$6\Delta_4 = 3n_{AB} + 4n_{BC} + 3n_{BD} + 3n_{AE}$$
$$+3n_{FC} + 3n_{GC} + 3n_{HD} + 3n_{EI}$$

To check this, one can patiently write out all six Δ_{ij} and sum them, or think about the number of times our six comparisons will use each arc. Similar reasoning shows that in Case 2

$$6\Delta_4 = 4n_{AB} + 3n_{BC} + 3n_{BD} + 4n_{AE}$$
$$+3n_{FE} + 3n_{GE} + 3n_{HD} + 3n_{CI}$$

We will refer to n_{AB} as a level one variable, n_{BC}, n_{BD}, and n_{AE} as level two variables, and the others as level three. Variables on different levels are independent. We have already derived all of the basic formulas for level one and two variables, but we need new formulas for the level three variables.

To compute the mean of n_{CF}, note that the time of the first coalescence T_3 has an exponential distribution with mean $1/\binom{4}{2} = 1/6$, and that mutations occur at rate $\theta/2$, so if we condition on the time T_3, the number of mutations is Poisson with mean $T_3\theta/2$. $E(n_{CF}|T_3) = T_3\,\theta/2$ and hence

(j)
$$En_{CF} = \frac{\theta}{2}ET_3 = \frac{\theta}{2}\cdot\frac{1}{6}$$

To compute the variance we recall that if Z has a Poisson distribution with mean λ, then $EZ^2 = \lambda + \lambda^2$ so

$$E(n_{CF}^2|T_3) = T_3\,\theta/2 + (T_3\,\theta/2)^2$$

Recalling that if X has an exponential distribution with mean μ then $EX^2 = 2\mu^2$, we have

(k)
$$E(n_{CF}^2) = \frac{\theta}{2} \cdot \frac{1}{6} + \frac{\theta^2}{4} \cdot \frac{2}{36}$$

and it follows that

(ℓ)
$$\text{var}(n_{CF}) = E(n_{CF}^2) - (En_{CF})^2 = \frac{\theta}{12} + \frac{\theta^2}{144}$$

Since n_{CF} and n_{CG} are conditionally independent given T_3, we have

$$E(n_{CF}\, n_{CG}|T_2) = \left(\frac{T_3\,\theta}{2}\right)^2$$

and hence

(m)
$$E(n_{CF}\, n_{CG}) = \frac{\theta^2}{4} \cdot \frac{2}{36} = \frac{\theta^2}{72}$$

From this and (j), it follows that

(n)
$$\text{cov}(n_{CF}, n_{CG}) = \frac{\theta^2}{72} - \left(\frac{\theta}{12}\right)^2 = \frac{\theta^2}{144}$$

Letting C_i denote case i, and using (b), (d), and (j),

$$E(\Delta_4|C_1) = \frac{\theta}{12}\left\{3\cdot 2 + 10 \cdot \frac{1}{3} + 12 \cdot \frac{1}{6}\right\} = \frac{17}{18}\theta$$

$$E(\Delta_4|C_2) = \frac{\theta}{2}\left\{4\cdot 2 + 10 \cdot \frac{1}{3} + 12 \cdot \frac{1}{6}\right\} = \frac{10}{9}\theta$$

Multiplying the first equation times $2/3$ and adding it to $1/3$ times the second,

$$E\Delta_4 = \left(\frac{2}{3}\cdot\frac{17}{18} + \frac{1}{3}\cdot\frac{20}{18}\right)\theta = \theta$$

in agreement with (4.5).

We will now use a similar strategy to compute $\text{var}(\Delta_4)^2$. Taking the expected value and noting that variables on different levels are independent gives

$$36\,\text{var}(\Delta_4^2|C_1) = 9\,\text{var}(n_{AB}) + 34\,\text{var}(n_{BC}) + 66\,\text{cov}(n_{BC}, n_{BD})$$
$$+36\,\text{var}(n_{CF}) + 108\,\text{cov}(n_{CF}, n_{CG})$$

Plugging in values from (b), (f), (h), (ℓ), and (n) gives

$$= 9(\theta + \theta^2) + 34\left(\frac{\theta}{6} + \frac{\theta^2}{36}\right) + 66\frac{\theta^2}{36} + 36\left(\frac{\theta}{12} + \frac{\theta^2}{144}\right) + 108\frac{\theta^2}{144}$$

$$= \left(\frac{53}{3}\right)\theta + \left(\frac{115}{9}\right)\theta^2$$

Similar reasoning for the case 2 formula gives

$$
\begin{aligned}
36 \operatorname{var}\left(\Delta_4^2 | C_2\right) & = 16 \operatorname{var}\left(n_{AB}\right) + 34 \operatorname{var}\left(n_{BC}\right) + 66 \operatorname{cov}\left(n_{BC}, n_{BD}\right) \\
& \quad + 36 \operatorname{var}\left(n_{CF}\right) + 108 \operatorname{cov}\left(n_{CF}, n_{CG}\right) \\
& = 36 \operatorname{var}\left(\Delta_4^2 | C_1\right) + 7 \operatorname{var}\left(n_{AB}\right)
\end{aligned}
$$

and plugging in values, we have

$$
36 \operatorname{var}\left(\Delta_4^2 | C_2\right) = \left(\frac{74}{3}\right)\theta + \left(\frac{178}{9}\right)\theta^2
$$

We cannot simply average the conditional variances to get the overall variance. However, using

$$
\operatorname{var}(Y) = E(\operatorname{var}(Y|X)) + \operatorname{var}(E(Y|X))
$$

with $X = i$ on C_i for $i = 1, 2$, we have

$$
\begin{aligned}
\operatorname{var}\left(\Delta_4\right) & = \frac{2}{3}\operatorname{var}\left(\Delta_4 | C_1\right) + \frac{1}{3}\operatorname{var}\left(\Delta_4 | C_2\right) \\
& \quad + \frac{2}{3}\left(E(\Delta_4 | C_1) - E\Delta_4\right)^2 \\
& \quad + \frac{1}{3}\left(E(\Delta_4 | C_2) - E\Delta_4\right)^2
\end{aligned}
$$

Plugging in our values gives

$$
\begin{aligned}
& = \frac{2}{3}\left[\frac{53}{108}\theta + \frac{115}{324}\theta^2\right] + \frac{1}{3}\left[\frac{74}{108}\theta + \frac{178}{324}\theta^2\right] \\
& \quad + \frac{2}{3}\left(\frac{17}{18}\theta - \theta\right)^2 + \frac{1}{3}\left(\frac{20}{18}\theta - \theta\right)^2
\end{aligned}
$$

which simplifies to

$$
(o) \qquad \operatorname{var}\left(\Delta_4\right) = \left(\frac{5}{9}\right)\theta + \left(\frac{23}{54}\right)\theta^2
$$

which agrees with (4.6) in the case $n = 4$.

Having calculated $\operatorname{var}\left(\Delta_n\right)$ for $n = 2, 3, 4$, we can now solve for U_2, U_3, and U_4. From (4.4) we have

$$
(p) \qquad U_2 = \theta + \theta^2
$$

To find U_3, we use $(\star)$ to conclude that

$$
3 \operatorname{var}\left(\Delta_3\right) = U_2 + 2U_3
$$

and then plug in (i) and (p) to get

$$
2\theta + \frac{5}{3}\theta^2 = \theta + \theta^2 + 2U_3
$$

Rearranging gives

$$
(q) \qquad U_3 = \frac{1}{2}\left(\theta + \frac{2}{3}\theta^2\right) = \frac{\theta}{2} + \frac{\theta^2}{3}
$$

To find U_4, we use $(\star)$ to conclude that

$$6 \operatorname{var}(\Delta_4) = U_2 + 4U_3 + U_4$$

and then plug in (o), (p), and (q) to get

$$\frac{10}{3}\theta + \frac{23}{9}\theta^2 = \theta + \theta^2 + 4\left(\frac{\theta}{2} + \frac{\theta^2}{3}\right) + U_4$$

Rearranging gives

(r) $$U_4 = \frac{\theta}{3} + \frac{2}{9}\theta^2$$

Substituting (p), (q), and (r) into $(\star)$ gives

$$\operatorname{var}(\Delta_n) = \binom{n}{2}^{-1}\left[\theta + \theta^2 + 2(n-2)\left(\frac{\theta}{2} + \frac{\theta^2}{3}\right)\right.$$
$$\left. + \frac{(n-2)(n-3)}{2} \cdot \frac{\theta}{3} + \frac{2\theta^2}{9}\right]$$

The term in square brackets is

$$\theta\left(\frac{6 + 6n - 12 + n^2 - 5n + 6}{6}\right) + \theta^2\left(\frac{9 + 6n - 12 + n^2 - 5n + 6}{9}\right)$$

Rearranging gives

$$\operatorname{var}(\Delta_n) = \binom{n}{2}^{-1}\left(\frac{n(n+1)}{6}\theta + \frac{n^2 + n + 3}{9}\theta^2\right)$$

which is the desired result. $\qquad\qquad\qquad\qquad\qquad\qquad\qquad\Box$

Nucleotide Diversity

Let μ be the mutation rate per nucleotide per generation. Using (2.13) we see that the probability that two nucleotides differ is

$$\frac{4N\mu}{1 + 4N\mu} \approx 4N\mu$$

since in most cases $4N\mu$ is small. This is called the *nucleotide diversity* and is denoted by π. Li and Sadler (1991) estimated π for humans by examining 49 genes. At fourfold degenerate sites (i.e., where no substitution changes the amino acid) they found $\pi = 0.11\%$ (i.e., $\pi = 0.0011$). At twofold degenerate sites (i.e., where only one of the three possible changes is synonymous), and nondegenerate sites, the values were 0.06% and 0.03% respectively. More recent studies have confirmed this. Harding et al. (1997) sequenced a 3 kb stretch including the β-globin gene in 349 chromosomes from nine populations in Africa, Asia, and Europe, revealing an overall nucleotide diversity of $\pi = 0.18\%$. Clark et al. (1998) and Nickerson et al. (1998) sequenced a 9.7 kb region near the lipoprotein lipase gene in 142 chromosomes finding an average nucleotide diversity of 0.2%.

In contrast, data compiled by Aquadro (1991) for various species of *Drosophila* give the following estimates for π

	D. pseudoobscura	D. simulans	D. melanogaster
Adh	0.026	0.015	0.006
Amy	0.019		0.008
rosy	0.013	0.018	0.005

Since $\pi = 4N\mu$, the differences in the value of π can be due to differences in N or in μ. Here N is not the physical population size, i.e., 6 billion for humans or an astronomical number for *Drosophila*, but instead is the "effective population size." To explain the need for this concept, we note that in the recent past the human population has grown exponentially and *Drosophila* populations undergo large seasonal fluctuations, so neither fits our assumption of a population of constant size. The effective population size will be defined precisely in Section 2.1. To illustrate its use in the current example, we note that current estimates (see Drake et al. 1998) of the mutation rate in humans are $\mu = 10^{-8}$ per nucleotide per generation. Setting $1.1 \times 10^{-3} = 4N \cdot 10^{-8}$ and solving gives $N_e = 27,500$.

Example 4.4. Single nucleotide polymorphisms (abbreviated SNPs and pronounced "snips") are nucleotides that are variable in a population but in which no allele has a frequency of more than 99%. If we restrict our attention to nucleotides for which there has been only one mutation then (3.6) can be used to estimate the number of SNPs in the human genome. Taking n to be the population size for humans and ignoring the case in which $m = n/2$, (3.6a) tells us that if $m < n - m$ the probability of having m of one allele and $n - m$ of the other is

$$\frac{n!}{\theta_{(n)}} \cdot \frac{\theta^2}{m(n-m)}$$

where $\theta = 4n\mu$ and μ is the mutation rate per nucleotide per generation (so in this case θ is what we have called π above). As noted above, the "effective size" of the human population is in the tens of thousands and $\mu \approx 1 \times 10^{-8}$, so $4N\mu$ is small and hence

$$\frac{n!}{\theta(\theta+1)\cdots(\theta+n-1)} \cdot \frac{\theta^2}{m(n-m)} \approx \frac{n\theta}{m(n-m)}$$

The probability that the less frequent allele is present in at least a fraction x of the population is then

$$\approx \frac{1}{n} \sum_{m=xn}^{n/2} \frac{\theta}{\frac{m}{n} \cdot \frac{n-m}{n}} \approx \int_x^{1/2} \frac{\theta}{y(1-y)} \, dy$$

$$= \theta \int_x^{1/2} \frac{1}{y} + \frac{1}{1-y} \, dy \theta \int_x^{1-x} \frac{\theta}{y} \, dy = \theta \ln\left(\frac{1-x}{x}\right)$$

in agreement with a computation of Kruglyak and Nickerson (2001). If we use their figure of $\pi = 1/1331$ and take $x = 0.01$, then we see that the density of SNPs is $\ln(99) = 4.59$ times π, or 1 every 289 bp. This means that the 3.2 billion nucleotides of the human genome contain more than 11 million SNPs.

Segregating Sites

Another quantity of interest in the infinite sites model is the number of *segregating sites*, S_n, in the sample of size n, that is, the number of positions where some pair of sequences differs. The results here are due to Watterson (1975). Let t_j be the amount of time in the coalescent during which there are j lineages. In (2.6) we showed that if N is large and time is measured in units of $2N$ generations, then t_j has approximately an exponential distribution with mean $2/j(j-1)$. The total amount of time in the tree for a sample of size n is

$$T_{tot} = \sum_{j=2}^{n} j t_j$$

Taking expected values, we have

(4.7) $$ET_{tot} = \sum_{j=2}^{n} j \cdot \frac{2}{j(j-1)} = 2 \sum_{j=2}^{n} \frac{1}{j-1}$$

so the expected number of segregating sites is

(4.8) $$ES_n = 2Nu \cdot ET_{tot} = \theta \sum_{i=1}^{n-1} \frac{1}{i}$$

where u is the per locus mutation rate and $\theta = 4Nu$.

Example 4.5. In the Aquadro and Greenberg data set $S = 44$, while

$$1 + \frac{1}{2} + \frac{1}{3} + \frac{1}{4} + \frac{1}{5} + \frac{1}{6} = 2.45$$

so our new estimate based on the number of segregating sites S_7 is

$$\theta = 44/2.45 = 17.96$$

compared with the previous estimate of 14.86 based on pairwise differences, Δ_7. Using our estimate of $N_e = 25,000$ for the human population, we can translate the estimate 17.96 for $4N_e(900\mu)$ into a mutation rate estimate of 2×10^{-7} per nucleotide per generation for the region of mtDNA studied by Aquadro and Greenberg (1983). This is higher than the rate of 10^{-8} we quoted earlier for nuclear DNA but is consistent with the observation that mitochondrial DNA evolves much more rapidly than nuclear DNA. (See Brown et al. 1979 and Miyata et al. 1982.)

To understand the variability in the estimator of the scaled mutation rate

$$\hat{\theta} = \frac{S_n}{\sum_{i=1}^{n-1} 1/i}$$

our next step is to show that

(4.9)
$$\text{var}\,(S_n) = \theta \sum_{i=1}^{n-1} \frac{1}{i} + \theta^2 \sum_{i=1}^{n-1} \frac{1}{i^2}$$

Proof. Let s_j be the number of segregating sites created when there were j lineages. While there are j lineages, we have a race between mutations happening at rate $2Nuj$ and coalescence at rate $j(j-1)/2$, so

$$P(s_j = k) = \left(\frac{\theta}{\theta + j - 1}\right)^k \frac{j-1}{\theta + j - 1}$$

This is a shifted geometric distribution with $p = (j-1)/(\theta + j - 1)$, so using (4.3) we have

$$
\begin{aligned}
\text{var}\,(s_j) &= \frac{1-p}{p^2} = \frac{\theta}{\theta + j - 1} \cdot \frac{(\theta + j - 1)^2}{(j-1)^2} \\
&= \frac{\theta^2 + (j-1)\theta}{(j-1)^2} = \frac{\theta}{j-1} + \frac{\theta^2}{(j-1)^2}
\end{aligned}
$$

Summing from $j = 2$ to n and letting $i = j - 1$ gives the result. □

The last proof is simple, but one can obtain additional insight and generality by starting with the observation that the distribution of $(S_n | T_{tot} = t)$ is Poisson with mean $t\theta/2$. From this it follows that

$$
\begin{aligned}
E(S_n) &= \frac{\theta}{2} ET_{tot} \\
\text{var}\,(S_n) &= E\{\text{var}\,(S_n | T_{tot})\} + \text{var}\,\{E(S_n | T_{tot})\} \\
&= \frac{\theta}{2} ET_{tot} + \frac{\theta^2}{4} \text{var}\,(T_{tot})
\end{aligned}
$$

The last result is valid for any genealogy. If we now use the fact that in the Wright-Fisher model $T_{tot} = \sum_{j=2}^{n} jt_j$, where the t_j are exponential with mean $2/j(j-1)$ and variance $4/j^2(j-1)^2$, then (4.9) follows and we see the source of the two terms.

(4.8) and (4.9) show that $\hat{\theta} = S_n/(\sum_{i=1}^{n-1} 1/i)$ is an unbiased estimator of θ with

$$\text{var}\,(\hat{\theta}) = \frac{\theta}{(\sum_{i=1}^{n-1} 1/i)} + \frac{\theta^2 \sum_{i=1}^{n} 1/i^2}{(\sum_{i=1}^{n-1} 1/i)^2}$$

For large n, the right hand side is $\sim \theta/\ln n$ so again there is very slow convergence to the limiting expected value $\theta = E\hat{\theta}$. The proof of (4.9) shows that

(4.10) $S_n = \sum_{j=2}^{n} s_j$ where the s_j are independent shifted geometrics with success probabilities $p = (j-1)/(\theta + j - 1)$.

Using the triangular array form of the central limit theorem, see for example (4.5) on page 116 of Durrett (1995), we have that as $n \to \infty$,

$$P\left(\frac{S_n - ES_n}{\sqrt{\text{var}\,(S_n)}} \le x\right) \to P(\chi \le x)$$

If one wants the exact distribution of S_n, one can use $S_n = S_{n-1} + s_n$ and (4.10) to conclude

(4.11) $\quad P(S_n = k) = \sum_{m=0}^{k} P(S_{n-1} = k - m) \left(\frac{\theta}{\theta + n - 1}\right)^m \frac{n-1}{\theta + n - 1}$

Tavaré (1984) has used this approach to obtain explicit expressions for the distribution of S_n. The result is very simple for $k = 0$. In that case

$$P(S_n = 0) = P(S_{n-1} = 0) \cdot \frac{n-1}{\theta + n - 1}$$

and iterating gives

(4.12) $\qquad P(S_n = 0) = \frac{(n-1)!}{(\theta + 1) \cdots (\theta + n - 1)}$

Example 4.6. Nachman, Bauer, Crowell, and Aquadro (1998) sequenced 11,365 bp from introns of seven X-linked genes in ten humans, one chimpanzee, and one orangutan. Two of these genes, interleukin-2 receptor γ chain (*Il2rg*) and iduronate sulphate sulphatase (*Ids*), showed no variation in humans even though 1147 bp were sequenced in the first case and 1909 bp were sequenced in the second. If we suppose an effective population size of 10,000 for humans and a per nucleotide mutation rate $\mu = 2 \times 10^{-8}$ then the nucleotide diversity is predicted to be $\pi = 4N_e\mu = 8 \times 10^{-4}$, or 0.08%, and we have mutation rates of $\theta = 0.92$ and $\theta = 1.53$ for the two regions. Using (4.12) now, we conclude that $P(S_{10} = 0)$ is 0.117 and 0.038, respectively. The second probability is less than 0.05. Indeed $P(S_{10} = 0) \le 0.05$ whenever $\theta \ge 1.378049$.

As a check on the mutation rates that we have assumed we note that the divergence between the human and the chimp sequence is 0.78% for *Il2rg* and 0.26% for *Ids*. If we assume the divergence took place 5 million years ago and use 20 years for the average of human and chimp generation times, then 500,000 generations separate the two sequences. (Recall that mutations occur on both branches of the genealogy.) The observed divergences translate into mutation rate estimates of 1.56×10^{-8} and 5.2×10^{-9}. Reducing the mutation rate estimate to $\mu = 1 \times 10^{-8}$ in the case of *Ids* makes our estimate of $P(S_{10} = 0) > 0.05$, so we are not 95% confident that this pattern is unusual.

Example 4.7. Aguadé, Miyashita, and Langley (1989) studied a 106 kb region encompassing the *yellow* gene and the *achaete-scute* complex that is located in a region of reduced recombination near the end of the X chromosome of *Drosophila melanogaster*. They digested the DNA using seven hexanucleotide-recognizing restriction enzymes, which cut the DNA at each occurrence of a sequence of six specific nucleotides. In the region they studied, there were 176 sites where one of the enzymes could cut the DNA. However, only 9 of the 176 sites were found to be polymorphic in the sample of size 64. As they argued on page 612 of their paper, this low level of polymorphism is very surprising.

By comparison with a number of other gene regions that had been studied, Aquadé, Miyashita, and Langley (1989) argued that the nucleotide diversity was $\pi = 0.005$. To translate this into a per locus mutation rate they multiplied by $2112 = 6 \times 176 \times 2$ to arrive at an estimate of $\theta = 4Nu$ of 10.56. The first factor in 2112 comes from the fact that the restriction enzymes look at six sites and will not work if one of the nucleotides is changed. The second factor is the observed number of places where the DNA was cut. The final factor of 2 comes from the fact that for a given sequence of six nucleotides there are 18 other sequences that differ from it at one nucleotide, and hence by 1 of 18 possible changes can be converted into a sequence that can be cut. In words, restriction sites can be destroyed or created by mutations and the two rates are the same, hence the factor of 2.

A short computer program shows that

$$\sum_{i=1}^{63} \frac{1}{i} = 4.728266 \qquad \sum_{i=1}^{63} \frac{1}{i^2} = 1.629186$$

Alternatively one can let $\gamma = 0.57721566\ldots$ be Euler's constant and use the approximations

$$\sum_{j=1}^{n-1} \frac{1}{i} \approx \ln n + \gamma \qquad \sum_{i=1}^{\infty} \frac{1}{i^2} = \frac{\pi^2}{6}$$

to arrive at values 4.7361 and 1.6449.

Using the exact values in (4.8) and (4.9) shows that if we accept this estimate of θ, then the mean and variance of the number of segregating sites are

$$E(S_{64}) = 49.9 \qquad \text{var}\,(S_{64}) = 49.9 + 181.6 = 231.5$$

The standard deviation of the distribution is $\sqrt{231.5} = 15.2$, so the observed value of 9 is $(49.9 - 9)/15.2 = 2.69$ standard deviations below the mean. For the normal distribution where a deviation this large is an event of probability 0.0036, so we conclude that this is very unlikely to have occurred by chance.

At this point, we must admit that the computations in the last paragraph are flawed since they use formulas that assume there is no recombination. The formula for the mean remains correct. The expected number of mutations that affect a single nucleotide is, by the reasoning for (4.8),

$$2N\mu\,ET_{tot} = 4N\mu \sum_{i=1}^{n-1} \frac{1}{i}$$

where μ is the mutation rate per nucleotide per generation, and multiplying by the number of nucleotides L gives the previous result. If, however, there was a lot of recombination, then the genealogies for the different nucleotides would be independent Poisson random variables. Since the variance of the Poisson is equal to its mean, the total variance of L nucleotides would be

(4.12)
$$\theta \sum_{i=1}^{n-1} \frac{1}{i}$$

i.e., the first term in (4.9).

With a positive but finite amount of recombination, the total time in the tree for different nucleotides is positively correlated, so the variance of the number of segregating sites will be intermediate between (4.12) and (4.8). The good news is that we have overestimated the variance and the test is conservative. This good news is also bad news. In the current example, the upper bound from (4.8) is 231.5 versus a lower bound of 49.9, so there is a potential for missing significant results.

1.5   Finite Sites, Four Nucleotides

As we noted at the beginning of the previous section when one is studying a locus with L nucleotides, the assumption of infinite sites will hold until there have been about $L^{1/2}$ substitutions. To go beyond this time scale, we need models that deal explicitly with the fact that there are only finitely many sites and four nucleotides. We begin with models of the evolution of a single nucleotide due to substitutions. Then we will use some of these models to analyze data.

Models

The first and simplest of these is the model of Jukes and Cantor (1969), which assumes that substitutions occur randomly among the four types of nucleotides and that in each generation a change from i to $j \neq i$ occurs with probability α. Let X_t be the state of the nucleotide at time t and define the transition probability by

$$p_{ij}(t) = P(X_t = j | X_t = i)$$

By considering what happens on the last step, we have

$$p_{ij}(t+1) = p_{ij}(t)(1 - 3\alpha) + \alpha \sum_{k \neq j} p_{ik}(t)$$

Since $\sum_{k \neq j} p_{ik}(t) = 1 - p_{ij}(t)$, rearranging gives

$$p_{ij}(t+1) - p_{ij}(t) = -4\alpha p_{ij}(t) + \alpha$$

Since α is small, it is convenient to reformulate things in continuous time and write

$$\frac{d}{dt} p_{ij}(t) = -4\alpha p_{ij}(t) + \alpha$$

The general solution to this differential equation is

$$p_{ij}(t) = \frac{1}{4} + \left(p_{ij}(0) - \frac{1}{4} \right) e^{-4\alpha t}$$

which we can check by differentiating.

$$\frac{d}{dt} p_{ij}(t) = -4\alpha \left(p_{ij}(0) - \frac{1}{4} \right) e^{-4\alpha t} = -4\alpha \left(p_{ij}(t) - \frac{1}{4} \right)$$

Since $p_{ij}(0)$ is either 1 or 0, there are only two cases

(5.1)
$$p_{ij}(t) = \begin{cases} 1/4 + 3/4 e^{-4\alpha t} & i = j \\ 1/4 - 1/4 e^{-4\alpha t} & i \neq j \end{cases}$$

Note that all the $p_{ij}(t) \to 1/4$ as $t \to \infty$, but if $i \neq j$ we have

$$p_{ii}(t) > 1/4 > p_{ij}(t)$$

As noted in our discussion of mitochondrial DNA in Example 3.1, the assumption that all nucleotide substitutions occur randomly is unrealistic since transitions are more common than transversions. To take this fact into account, Kimura (1980) proposed a two-parameter model. If we let q_{ij} be the rate at which jumps from i to j occur and let $q_{ii} = -\sum_{j \neq i} q_{ij}$ then the transition rate matrix q_{ij} for the two-parameter model can be written as

	A	G	C	T
A	$-\alpha - 2\beta$	α	β	β
G	α	$-\alpha - 2\beta$	β	β
C	β	β	$-\alpha - 2\beta$	α
T	β	β	α	$-\alpha - 2\beta$

In our genetics application $\alpha > \beta$, and indeed α is about 20 times as large as β. Our convention concerning the diagonal entries in the matrix q_{ij} is the standard one in Markov chain theory since it allows us to write

$$(5.2) \qquad \frac{d}{dt}p_{ij}(t) = \sum_k p_{ik}(t)q_{kj}$$

Proof. Reasoning as in the Jukes-Cantor model

$$p_{ij}(t+1) = p_{ij}(t)(1 + q_{jj}) + \sum_{k \neq j} p_{ik}(t)q_{kj}$$

so we have $p_{ij}(t+1) - p_{ij}(t) = \sum_k p_{ik}(t)q_{kj}$. □

An almost identical argument, left to the reader, shows

$$(5.3) \qquad \frac{d}{dt}p_{ij}(t) = \sum_k q_{ik}p_{kj}(t)$$

This and (5.2) are Kolmogorov's forward and backward differential equations.

Suppose without loss of generality that $i = A$. If we combine states A and G into a superstate u (for purine), and combine states C and T into a superstate y (for pyrimidine), then the combined chain makes transitions as follows

	u	y
u	-2β	2β
y	2β	-2β

To solve this equation we note that (5.2) implies

$$\frac{d}{dt}p_{uu}(t) = -2\beta p_{uu}(t) + 2\beta p_{uy}(t)$$

$$\frac{d}{dt}p_{uy}(t) = 2\beta p_{uu}(t) - 2\beta p_{uy}(t)$$

Taking differences gives

$$\frac{d}{dt}(p_{uu}(t) - p_{uy}(t)) = -4\beta(p_{uu}(t) - p_{uy}(t))$$

so we have $p_{uu}(t) - p_{uy}(t) = e^{-4\beta t}$. Since $p_{uu}(t) + p_{uy}(t) = 1$,

$$(\star) \qquad p_{uu}(t) = 1/2 + (1/2)e^{-4\beta} \qquad p_{uy}(t) = 1/2 - (1/2)e^{-4\beta}$$

Symmetry dictates that $p_{AC}(t) = p_{AT}(t) = (1/2)p_{uy}(t)$. To complete the solution, we note that using (5.2) with the 4 by 4 matrix of transition rates gives

$$\frac{d}{dt}(p_{AA}(t) - p_{AG}(t)) = -(2\alpha + 2\beta)(p_{AA}(t) - p_{AG}(t))$$

so we have $p_{AA}(t) - p_{AG}(t) = e^{-2(\alpha+\beta)t}$ and using ($\star$) it follows that

(5.4) *The transition probability of Kimura's two-parameter model is*

$$\begin{aligned} p_{AA}(t) &= 1/4 + (1/4)e^{-4\beta t} + (1/2)e^{-2(\alpha+\beta)t} \\ p_{AG}(t) &= 1/4 + (1/4)e^{-4\beta t} - (1/2)e^{-2(\alpha+\beta)t} \\ p_{AC}(t) &= 1/4 - (1/4)e^{-4\beta t} \\ p_{AT}(t) &= 1/4 - (1/4)e^{-4\beta t} \end{aligned}$$

Again all $p_{ij}(t) \to 1/4$ as $t \to \infty$, and we have

$$p_{AA}(t) > 1/4 > p_{AC}(t), p_{AT}(t)$$

However, we will have $p_{AG}(t) > 1/4$ if $(1/4)e^{-4\beta t} > (1/2)e^{-2(\alpha+\beta)t}$, which occurs if $1/2 > e^{2(\alpha-\beta)t}$ or $t > (\ln 2)/(\alpha - \beta)$.

Kimura's two-parameter model differentiates between transitions and transversions but in equilibrium all four bases have equal frequencies. However, in the heavy strand of human mtDNA that we are about to consider, the frequencies of nucleotides are

A	T	G	C
0.247	0.313	0.302	0.139

This problem can be addressed with Kimura's (1981) six-parameter model, which has transition rates

	A	G	C	T
A	$-2\alpha - \gamma_1$	γ_1	α	α
G	δ_1	$-2\alpha - \delta_1$	α	α
C	β	β	$-2\beta - \gamma_2$	γ_2
T	β	β	δ_2	$-2\beta - \delta_2$

The first step in analyzing this chain is to determine its stationary distribution, i.e., the vector π_i with $\sum_i \pi_i p_{ij}(t) = \pi_j$ for all t. For this we need the following fact

(5.5) π *is a stationary distribution if and only if* $\sum_i \pi_i q_{ij} = 0$.

In words, if we write π as a row vector and multiply it by the matrix q, then $\pi q = (0, 0, \ldots 0)$.

Proof. To begin, we note that if π is a stationary distribution, (5.2) implies

$$0 = \frac{d}{dt} \sum_i \pi_i p_{ij}(t) = \sum_k \sum_i \pi_i p_{ik}(t) q_{kj} = \sum_k \pi_k q_{kj}$$

In the other direction, (5.3) implies

$$\frac{d}{dt} \sum_i \pi_i p_{ij}(t) = \sum_k \sum_i \pi_i q_{ik} p_{kj}(t) = 0 \qquad\qquad \square$$

To begin to guess the stationary distribution, we can observe that the first step in the analysis of the two-parameter model works here. If we combine states A and G into a superstate u, and combine states C and T into a superstate y, then the combined chain makes transitions as follows

$$
\begin{array}{c c c}
 & u & y \\
u & -2\alpha & 2\alpha \\
y & 2\beta & -2\beta
\end{array}
$$

Using (5.5) it is easy to see that this chain has stationary distribution

$$\pi_u = \frac{\beta}{\beta + \alpha} \qquad \pi_v = \frac{\alpha}{\beta + \alpha}$$

Using this as a starting point, one can guess that the stationary distribution for the six-parameter chain is

$$\pi_A = \frac{\beta}{\beta + \alpha} \cdot \frac{\alpha + \delta_1}{2\alpha + \gamma_1 + \delta_1} \qquad \pi_G = \frac{\beta}{\beta + \alpha} \cdot \frac{\alpha + \gamma_1}{2\alpha + \gamma_1 + \delta_1}$$

$$\pi_C = \frac{\alpha}{\beta + \alpha} \cdot \frac{\alpha + \delta_2}{2\alpha + \gamma_2 + \delta_2} \qquad \pi_T = \frac{\alpha}{\beta + \alpha} \cdot \frac{\alpha + \gamma_2}{2\alpha + \gamma_2 + \delta_2}$$

To check the first of the four conditions in (5.5), we note that

$$-(2\alpha + \gamma_1)\frac{\alpha + \delta_1}{2\alpha + \gamma_1 + \delta_1} + \delta_1 \frac{\alpha + \gamma_1}{2\alpha + \gamma_1 + \delta_1} = -\alpha$$

so the dot product of the stationary distribution and the first column of the q matrix is

$$\frac{\beta}{\beta + \alpha}(-\alpha) + \frac{\alpha}{\beta + \alpha}(\beta) = 0$$

The remaining computations are similar and are left to the reader.

To solve for the transition probability of the six parameter chain, Gojobori, Ishii, and Nei (1982) used matrix theory to conclude that

$$(5.6) \qquad\qquad p_{ij}(t) = \pi_i + \sum_{k=1}^{3} u_i^k v_j^k e^{-\lambda_k t}$$

where u^k and v^k are the left and right eigenvectors corresponding to the eigenvalues

$$\lambda_1 = -2(\alpha + \beta) \quad \lambda_2 = -(2\alpha + \gamma_1 + \delta_1) \quad \lambda_3 = -(2\alpha + \gamma_2 + \delta_2)$$

That is $u^k q = \lambda_k u^k$ and $qv^k = \lambda_k$. We refer the reader to their paper for the eigenvectors and further details.

A simpler way to achieve the observed frequencies of the four nucleotides $\pi_A, \pi_G, \pi_C, \pi_T$ is the *equal input model* of Felsenstein (1981) and Tajima and Nei (1982). In this case, the transition matrix is α times

$$
\begin{array}{c|cccc}
 & A & G & C & T \\
\hline
A & \pi_A - 1 & \pi_G & \pi_C & \pi_T \\
G & \pi_A & \pi_G - 1 & \pi_C & \pi_T \\
C & \pi_A & \pi_G & \pi_C - 1 & \pi_T \\
T & \pi_A & \pi_G & \pi_C & \pi_T - 1
\end{array}
$$

One can describe this chain in words as: stay at the current site i for an exponential amount of time with mean $1/\alpha$ and then take a jump according to the distribution π. With probability π_i one lands back at the same place and no visible change occurs. It is easy to use (5.5) to check that the stationary distribution is $(\pi_A, \pi_G, \pi_C, \pi_T)$. Since after the first attempted jump the chain is in the stationary distribution,

$$(5.7) \qquad p_{ij}(t) = e^{-\alpha t} I_{ij} + (1 - e^{-\alpha t}) \pi_j$$

where $I_{ij} = 1$ if $i = j$ and $= 0$ if $i \neq j$ is the identity matrix.

The last model does not distinguish between transitions and transversions. To do this, Hasegawa, Kishino, and Yano (1985) introduced the following model:

$$
\begin{array}{c|cccc}
 & A & G & C & T \\
\hline
A & -\alpha\pi_G - \beta\pi_Y & \alpha\pi_G & \beta\pi_C & \beta\pi_T \\
G & \alpha\pi_A & -\alpha\pi_A - \beta\pi_Y & \beta\pi_C & \beta\pi_T \\
C & \beta\pi_A & \beta\pi_G & -\alpha\pi_T - \beta\pi_R & \alpha\pi_T \\
T & \beta\pi_A & \beta\pi_G & \alpha\pi_C & -\alpha\pi_C - \beta\pi_R
\end{array}
$$

where $\pi_Y = \pi_T + \pi_C$ and $\pi_R = \pi_A + \pi_G$ are the equilibrium probabilities of pyrimidines and purines. At first, it is not clear that the stationary distribution is $(\pi_A, \pi_G, \pi_C, \pi_T)$. To check this, we can use the following

(5.8) A sufficient condition for π to be a stationary distribution is $\pi_i q_{ij} = \pi_j q_{ji}$.

Proof. $\sum_i \pi_i q_{ij} = \pi_j \sum_i q_{ji} = 0$ since each row sums to 0. $\qquad \square$

In words, the condition in (5.8) says that the rate at which probability mass jumps from i to j is exactly balanced by the rate at which it jumps from j to i. Markov chains that satisfy the conditions in (5.8) are said to be *reversible* since that condition implies

$$\pi_i p_{ij}(t) = \pi_j p_{ji}(t)$$

In words, a movie of the process in equilibrium looks the same going forwards or backwards in time. The Jukes-Cantor model and Kimura's two-parameter model are symmetric $(p_{ij}(t) = p_{ji}(t))$ and hence reversible with $\pi_i = 1/4$. Kimura's six-parameter model is not reversible in general since

$$\frac{\pi_A \, q_{AG}}{\pi_G \, q_{GA}} = \frac{(\alpha + \delta_1)\gamma_1}{(\alpha + \gamma_1)\delta_1} \neq 1$$

unless $\delta_1 = \gamma_1$.

Hasegawa, Kishino, and Yano analyzed their chain by using the eigenvalue-eigenvector formula (5.6). The eigenvalues are

$$\lambda_1 = -\beta \qquad \lambda_2 = -(\pi_Y \beta + \pi_R \alpha) \qquad \lambda_3 = -(\pi_Y \alpha + \pi_R \beta)$$

while the eigenvectors are

$$u^1 = \begin{pmatrix} -\pi_Y \pi_A \\ -\pi_Y \pi_G \\ \pi_R \pi_C \\ \pi_R \pi_T \end{pmatrix} \qquad u^2 = \begin{pmatrix} 1 \\ -1 \\ 0 \\ 0 \end{pmatrix} \qquad u^3 = \begin{pmatrix} 0 \\ 0 \\ 1 \\ -1 \end{pmatrix}$$

$$v^1 = \begin{pmatrix} 1/\pi_R \\ 1/\pi_R \\ -1/\pi_Y \\ -1/\pi_Y \end{pmatrix} \qquad v^2 = \begin{pmatrix} \pi_G/\pi_R \\ -\pi_A/\pi_R \\ 0 \\ 0 \end{pmatrix} \qquad v^3 = \begin{pmatrix} 0 \\ 0 \\ \pi_T/\pi_Y \\ -\pi_C/\pi_Y \end{pmatrix}$$

The second and third are easy to see. To check the first ones we note that the dot product of u^1 with the first column of q is

$$\beta \pi_Y \pi_Y \pi_A + \beta \pi_A \pi_R \pi_C + \beta \pi_A \pi_R \pi_T = \beta \pi_Y \pi_A$$

since $\pi_C + \pi_T = \pi_Y$ and $\pi_Y + \pi_R = 1$. The other three columns are similar. As for v^1, its dot product with the first row of q is

$$-\frac{\beta \pi_Y}{\pi_R} - \frac{\beta \pi_Y}{\pi_Y} = -\frac{\beta(\pi_Y + \pi_R)}{\pi_R} = -\frac{\beta}{\pi_R}$$

At this point, we may have exhausted the reader (and the author) but not the possibilities for transition matrices. See Zharkikh (1994) for a survey that describes some other possibilities.

Data Analysis

In this subsection we will use some of the evolutionary distances to analyze a data set. We will restrict our attention to the simpler ones for which explicit formulas can be derived. It is fairly straightforward to develop numerical methods to implement the more complicated ones. The most basic statistic for estimating the evolutionary distance between two sequences under study is the proportion of identical nucleotides. The expected value of this proportion is equal to the probability that a nucleotide is the same in the two sequences. Let us start by supposing that the most recent common ancestor occurred t generations ago and at that time the nucleotide at a given site was A. Taking into account that the descendant nucleotide could be A, T, C, or G in each of the two sequences, we see that the probability that the nucleotides in the two sequences today are identical is

$$I(t) = p_{AA}^2(t) + p_{AT}^2(t) + p_{AC}^2(t) + p_{AG}^2(t)$$

If the transition probability is symmetric, i.e., has $p_{ij}(t) = p_{ji}(t)$, we can write the last formula as

(5.9)
$$I(t) = \sum_k p_{Ak}(t) p_{kA}(t) = p_{AA}(2t)$$

since in order to go from A to A in $2t$ units, we must first go from A to some k in the first t units and then from that k to A in the last t units of time.

Using (5.9) with (5.1), it follows that for the Jukes-Cantor (1969) model

(5.10)
$$I(t) = \frac{1}{4} + \frac{3}{4} e^{-8\alpha t}$$

and this is independent of the starting nucleotide. Kimura's two parameter model is also symmetric, so using (5.9) with (5.4) gives

(5.11)
$$I(t) = 1/4 + (1/4)e^{-8\beta t} + (1/2)e^{-4(\alpha+\beta)t}$$

which is again independent of the starting nucleotide.

In the models where the equilibrium frequencies of the four nucleotides are not equal, we define $I(t)$ by averaging over the equilibrium frequencies:

$$I(t) = \sum_i \pi_i \sum_j p_{ij}^2(t)$$

In the reversible models $\pi_i p_{ij}(t) = \pi_j p_{ji}(t)$, and this may be rewritten as

$$I(t) = \sum_j \sum_i \pi_j p_{ji}(t) p_{ij}(t) = \sum_j \pi_j p_{jj}^2(t)$$

Although the last formula is compact, we will not use it to analyze the equal input model but instead follow the original approach of Tajima and Nei (1984). Let $y_{ij}(t)$ be the fraction of positions where there is an i in the first sequence and a j in the second. Using (5.7)

$$
\begin{aligned}
y_{ij}(t) &= \sum_k \pi_k p_{ki}(t) p_{kj}(t) \\
&= \sum_k \pi_k \Big\{ e^{-2\alpha t} I_{kj} I_{ki} + e^{-\alpha t}(1 - e^{-\alpha t}) \pi_i I_{kj} \\
&\quad + e^{-\alpha t}(1 - e^{-\alpha t}) \pi_j I_{ki} + (1 - e^{-\alpha t})^2 \pi_i \pi_j \Big\}
\end{aligned}
$$

When $i \neq j$, the first term in the sum is always 0, while the second and third sum to the same thing, so the above simplifies to

$$2e^{-\alpha t}(1 - e^{-\alpha t})\pi_i\pi_j + (1 - 2e^{-\alpha t} + e^{-2\alpha t})\pi_i\pi_j = \pi_i\pi_j(1 - e^{-2\alpha t})$$

Summing over $i \neq j$, we have

$$(5.12) \qquad 1 - I(t) = (1 - e^{-2\alpha t}) \sum_{i \neq j} \pi_i \pi_j = (1 - e^{-2\alpha t})(1 - \sum_k \pi_k^2)$$

Our problem is to use the observed fraction of differences p between two sequences to estimate the number of substitutions k that have actually occurred. If we adopt the Jukes-Cantor model, then (5.10) implies

$$p = \frac{3}{4}\left(1 - e^{-8\alpha t}\right)$$

and solving we have

$$8\alpha t = -\ln\left(1 - \frac{4p}{3}\right)$$

In the Jukes-Cantor model, we expect $3\alpha t$ substitutions by time t in each lineage so $Ek = 2(3\alpha t)$ and we estimate k by

$$(5.13) \qquad \hat{k} = -\frac{3}{4}\ln\left(1 - \frac{4p}{3}\right)$$

In the equal input model, p is given by (5.7). The expected number of substitutions between two sequences is

$$(5.14) \qquad Ek = 2\sum_i \pi_i \cdot \alpha(1 - \pi_i)t = 2(1 - \sum_i \pi_i^2)\alpha t$$

since substitutions are attempted at a total rate α but only result in a visible change with probability $1 - \pi_i$ for the ith nucleotide. Writing $h = 1 - \sum_i \pi_i^2$ for the heterozygosity (the probability that two randomly chosen nucleotides are different), (5.12) and (5.14) become $p = h(1 - e^{-2\alpha t})$ and $Ek = 2h\alpha t$, so $p = h(1 - e^{-Ek/h})$ and we can solve to get

$$(5.15) \qquad \hat{k} = -h\ln(1 - p/h)$$

When each $\pi_i = 1/4$, the equal input model reduces to the Jukes-Cantor model. In this case $h = 3/4$ and (5.15) reduces to (5.13).

In order to use Kimura's two parameter model, we will look separately at the frequency of transitional and transversional changes between the two sequences and call them q and r. The first step is to compute the number of such changes that we expect. Reversing the flow of time from the ancestral sequence to sequence 2:

ancestral sequence

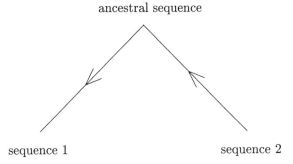

sequence 1   sequence 2

we can see that the probability of a transition or transversion between two sequences that have evolved for t units of time from a common ancestor is the same as that for one sequence that has evolved for $2t$ units of time. Using (5.4) now and letting Q and R denote the expected values of q and r, we conclude that

$$
\begin{aligned}
Q &= p_{AG}(2t) = 1/4 + (1/4)e^{-8\beta t} - (1/2)e^{-4(\alpha+\beta)t} \\
R &= p_{AC}(2t) + p_{AT}(2t) = 1/2 - (1/2)e^{-8\beta t}
\end{aligned}
$$

A little algebra shows

$$
\begin{aligned}
1 - 2Q - R &= e^{-4(\alpha+\beta)t} \\
1 - 2R &= e^{-8\beta t}
\end{aligned}
$$

The expected number of substitutions on each lineage is $(\alpha + 2\beta)t$, so we have $Ek = (2\alpha + 4\beta)t$ and can estimate k by

$$
\hat{k} = -\frac{1}{2}\ln(1 - 2q - r) - \frac{1}{4}\ln(1 - r)
$$

Example 5.1. We will now apply the methods above to the sequence of the mRNA for the somatotropin gene. Somatotropin is a growth hormone. In childhood, deficiency of somatotropin results in dwarfism. Seeburg et al. (1977) gives the sequence for rat, while Martial et al. (1979) gives the sequence for human. Alignment of the two sequences of amino acids indicates that they are separated by three insertion/deletion events. Of the 213 amino acids that can be compared, 74, or 34.7%, are different.

If we include the final stop codon, which is UAG in each sequence, then 214 triplets of nucleotides can be compared. The first thing we this done is simply to count the use of the four nucleotides at each of the three codon positions and compute the heterozygosity.

position	A	G	C	U	h
first	0.238	0.257	0.308	0.196	0.744
second	0.320	0.161	0.224	0.294	0.735
third	0.102	0.329	0.434	0.156	0.669

With this done, we are ready to count the changes that have occurred and compute the three genetic distances considered above: Jukes-Cantor (JC), equal input (EI), and two parameter (2P).

	first	second	third
transitions	28	24	27
transversions	20	8	31
p	0.221	0.150	0.366
JC	0.261	0.168	0.502
EI	0.261	0.168	0.530
2P	0.240	0.162	0.481
3P	0.26	0.18	0.53
6P	0.28	0.18	0.75

The last two rows are from Kimura (1981). The last (6P) is the six-parameter model we have considered above. The next to last (3P) is a three-parameter model in which there are different rates for the transversions that change the strength of the hydrogen bond ($A \rightarrow C$, $U \rightarrow G$, $C \rightarrow A$, $G \rightarrow U$).

The estimates from the various methods are similar except for the six parameter model at third position which is about 30% larger than the others. Note the striking difference in the rates at the three positions. This is what we would expect from the genetic code. Substitutions at the third position are often synonymous, while those at the second position never are, and those at first position are rarely so. Using the fact that humans and rats diverged about 80 million years ago and choosing 0.53 as the number of substitutions per nucleotide at the third position, we can estimate the mutation rate at that position as $0.53/(8 \times 10^7) = 6.6 \times 10^{-9}$ per year.

2
Neutral Complications

2.1 Nonconstant Population Size

In some cases, such as the human population, it is clear that the population size has not stayed constant in time. This motivates the consideration of a version of the Wright-Fisher model in which the number of diploid individuals in generation t is $N(t)$, but the rest of the details of the model stay the same. That is, in the case of no mutation, generation t is built up by choosing with replacement from generation $t - 1$. Reversing time leads as before to a coalescent.

To begin to develop some familiarity with this process, we will compute the probability that the lineages of two genes sampled at time 0 do not coalesce before generation $t < 0$. Since this occurs if and only if we avoid coalescence at each step, the probability is

$$(1.1) \qquad \prod_{s=t}^{-1} \left(1 - \frac{1}{2N(s)}\right) \approx \exp\left(-\sum_{s=t}^{-1} \frac{1}{2N(s)}\right)$$

where we have used $1 - x \approx e^{-x}$. Consider for concreteness

Example 1.1. Exponentially growing population. Let $N(s) = N_0 e^{\rho s}$ for $0 \geq s \geq s_0$, where $s_0 = -\rho^{-1} \ln(N_0)$ is defined so that $N(s_0) = 1$. A concrete example of this can be found in the work of Harding et al. (1997), who used $N_0 = 18,807$ and $\rho = 0.7/2N_0 = 1.861 \times 10^{-5}$ as a best fit model for data from the β-globin locus in the human population. When

$N(s) = N_0 e^{\rho s}$, the right-hand side of (1.1) can be approximated by

$$\exp\left(-\int_{s=t}^{0} \frac{e^{-\rho s}}{2N_0}\, ds\right) = \exp\left(-\frac{e^{-\rho t} - 1}{2\rho N_0}\right)$$

In the concrete example considered above, the right-hand side is

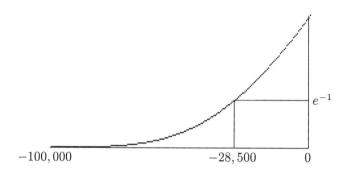

To check the graph, we note that $2\rho N_0 = 0.7$ so the right-hand side is e^{-1} when $t = -\rho^{-1}\ln(1 + 2\rho N_0) = -28,500$. When x is small, $e^{-x} \approx 1 - x$, so the right-hand side $\approx 1 - (e^{-\rho t} - 1)/0.7 \approx 1 + \rho t/0.7 = 1 + t/2N_0$ i.e., a straightline that would hit 0 at $-2N_0 = 37,614$. At the other extreme $s_0 = -528,850$ but as the graph shows, almost all of the coalescence has occurred by time $-75,000$.

The shape of the coalescence curve may surprise readers who have heard the phrase that genealogies in exponentially growing populations will tend to be *star-shaped*. That is, all of the coalescence tends to occur at the same time. Results of Slatkin and Hudson (1991) show that this is true provided $2N_0\rho$ is large while in our first example $2N_0\rho = 0.7$. Consider now a situation in which $N_0 = 100,000$ and $\rho = 5 \times 10^{-4}$ so $2N_0\rho = 10$.

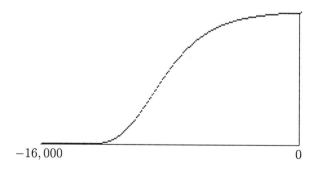

The distribution is now more concentrated but there still is a considerable amount of variability.

To further understand the nature of the phylogenies in a population of variable size, we note that when there are k lineages at time $s + 1$ a coalescence will occur at time s with probability

$$\binom{k}{2}/N(s) + O(1/N(s)^2)$$

From this it follows that if we represent the time interval $[s, s + 1]$ as a segment of length $1/N(s)$ then on the new time scale our process is almost the continuous time coalescent in which k lineages coalesce after an exponentially distributed amount of time with mean $1/\binom{k}{2}$. This idea, which is due to Kingman (1982b), see page 104, allows us to reduce our computations for a population of variable size at times $t \le s \le 0$ to one for the ordinary coalescent run for an amount of time

$$(1.2) \qquad\qquad \tau = \sum_{s=t}^{-1} \frac{1}{2N(s)}$$

Biologists have a different way of saying this. Returning to (1.1), we see that the probability of no coalescence in $[t, 0]$ is

$$\prod_{s=t}^{-1}\left(1 - \frac{1}{2N(s)}\right) \approx 1 - \sum_{s=t}^{-1}\frac{1}{2N(s)}$$

If we let $1/N_e = (1/t)\sum_{s=t}^{-1} 1/N(s)$ be the geometric mean of $N(-1), \ldots N(t)$, then the above is

$$= 1 - \frac{t}{2N_e} \approx \left(1 - \frac{1}{2N_e}\right)^t$$

i.e., the answer for a population of constant size N_e.

The N_e we have defined here is one example of the *effective population size*, one that will be called the *inbreeding effective population size* below. In general, the effective size of a population for a given statistic is the constant population size with the same value of that statistic. There are several statistics we can look at:

(i) the probability, π_2, that two genes picked at random are descendents of the same parent gene $= 1/2N$

(ii) the expected coalescence time, ET_2, of two lineages $= 2N$

(iii) the largest eigenvalue smaller than 1, $\lambda_{max} = 1 - 1/2N$

(iv) var $(x_{t+1}|x_t) = x_t(1 - x_t)/2N$, where $x_t =$ the fraction of A alleles

Each of these statistics leads to a different notion of effective population size.

$N_e^i =$ the inbreeding effective population size $(2\pi_2)^{-1}$

$N_e^c =$ the coalescence effective population size $ET_2/2$

$N_e^e =$ the eigenvalue effective population size $\frac{1}{2}(1 - \lambda_{max})^{-1}$

$N_e^v =$ the variance effective population size $\frac{x_t(1-x_t)}{\text{var}\,(x_{t+1}|x_t)}$

To illustrate these notions, we will begin with

Example 1.2. Periodically varying population. Suppose that the population size $N(s)$ cyclically assumes the values $N_1, N_2, \ldots N_k$. Using the computation above and generalizing the defintion of N_e^i to the periodic case, we have

$$\prod_{s=1}^{k}\left(1 - \frac{1}{2N(s)}\right) = \left(1 - \frac{1}{2N_e^i}\right)^k$$

When the population sizes are large, this implies

$$\frac{k}{2N_e^i} \approx \sum_{s=1}^{k}\frac{1}{2N(s)}$$

and we once again arrive at the geometric mean

$$(1.3) \qquad N_e^i \approx k/\sum_{s=1}^{k}\frac{1}{N(s)}$$

For a concrete example, suppose we have a population size that increases from 10 to 100 to 1000 and then crashes back to 10 again to repeat the cycle. Then it has effective population size

$$3\left/\left(\frac{1}{10} + \frac{1}{100} + \frac{1}{1000}\right)\right. = \frac{3000}{111} = 27.0270$$

Since there is a constant probability per cycle of coalescence, the coalescence effective population size is the same as the inbreeding effective population size. To compute the eigenvalue effective population size, we iterate the result for the Wright-Fisher model to conclude that if $X_t =$ the number of A alleles, then

$$E(X_{t+k}(2N_i - X_{t+k})|X_t) = X_t(2N_i - X_t)\prod_{j=1}^{k}\left(1 - \frac{1}{2N_j}\right)$$

This calculation identifies $m(2N_i - m)$ as an eignevector for the chain. Since it is strictly positive, matrix theory tells us that it is the eigenvalue associated with the largest eigenvalue < 1 so

$$\prod_{s=1}^{k} \left(1 - \frac{1}{2N(s)}\right) = (1 - (2N_e^e)^{-1})^k$$

This shows $N_e^e = N_e^i$. One can also compute the variance effective population size and show that it is essentially equal to the harmonic mean (see page 110 of Ewens 1979). However this notion is difficult to apply in some settings so we will systematically ignore it here.

For our next example, we will consider

Example 1.3. Two-sex model. Suppose that in any generation there are N_1 diploid males and N_2 diploid females with $N_1 + N_2 = N$ and that each diploid offspring gets one gene chosen at random from the male population and one chosen at random from the female population. To compute the inbreeding effective population size we note that two genes taken at random from the population will have identical parent genes if both are descended from the same male gene or both from the same female gene. Taking the two cases into account, the probability of identical parentage is thus

$$\pi_2 = \frac{N(N-1)}{2N(2N-1)} \left\{ (2N_1)^{-1} + (2N_2)^{-1} \right\}$$

From this it follows that

$$(1.4) \qquad N_e^i = (2\pi_2)^{-1} \approx \frac{2}{(2N_1)^{-1} + (2N_2)^{-1}} = \frac{4N_1 N_2}{N_1 + N_2}$$

For a concrete example, consider a herd of cattle where each generation has 10 bulls and 1000 cows. In this case

$$N_i^e = \frac{4 \cdot 10 \cdot 1000}{1010} = 39.6$$

In general, if $N_1 \ll N_2$ then $N_i^e \approx 4N_1$.

To compute the eigenvalue effective population size, we cheat and look up the answer on page 107 of Ewens (1979). As we noted above, it is sufficient to find some function $Y(X_1, X_2)$ that is 0 on the absorbing states of the system but positive otherwise and has

$$E(Y(X_1(t+1), X_2(t+1))|X_1(t), X_2(t)) = \lambda Y(X_1(t), X_2(t))$$

As Ewens says, "in the present case it is found, after much labor, that a suitable function is"

$$\begin{aligned}
Y(X_1, X_2) &= C\left\{ X_1(2N_1 - X_1)(2N_1)^{-2} + X_2(2N_2 - X_2)(2N_2)^{-2} \right\} \\
&\quad + \left\{ 1 - (X_1 - N_1)(X_2 - N_2)N_1^{-1}N_2^{-1} \right\}
\end{aligned}$$

where $C = \{1 + (1 - 2N_1^{-1} - 2N_2^{-1})\}/4$. With this definition, the eigenvalue becomes

$$\lambda = \frac{1}{2}[1 - (4N_1)^{-1} - (4N_2)^{-1} + \{1 + N^2(4N_1N_2)^{-2}\}^{1/2}]$$

When N_1N_2/N is large, $\{1 + N^2(4N_1N_2)^{-2}\}^{1/2} \approx 1 + N^2/2(4N_1N_2)^2$ it follows that

(1.5) $\lambda \approx 1 - (N_1 + N_2)/(8N_1N_2)$

and hence $N_e^e = \frac{1}{2}(1 - \lambda)^{-1} \approx 4N_1N_2/(N_1 + N_2)$.

For our third exmple, we will consider

Example 1.4. Kruglyak's (1999) model of the human population expansion. Humans expanded out of Africa about 100,000 years ago. Assuming a generation time of 20 years, this translates into $T = 5,000$ generations. If we assume that the population had size 10,000 before expansion and use a figure of 6 billion for the population size today, then therate of expansion found by solving the equation

$$e^{5000\rho} = (6 \times 10^9)/(10,000)$$

is $\rho = (\ln(6 \times 10^5))/5000 = 0.00266$. Using (1.2) we see that genealogies in $[0, T]$ correspond to the coalescent run for time

$$\tau = \sum_{t=0}^{T-1} \frac{1}{20,000e^{\rho t}} \approx \frac{1}{20,000} \int_0^T e^{-\rho t}\, dt$$

$$= \frac{1 - e^{-\rho T}}{20,000\rho} \approx \frac{1}{2N_0\rho} = \frac{1}{52.2} = 0.01916$$

since $e^{-\rho T} = 1/(6 \times 10^5)$.

The definitions N_e^i and N_e^e do not make sense in this context due to the temporal inhomogeneity. If we consider two particles, then the probability of no coalescence before time 0 as we work back from the present time T is

$$P(T_1 > 0.01916) = e^{-0.01916} = 0.9810$$

When the two lineages do not coalesce before time 0, then they are two lineages in a population of constant size 10,000 and hence require an additional amount of time with mean 20,000 to coalesce. Ignoring the possibility of coalescence before time 0, which will introduce only a small error, we conclude that the expected coalescence time of two lineages is 25,000. This is the same as the expected time in a population of constant size 12,500, so $N_e^c = 12,500$.

If we now consider three particles, then there are three pairs trying to coalesce so

$$P(T_2 > 0.01916) = e^{-3 \cdot 0.01916} = 0.9441$$

When none of the three lineages coalesce before time 0, the time to the first coalescence will require an average of $2N/3 = 13,000$ generations and then the final coalescence will require another 20,000 generations on the average. From this we can see that the genealogy is not star shaped. Indeed, to a good first approximation, the effect of population expansion has been simply to add 5,000 generations to the end of each lineage in the ordinary coalescent.

The lengthening of the tips of the genealogical tree in Kruglyak's model results in an excess of mutations that have one representative. This should remind the reader of the Aquadro and Greenberg data set. Before we tackle the thorny question: "Do the patterns of variation in human mitochondrial DNA show signs of the human population expansion?", we will introduce two more demographic scenarios.

Example 1.5. Sudden population expansion. Let $N(t) = N_1$ for $-t_1 < t \le 0$, $N(t) = N_2$ for $t \le -t_1$, where N_1 is much larger than N_2.

DiRienzo et al. (1994) used a sudden expansion model with $t_1 = 5,000$ generations, $N_1 = 10^7$ and $N_2 = 10^3$, to model the Sardinian population. As the authors say "this model represents a drastic bottleneck in the population's size that results in a starlike gene genealogy." To check this for their sample of size 46, note that the initial probability of coalescence per generation is

$$\frac{46 \cdot 45}{2} \cdot \frac{1}{2 \cdot 10^7} = 5.175 \times 10^{-5}$$

so the expected number of coalescence events in 5000 generations is 0.25875. Of course, once the 46 (or 45) lineages reach time -5000 and the population size drops to 1,000, the remainder of the coalescence will take an average of

$$2000 \cdot \left(2 - \frac{1}{46} \right) = 3956 \quad \text{generations}$$

Since this number is almost as large as the original 5000 we see that even in this extreme scenario the genealogies are not quite star-shaped.

Example 1.6. Bottleneck. Consider now a situation in which a population has a constant size for a long time, undergoes a sudden reduction, and then slowly grows back to a possibly new equilibrium value. For an extreme example, suppose that a single inseminated female from a large population migrates into an unoccupied geographical location and establishes a new colony followed by a rapid population growth in the new environment. This process is believed to have occurred repeatedly in the evolution of Hawaiian *Drosophila* species.

To study the effect of bottlenecks on genetic variability in populations, we will follow Nei, Maruyama, and Chakraborty (1975) and consider J_t = the expected homozygosity in generation t. Letting v denote the mutation rate per locus per generation, we have

(1.6) $$J_t = (1-v)^2 \left[\frac{1}{2N_{t-1}} + \left(1 - \frac{1}{2N_{t-1}}\right) J_{t-1} \right]$$

Iterating this relationship, we find

$$J_t = \sum_{j=1}^{t} \frac{(1-v)^{2j}}{2N_{t-j}} \prod_{i=1}^{j-1} \left(1 - \frac{1}{2N_{t-i}}\right)$$
$$+ J_0 (1-v)^{2t} \prod_{i=1}^{t} \left(1 - \frac{1}{2N_{t-i}}\right)$$

where $\prod_{i=1}^{0} z_i = 1$ by convention. This formula can be derived directly by breaking things down according to the generation $t-j$ on which coalescence occurs, with the last term giving the probability of no coalescence. When v is small and the N_r's are large, this can be approximated by

$$J_t = \sum_{j=1}^{t} \frac{1}{2N_{t-j}} \exp\left(-2vj - \sum_{i=1}^{j-1} \frac{1}{2N_{t-i}}\right)$$
$$+ J_0 \exp\left(-2vt - \sum_{i=1}^{t} \frac{1}{2N_{t-i}}\right)$$

Changing variables $k = t - j$ and $\ell = t - i$, we have

$$J_t = \sum_{k=0}^{t-1} \frac{1}{2N_k} \exp\left(-2v(t-k) - \sum_{\ell=k+1}^{t-1} \frac{1}{2N_\ell}\right)$$
$$+ J_0 \exp\left(-2vt - \sum_{\ell=0}^{t-1} \frac{1}{2N_\ell}\right)$$

Converting the sums into integrals gives

(1.7) $$J_t = \int_0^t \frac{1}{2N_s} \exp\left(-2v(t-s) - \int_s^t \frac{1}{2N_u} du\right) ds$$
$$+ J_0 \exp\left(-2vt - \int_0^t \frac{1}{2N_s} ds\right)$$

This corrects an error in formula (5) of Nei, Maruyama, and Chakraborty (1975). They have

$$-2vs - \int_0^s \frac{1}{2N_u} du$$

in the exponential on the first line. To see that this cannot be correct, consider a situation in which $N(s) = N$ is constant for $t/2 \le s \le t$. In this case, if t is large then J_t should be almost the same as for a population of constant size N.

If we consider a periodic population, i.e., one in which $N_s = N_{s+k}$ and define the harmonic mean by

$$\frac{1}{\hat{N}} = \frac{1}{k} \sum_{s=0}^{k-1} \frac{1}{N_s}$$

then the above becomes

$$J_t = \frac{1}{2\hat{N}} \int_0^t \exp\left(-\frac{4v\hat{N}+1}{2\hat{N}}(t-s)\right) ds + J_0 \exp\left(-\frac{4v\hat{N}+1}{2\hat{N}}t\right)$$

Evaluating the integral gives

$$(1.8) \qquad J_t = \frac{1}{4\hat{N}v+1} + \left(J_0 - \frac{1}{4\hat{N}v+1}\right) \exp\left(-\frac{4v\hat{N}+1}{2\hat{N}}t\right)$$

This result, which also holds for a constant population size, shows that the expected homozygosity, J_t, converges exponentially fast to its limiting value. This calculation gives another indication that for a periodically varying population the effective population size is the harmonic mean of the population sizes. A little thought reveals that this conclusion is also valid for a population with randomly fluctuating sizes if we let $1/\hat{N} = E(1/N_s)$.

For a concrete example of the use of our formulas for J_t, consider

Example 1.7. Logisitic population growth. Let $N_t = K/(1 + Ce^{-rt})$, where K is the equilibrium population size, $C = (K - N_0)/N_0$, and r is the intrinsic growth rate. With the Hawaiian *Drosophila* example in mind, Nei, Maruyama, and Chakraborty took $N_0 = 2$, $v = 10^{-8}$, and $K = 4 \times 10^6$. $N_0 = 2$ indicates the founding of the population by a single inseminated female. The mutation rate was chosen based on experimental evidence. The population size was then chosen so that the heterozygosity

$$H_0 = \frac{4Nv}{4Nv+1} = \frac{0.16}{1.16} = 0.138$$

matches that observed in nature. We do not have much information about the intrinsic growth rate r, so as Nei, Maruyama, and Chakraborty did, we will consider several values of r ranging from 0.1 to 1. $N_0 = 2 \ll K$ so $C \approx K/2$. Thus, when $r = 0.1$ it takes $t = 10\ln(K/2) = 145$ generations for the population to reach size $K/2$ and $t = 10\ln(5K) = 161$ generations to reach size $K/1.1$.

To begin to evaluate (1.7), we note that $\frac{1}{N_u} = \frac{1}{K} + \frac{1}{2}e^{-ru}$. Inserting this into (1.7) leads to an ugly expression with two levels of exponentials. Because of this and the fact that the approximations that led to (1.7) are not valid when $N(s)$ is small, we use the recursion (1.6) to evaluate J_t. The next graph gives the values of J_t for $0 \le t \le 50$ and $r = 1.0, 0.5, 0.2, 0.1$.

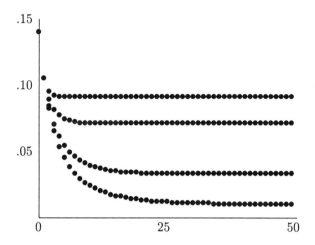

If we continue to iterate up to time 300 then the values change by very little.

	$r = 1.0$	$r = 0.5$	$r = 0.2$	$r = 0.1$
50	0.089022	0.069016	0.031176	0.008346
100	0.089022	0.069015	0.031174	0.008201
150	0.089021	0.069015	0.031174	0.008200
200	0.089021	0.069015	0.031174	0.008200
250	0.089020	0.069014	0.031174	0.008200
300	0.089020	0.069014	0.031173	0.008199

At time 300, we have $N_t = 3,999,999.17$ when $r = 0.1$. Since N_t increases with r or with t we see that for $t \ge 300$, $N_t \approx K = 4,000,000$. Using this in (1.7), we see that for $t \ge 300$

$$
J_t \approx \int_{300}^{t} \frac{1}{2K} \exp\left(-\left(2v + \frac{1}{2K}\right)(t - s)\right) ds
$$
$$
+ J_{300} \exp\left(-\left(2v + \frac{1}{2K}\right)(t - 300)\right)
$$

Evaluating the integral and letting $\gamma = 2v + 1/2K = 1.45 \times 10^{-7}$ we have

$$
J_t \approx \frac{1}{4Kv + 1}\left(1 - \exp^{-\gamma(t-300)}\right) + J_{300} \exp^{-\gamma(t-300)}
$$

This shows that J_t eventually returns to the equilibrium value $1/(4Kv+1)$. However, the time required is a mutliple of $1/\gamma = 6,896,551$ generations.

Example 1.8. Human mitochondrial DNA. Cann, Stoneking, and Wilson (1987) collected mtDNA from 147 people drawn from five geographic populations and analyzed them using 12 restriction enyzmes, finding 398 mutations. Their analysis found 133 different patterns. Adding in the pattern associated with the reference sequence of human mtDNA from Anderson (1981), they built a parsimony tree using the computer program PAUP designed by David Swofford. Noting that one of the two primary branches leads exclusively to mtDNA types, while the second primary branch also leads to African mtDNA types, they suggested that Africa was the likely source of the mtDNA gene pool.

To assign a time scale to the tree, they first used their data and previous sources to argue that the mean rate of mtDNA divergence for humans lies between 2 and 4 percent per million years; see Stoneking, Bhatia, and Wilson (1986). Using their tree, they concluded that the average divergence between the African group and the rest of the sample was 0.57%, giving an estimate of 140,000 to 290,000 years for the date of the common ancestor. Similar results were obtained in two other studies by Vigilant et al. (1989) and Horai and Hayasaka (1990).

The next figure shows the distribution of the number of differences when all possible pairs of the 147 data points are compared. The x-axis gives the number of differences, while the y-axis gives the number of pairwise comparisons with that number of differences.

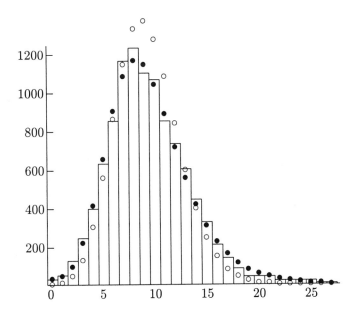

The circles show the best fitting a Poisson distribution, which has mean 9.2. The idea behind fitting the Poisson distribution is that if there is rapid population growth then the genealogy tends to be star-shaped, and if the genealogy were exactly star-shaped

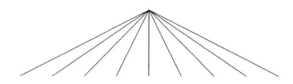

then the number of pairwise differences between two individuals would have exactly a Poisson distribution.

Rogers and Harpending (1992) took a more sophisticated approach to fitting the data on pairwise differences, resulting in the fit given by the black dots. Their starting point was a result of Li (1977), which we will now derive. Shifting the time of the expansion to 0 for convenience we suppose $N(s) = N_0$ for $s < 0$, $N(s) = N_1$ for $s \geq 0$. Consider the situation $2N_1 t$ units of time after the population expansion, use the infinite sites model for the mutation process, and let $F_i(t)$ be the probability that two randomly chosen individuals differ at i sites. Breaking things down according to the time to coalescence of two lineages, which in a population of constant size N_1 has an exponential distribution with mean 1, and recalling that mutations occur on each lineage at rate $2N_1 u = \theta_1/2$, we have

$$F_i(t) = \int_0^t e^{-s} e^{-\theta_1 s} \frac{(\theta_1 s)^i}{i!}\, ds + e^{-t} \sum_{j=0}^i e^{-\theta_1 t} \frac{(\theta_1 t)^j}{j!} F_{i-j}(0)$$

where $F_k(0) = \theta_0^k/(1+\theta_0)^{k+1}$ is the probability that two individuals at time 0 differ at k sites.

To convert this into the form given in Li's paper, we note that the equilibrium probability of i differences is

$$\hat{F}_i = \int_0^\infty e^{-s} e^{-\theta_1 s} \frac{(\theta_1 s)^i}{i!}\, ds = \frac{\theta_1^i}{(1+\theta_1)^{i+1}}$$

where the second equality follows by recalling the formula for the ith moment of the exponential distribution or by integrating by parts i times. Noticing that in a population of constant size N_1 if the two lineages do not coalesce before time t then the number of mutations that occur after time t before coalescence has distribution $\hat{F}_k$, we have

$$\hat{F}_i = \int_0^t e^{-s} e^{-\theta_1 s} \frac{(\theta_1 s)^i}{i!}\, ds + e^{-t} \sum_{j=0}^i e^{-\theta_1 t} \frac{(\theta_1 t)^j}{j!} \hat{F}_{i-j}$$

Subtracting this from the corresponding formula for $F_i(t)$ we have

$$F_i(t) = \hat{F}_i + e^{-t} \sum_{j=0}^{i} e^{-\theta_1 t} \frac{(\theta_1 t)^j}{j!} (F_{i-j}(0) - \hat{F}_{i-j})$$

Introducing the scaled time variable $\tau = \theta_1 t$, Rogers and Harpending found the best parameters to fit the data of Cann, Stoneking, and Wilson (1987) were as follows: $\theta_0 = 2.44$, $\theta_1 = 410.69$, $\tau = 7.18$. The predicted values given by the black dots in the figure give a much better fit to the data than the Poisson distribution. Of course, the Rogers and Harpending model has three parameters compared to one for the Poisson distribution.

To relate the fitted parameters to data, we must estimate u, which is the mutation rate in the region under study. Using the data of Cann, Stoneking, and Wilson (1987), Rogers and Harpending calculate that u is between 7.5×10^{-4} and 1.5×10^{-3}. The estimate $\hat{\tau} = 7.18$ implies that the population expansion began some $2N_1 t = \tau/2u$, or 2400–4800 generations ago. Assuming a generation time of 25 years, this translates into 60,000–120,000 years. The estimate of θ_0 puts the initial population at $\theta_0/4u$, or 400–800 females, and that of θ_1 puts the population after expansion at $\theta_1/4u$ or 68,500–137,000 females. The first prediction conflicts with the widely held belief, see Takahata (1995), that an effective population size of 10,000 individuals has been maintained for at least the last half million years.

Example 1.9. While studies of mtDNA show signs of a human population expansion, studies of nuclear DNA in general do not. Harding et al. (1997) have studied a 3 kb region on chromosome 11 encompassing the β-globin gene in nine populations from Africa, Asia, and Europe. Eliminating sequences that showed evidence of recombination they used methods of Griffiths and Tavaré (1994ab) to give a maximum-likelihood estimate of the genealogical tree, which has a most recent common ancestor 800,000 years ago. At first this may seem to disagree with the estimate of 200,000 years for mitochondrial eve, but mtDNA is haploid and maternally inherited, so the effective population size (and hence coalescence time) for nuclear genes is four times as large.

Maximum-likelihood estimates of the scaled mutation rate θ were made with a model of exponential growth for comparison with a constant-size model. The best fitting population model had $\theta = 4.5$ and a population size $18,087 e^{-0.7t}$ at $2N_0 t$ generations into the past. (See Example 1.1.) An improved fit compared with the constant population size model must occur because of the addition of a parameter to the model, but this improvement was not judged to be significant by a log-likelihood test ratio. Harding et al. (1997) concluded that any population size expansion has been too recent to be detectable in the surveyed patterns of β-globin diversity.

2.2 Recombination

In this section, we will investigate the effects of recombination, the reciprocal exchange of genetic material between a pair of homologous chromosomes. We begin with the simplest situation of two loci. To motivate the definition of the process, think of two genes or two exons of a single gene separated by a stretch of noncoding sequence. In this case, recombination within one of the gene regions is rare so, for a first approximation, we can assume that all of the recombination events occur between the two gene regions with a probability r per generation.

Ignoring the numbering of the copies, the possible states of the system are

$$
\begin{array}{cl}
(a)\,(a)\,(b)\,(b) & 0 \\
(a\,b)\,(a)\,(b) & 1 \\
(a\,a)\,(b)\,(b) & \Delta_{2,1,1} \\
(b\,b)\,(a)\,(a) & \Delta_{2,1,1} \\
(a\,b)\,(a\,b) & 2 \\
(a\,a)\,(b\,b) & \Delta_{2,2} \\
(a\,a\,b)\,(b) & \Delta_{3,1} \\
(a\,b\,b)\,(a) & \Delta_{3,1} \\
(a\,a\,b\,b) & \Delta_{4}
\end{array}
$$

Here the parentheses indicate the lineages that are in one individual. The second column gives our abbreviations for the states. The numbers 2, 1, and 0 indicate the number of ab pairs in the configuration. The Δs are configurations where one coalescence has occurred and we are waiting for the other one. To check that we have listed all of the possible configurations note that 4 can be written as 4, $3+1$, $2+2$, $2+1+1$, or $1+1+1+1$ and then the number of ways that the parentheses can be filled in are 1, 2, 2, 3, or 1 for a total of 10 possibilities.

Considering the Wright-Fisher model, speeding up time by a factor of $2N$, and letting $\rho = 2Nr$, the rates become

	2	1	0	$\Delta_{2,1,1}$	$\Delta_{3,1}$	$\Delta_{2,2}$	Δ_4	total
2		2ρ					1	$2\rho+1$
1	1		ρ		2			$\rho+3$
0		4		2				6

We ignore transitions out of the Δ states since from any of them the time to coalescence of the remaining pair is exponential with mean 1.

Let T_a be the time of the coalescence of the two copies of a and let T_b be the time of the coalescence of the two copies of b. The first thing we want to compute is $h(i)$, the probability that $T_a = T_b$ when we start from state i.

(2.1) If we let $R = 4Nr$, then

$$h(2) = \frac{R + 18}{R^2 + 13R + 18}$$

To check that this is reasonable note that if $R = 0$ then $h(2) = 1$, while if R is large then $h(2) \approx 1/R$.

Proof of (2.1). By considering what can happen on one step and using the table of rates above:

$$h(2) = \frac{2\rho}{2\rho + 1}h(1) + \frac{1}{2\rho + 1} \cdot 1$$

$$h(1) = \frac{1}{\rho + 3}h(2) + \frac{\rho}{\rho + 3}h(0)$$

$$h(0) = \frac{4}{6}h(1)$$

Rearranging the second equation, and then using the third equation,

$$h(2) = (\rho + 3)h(1) - \rho h(0)$$

$$= \left((\rho + 3) - \frac{2\rho}{3}\right)h(1) = \frac{\rho + 9}{3}h(1)$$

Using this in the first equation, we have

$$h(2) = \frac{2\rho}{2\rho + 1} \cdot \frac{3}{\rho + 9}h(2) + \frac{1}{2\rho + 1}$$

Multiplying each side by $2\rho + 1$, we have

$$\left(2\rho + 1 - \frac{6\rho}{\rho + 9}\right)h(2) = 1$$

Since $(2\rho + 1)(\rho + 9) = 2\rho^2 + 19\rho + 9$, it follows that

$$h(2) = \frac{\rho + 9}{2\rho^2 + 13\rho + 9}$$

Setting $R = 4Nr = 2\rho$ converts the above to

$$h(2) = \frac{R/2 + 9}{R^2/2 + 13R/2 + 9} = \frac{R + 18}{R^2 + 13R + 18} \qquad \square$$

Our next goal is to compute the covariance of T_a and T_b. Somewhat surprisingly, the new formula is exactly the same as the old one

(2.2) If we let $R = 4Nr$, then

$$\text{cov}(T_a, T_b) = \frac{R + 18}{R^2 + 13R + 18}$$

Proof. Since $ET_a = ET_b = 1$ we have

$$\text{cov}\,(T_a, T_b) = ET_a T_b - ET_a ET_b = ET_a T_b - 1$$

Let $u(i) = E_i(T_a T_b)$. To get an equation for $u(i)$, let J be the time of the first jump, and let X_J be the state at time J

$$
\begin{aligned}
E(T_a T_b | J, X_J) &= E((T_a - J + J)(T_b - J + J) | J, X_J) \\
&= E((T_a - J)(T_b - J) | J, X_J) + JE(T_a - J | J, X_J) \\
&\quad + JE(T_b - J | J, X_J) + J^2
\end{aligned}
$$

Let $v_a(X_J)$ and $v_b(X_J)$ be 1 if coalescence has not occurred and 0 if it has. Noting that J is independent of X_J and taking the expected value gives

$$u(i) = E_i u(X_J) + E_i J \cdot (E_i v_a(X_J) + E_i v_b(X_J)) + E_i J^2$$

If J is exponential with rate λ then $EJ = 1/\lambda$ and $EJ^2 = 2/\lambda^2$. Using this with our table of rates gives

$$
\begin{aligned}
u(2) &= \frac{2\rho}{2\rho + 1}\left(u(1) + 2 \cdot \frac{1}{2\rho + 1}\right) \\
&\quad + \frac{1}{2\rho + 1}\left(u(\Delta_4) + 0 \cdot \frac{1}{2\rho + 1}\right) + \frac{2}{(2\rho + 1)^2}
\end{aligned}
$$

$$
\begin{aligned}
u(1) &= \frac{\rho}{\rho + 3}\left(u(0) + 2 \cdot \frac{1}{\rho + 3}\right) \\
&\quad + \frac{1}{\rho + 3}\left(u(2) + 2 \cdot \frac{1}{\rho + 3}\right) \\
&\quad + \frac{2}{\rho + 3}\left(u(\Delta_{3,1}) + 1 \cdot \frac{1}{\rho + 3}\right) + \frac{2}{(\rho + 3)^2}
\end{aligned}
$$

$$
\begin{aligned}
u(0) &= \frac{4}{6}\left(u(1) + 2 \cdot \frac{1}{6}\right) \\
&\quad + \frac{2}{6}\left(u(\Delta_{2,1,1}) + 1 \cdot \frac{1}{6}\right) + \frac{2}{6^2}
\end{aligned}
$$

Since $u = 0$ for any Δ state, the last equation says

$$u(0) = \frac{2}{3}u(1) + \frac{8 + 2 + 2}{36} = \frac{2}{3}u(1) + \frac{1}{3}$$

Rearranging the second equation and then substituting the previous one gives

$$(\rho + 3)u(1) = \rho\left(\frac{2}{3}u(1) + \frac{1}{3}\right) + u(2) + \frac{2\rho + 6}{\rho + 3}$$

Moving the $u(1)$ from the right to the left and then dividing gives

$$u(1) = \frac{3}{\rho + 9} \cdot \left(u(2) + 2 + \frac{\rho}{3}\right) = \frac{3}{\rho + 9}u(2) + \frac{\rho + 6}{\rho + 9}$$

Rearranging the first equation and then inserting the previous one

$$
\begin{aligned}
u(2) &= \frac{2\rho}{2\rho+1}u(1) + \frac{4\rho+2}{(2\rho+1)^2} \\
&= \frac{2\rho \cdot 3}{(2\rho+1)(\rho+9)}u(2) + \frac{2\rho(\rho+6)}{(2\rho+1)(\rho+9)} + \frac{2}{2\rho+1}
\end{aligned}
$$

Noting that $(2\rho+1)(\rho+9) = 2\rho^2 + 19\rho + 9$, we have

$$(2\rho^2 + 13\rho + 9)u(2) = 2\rho^2 + 12\rho + 2\rho + 18$$

so $u(2) = 1 + (\rho+9)/(2\rho^2 + 13\rho + 9)$ and it follows that

$$\text{cov}\,(T_a, T_b) = \frac{\rho+9}{2\rho^2 + 13\rho + 9}$$

Changing variables $\rho = R/2$ leads as before to the answer.   □

m locus model

Generalizing from two loci, consider m linearly arranged loci, each of which follows the infinite sites model. As before we can think of this as m exons separated by $m-1$ introns. However, we will also use this model and let $m \to \infty$ to get a model of a segment of DNA where recombination can occur between any two adjacent loci. The number of mutations per generation per locus is assumed to have a Poisson distribution with mean u/m. Recombination does not occur within subloci, but occurs between adjacent subloci at rate $r/(m-1)$ per generation per gamete. With this assumption, the recombination rate between the most distant subloci is r.

Let S_j be the number of segregating sites in the jth locus in a sample of two alleles. If we let $\theta = 4Nu$, then it follows from (4.9) in Chapter 1 that

$$\text{var}\,(S_j) = \frac{\theta}{m} + \left(\frac{\theta}{m}\right)^2$$

Let T_i be the coalescence time of the two copies of locus i. This distribution of S_i given T_i is Poisson with mean $(\theta/m)T_i$ so

$$E(S_i|T_i) = \frac{\theta}{m}T_i$$

S_i, S_j are conditionally independent given T_i and T_j so

$$E(S_iS_j|T_i, T_j) = \left(\frac{\theta}{m}\right)^2 T_iT_j$$

and $\text{cov}\,(S_i, S_j) = (\theta/m)^2 \,\text{cov}\,(T_i, T_j)$. Now

$$\text{var}\,(S) = \sum_{i=1}^{m} \text{var}\,(S_j) + \sum_{1 \le i \ne j \le m} \text{cov}\,(S_i, S_j)$$

Using (2.2) and writing $f(x) = (x + 18)/(x^2 + 13x + 9)$, we see that the variance of the total number of segregating sites is

$$
(2.3) \qquad \text{var}\,(S) = \theta + \frac{\theta^2}{m} + 2\frac{\theta^2}{m^2} \sum_{j=1}^{m-1} (m - j)f\left(\frac{jR}{m-1}\right)
$$

where $R = 4Nr$. Letting $m \to \infty$, setting $y = j/m$, and noting that the sum approximates an integral, we see that for the infinite sites model

$$
(2.4) \qquad \text{var}\,(S) = \theta + 2\theta^2 \int_0^1 (1 - y)f(yR)\,dy
$$

Changing variables $y = z/R$, $dy = dz/R$, we can write this in a way that matches formula (4) in Hudson (1983):

$$
\text{var}\,(S) = \theta + \frac{2\theta^2}{R^2} \int_0^R f(z)(R - z)\,dz
$$

Still considering a sample of size 2, let $\bar{T} = \frac{1}{m}\sum_{i=1}^m T_i$ be the average coalescence time in the m locus model. Clearly $E\bar{T} = ET_i = 1$. Using (2.3) we can compute $\text{var}\,(\bar{T})$. We begin by recalling that

$$
\text{var}\,(S) = E[\,\text{var}\,(S|\bar{T})] + \text{var}\,[E(S|\bar{T})]
$$

Since the distribution of S given $\bar{T}$ is Poisson with mean $\theta\bar{T}$ it follows that

$$
\text{var}\,(S) = E(\theta\bar{T}) + \text{var}\,(\theta\bar{T}) = \theta + \theta^2\,\text{var}\,(\bar{T})
$$

Using this with (2.3) it follows that

$$
(2.5) \qquad \text{var}\,(T) = \frac{1}{m} + \frac{2}{m^2} \sum_{j=1}^{m-1} (m - j)f\left(\frac{jR}{m-1}\right)
$$

Larger sample sizes

Consider a sample of size n in the m locus model. Let τ_i be the total time in the tree for the ith locus and $\bar{\tau} = \frac{1}{m}\sum_{i=1}^m \tau_i$. Since the distribution of S given $\bar{\tau}$ is Poisson with mean $(\theta/2)\bar{\tau}$ it follows that

$$
(2.6) \qquad ES = \frac{\theta}{2}E\bar{\tau} = \theta \sum_{i=1}^{n-1} \frac{1}{j}
$$

The variance of S presents considerably more difficulty. Consider for the moment a two-locus model. When $R = 0$, formula (4.9) in Chapter 1 implies that

$$
\text{var}\,(S) \;=\; \theta \sum_{i=1}^{n-1} \frac{1}{i} + \theta^2 \sum_{i=1}^{n-1} \frac{1}{i^2}
$$

$$\text{var}(S_i) = \frac{\theta}{2} \sum_{i=1}^{n-1} \frac{1}{i} + \left(\frac{\theta}{2}\right)^2 \sum_{i=1}^{n-1} \frac{1}{i^2}$$

Since $\text{var}(S) = 2\text{var}(S_i) + 2\text{cov}(S_1, S_2)$, it follows that

(2.7)
$$\text{cov}(S_1, S_2) = \left(\frac{\theta}{2}\right)^2 \sum_{i=1}^{n-1} \frac{1}{i^2}$$

A look at (2.2) inspires the guess

$$\text{cov}(S_1, S_2) \approx \left(\frac{\theta}{2}\right)^2 \sum_{i=1}^{n-1} \frac{1}{i^2} \cdot \frac{R+18}{R^2 + 13R + 18}$$

Simulations in Hudson (1983), see his Figure 2, suggest that this approximation is quite good. In fact, the approximation is always within the 95% confidence bars based on the simulation.

Kaplan and Hudson (1985) develop equations that can be solved to find what they call $V(n, m)$, the variance of the number of segregating sites in a sample of size n in the m-locus model, and $F(n, m)$, the probability that there are no segregating sites. Analytical results for the quantities are difficult and messy, but it is reasonably easy to simulate the process. For simplicity we will consider only the case of two loci. Before describing the algorithm some definitions are necessary. Generation t signifies the population t generations before the present. We consider a sample of size n from the current population (generation 0). Those gametes of generation t that contain genetic material at either locus that is directly ancestral to genetic material of the sampled gametes will be referred to as ancestral gametes of generation t. Let $g(t)$ be the number of such gametes.

If any two ancestral gametes of generation t have a common ancestor in generation $t + 1$, we say that the event CA (coalescence) has occurred in generation $t + 1$.

If an ancestral gamete contains copies of both loci then with probability r, the gamete is a recombinant descendent of two ancestral gametes in generation $t + 1$. In this case, we say that the event RE (recombination) has occurred.

Let $d(t)$ be the number of ancestral gametes that contain copies of both loci. The algorithm starts at the present and proceeds backwards in time generating the times t_k of successive CA and RE events. $t_0 = 0$. If time is written in units of $4N$ generations, then $t_{k+1} - t_k$ has an exponential distribution with rate $\lambda(t_k) = Rd(t_k) + g(t_k)(g(t_k) - 1)$.

The event is RE with probability $Rd(t_k)/\lambda(t_k)$. In this case we pick one of the $d(t_k)$ gametes that contain copies of both loci to split.

The event is CA with probability $g(t_k)(g(t_k) - 1)/\lambda(t_k)$. In this case we pick one pair of ancestral gametes to coalesce.

Of course, after either of these events, we must compute the new values of $g(t_{k+1})$ and $d(t_{k+1})$. At each CA event, the coalescent tree for each locus is updated. When we finally reach the point at which there is only one individual, then we can move forward in time assigning mutations to the branches as in the ordinary coalescent. See Hudson (1991).

The details of the m locus model are similar to those above. One can deal directly with the infinite sites limit by representing the locus as the interval $[0, 1]$ and choosing recombinations uniformly on the interval. In this case the bookkeeping gets quite complicated. See Section 5.2 of Hudson (1983) or Griffiths and Marjoram (1997) for more details.

Estimating R

Suppose that there are two alleles, A and a, at site i and two alleles, B and b, at site j. As we observed in the analysis of Example 3.1 in Chapter 1, if all four gametic types AB, Ab, aB, and ab are present, then the two sites must have different genealogies. In this case, we can infer that there must have been a recombination in between i and j, and we set $d(i, j) = 1$. Otherwise $d(i, j) = 0$. To compute the minimal number of recombinations implied by the sample, R_M we represent the (i, j) with $d(i, j) = 1$ as an open interval and apply the following algorithm:

1. Delete all (m, n) that contain another interval (i, j).

2. Let (i_1, j_1) be the first interval not disjoint from all the others. If (m, n) has $i_1 < m < j_1$ then delete (m, n). Repeat until done.

It should be clear from 1 that for each i we only have to locate $j_i = \min\{j > i : d(i, j) = 1\}$. An example should help clarify the procedure. Following Hudson and Kaplan (1985) we will analyze Kreitman's (1983) data on the alcohol dehydrogenase locus of *Drosophila melanogaster*. On the next page, F and S indicate the fast and slow alleles that are caused by the substitution at the starred position. The first sequence is a reference sequence, the other 11 are the data. Here we have ignored the six sites at which there have been insertions and/or deletions.

	ref	1S	2S	3S	4S	5S	6S	1F	2F	3F	4F	5F
1	C	.	.	.	.	.	.	.	T	T	T	T
2	C	.	.	.	.	.	.	.	G	G	G	G
3	G	.	C	.	.	.	C	C	C	C	C	C
4	C	.	.	.	.	A	.	.	A	A	A	A
5	A	.	.	.	.	G	.	.	G	G	G	G
6	A	.	.	.	.	.	.	.	.	.	.	G
7	T	.	.	.	.	.	.	.	.	.	.	G
8	A	.	.	.	.	.	.	.	.	.	.	G
9	T	A	.	.	.	A	.	.	A	A	A	A
10	G	T	.	.	.	.	.	.	.	.	.	.
11	G	.	.	.	.	T	.	.	T	T	T	.
12	G	.	.	.	.	C	.	.	C	C	C	.
13	C	.	.	.	.	.	.	.	G	G	G	.
14	G	.	.	.	.	.	.	.	.	.	.	T
15	C	.	.	.	.	A	.	.	.	.	.	.
16	T	.	.	.	.	G	G	G	G	G	G	G
17	A	.	.	.	G	G	.	.	.	.	.	.
18	C	.	.	.	T	T	.	.	.	.	.	.
19	C	T	T	.	.	.	.	.	.	.	.	.
20	C	T	T	.	.	.	.	.	.	.	.	.
21	C	.	.	.	.	.	.	.	.	.	.	A
22	C	A	A	.	.	.	.	.	.	.	.	.
23	G	C	C	.	.	.	.	.	.	.	.	.
24	G	A	A	.	.	.	.	.	.	.	.	.
25	A	.	.	.	.	.	.	.	.	.	.	G
26	A	T	T	.	.	.	.	.	.	.	.	.
27	T	A	A	.	.	.	.	.	.	.	.	.
28	C	A	A	.	.	.	.	.	.	.	.	.
29	T	C	C	.	.	.	.	.	.	.	.	.
30	C	.	.	.	.	.	.	.	G	G	G	G
31	C	.	.	.	.	.	T	T	T	T	T	T
32*	A	.	.	.	.	.	.	C	C	C	C	C
33	C	.	.	.	.	.	T	T	T	T	T	T
34	T	.	.	.	.	.	.	C	C	C	C	C
35	A	.	.	.	.	.	C	C	C	C	C	C
36	G	.	.	A	A	.	A	.	.	.	.	.
37	A	.	.	.	.	C	C	C	C	C	C	C
38	C	.	.	.	.	.	.	.	G	G	G	.
39	A	.	.	.	T	.	.	.	.	.	.	.
40	G	.	.	.	A	.	.	.	.	.	.	.
41	C	.	.	T	.	.	.	.	.	.	.	.
42	C	.	.	.	.	.	T	.	.	.	.	.
43	T	.	.	A	.	.	.	.	.	.	.	.

The first stage is to find (i, j_i) for $1 \leq i \leq 43$. In doing this we can ignore sites 6, 7, 8, 10, 14, 15, 21, 25, and 39–43, which have only one mutation. Note that 13, 19–30, 32, 34, and 37–38 were all consistent with all of the rows that followed so they did not produce intervals. The remaining (i, j_i) pairs are as follows:

$$
\begin{array}{ccc}
 & (1,11) & (2,11) & \mathbf{(3,4)} \\
 & (4,17) & (5,17) & \mathbf{(9,16)} \\
 & (11,17) & (12,17) & \mathbf{(16,17)} \\
(17,36) & (18,36) & (31,36) & (33,36) & \mathbf{(35,36)} \\
 & & & & \mathbf{(36,37)}
\end{array}
$$

On each row, the interval at the end in boldfaced type is a subset of the previous intervals. The five intervals in boldface are disjoint so $R_M = 5$. This conflicts with the value $R_M = 4$ reported by Hudson and Kaplan (1985); however, one can verify the five comparisons in the table above and in the original data of Kreitman (1983).

R_M is a lower bound on the number of recombinations. To estimate how many escaped detection, Hudson and Kaplan (1985) turned to simulation. The number of segregating sites is $S = 43$, so $\theta = 4Nu$ can be estimated by

$$
S \Big/ \sum_{i=1}^{10} 1/i = \frac{43}{2.928968} = 14.68
$$

If $\theta = 15$, the average values of R_M were 3.7 for $R = 10$, 5.5 for $R = 20$, and 8.8 for $r = 50$. Interpolating suggests $R \approx 18$. To get a confidence interval for R, Hudson and Kaplan (1985) did further simulations with a fixed number of segregating sites to argue that R should be between 5 and 150.

Hudson (1987) took a different approach to estimating R based on $k_{\ell m}$, the number of pairwise differences between the ℓth and mth sequences. Let

$$
S_k^2 = \frac{1}{n^2} \sum_{\ell=1}^{n} \sum_{m=1}^{n} (k_{\ell m} - \bar{k})^2 \quad \text{where} \quad \bar{k} = \frac{1}{n^2} \sum_{\ell=1}^{n} \sum_{m=1}^{n} k_{\ell m}
$$

Let p_{ia} be the sample frequency of allele a at the ith site and let $h_i = 1 - \sum_a p_{ia}^2$ be the sample estimate of the heterozygosity. Let q_{ab}^{ij} be the sample frequency of gametes with allele a at site i and allele b at site j, and let

$$
D_{ab}^{ij} = q_{ab}^{ij} - p_{ia} p_{jb}
$$

be the sample estimate of the linkage disequilibrium. Letting s be the number of sites, Brown, Feldman, and Nevo (1980) have shown that

$$S_k^2 = \sum_{i=1}^{s} h_i - \sum_{i=1}^{s} h_i^2 + 2 \sum_{i=1}^{s-1} \sum_{j=i+1}^{s} \sum_a \sum_b [2p_{ia}p_{jb}D_{ab}^{ij} + (D_{ab}^{ij})^2]$$

Using this formula, Hudson (1987) showed that

$$E\left(S_k^2 - \sum_{i=1}^{s} h_i + \sum_{i=1}^{s} h_i^2\right) = \theta^2 g(R, n)$$

where $g(R, n) = (2/R^2) \int_0^R f(z)(R - z)\, dz$ and

$$f(z) = \frac{1}{z^2 + 13z + 18} \cdot \left[(z + 14) + \frac{z(z + 12)}{n} + \frac{(z + 2)(z + 13)}{n^2} + \frac{2(z + 6)}{n^3}\right]$$

Using $\hat{\theta} = \frac{n}{n-1} \sum_{i=1}^{s} h_i = \frac{2}{n(n-1)} \sum_{\ell \neq m} k_{\ell m}$ to estimate θ, Hudson (1987) defined his estimator of R, which we will call $\hat{R}_k$, by solving

$$g(\hat{R}_k, n) = E\left(S_k^2 - \sum_{i=1}^{s} h_i + \sum_{i=1}^{s} h_i^2\right) / \hat{\theta}^2$$

Using this new estimator, Hudson (1987) reanalyzed the Kreitman data using the 43 polymorphic sites and 4 of the length polymorphisms where the only variation is the length of the sequence. He calculated $\hat{\theta} \sim 16$, $S_k^2 = 83.6$, and $\hat{R} \sim 25$. Additional simulations suggested that $[0, 80]$ was a 95% confidence interval for R.

A decade later, Wakeley (1997) introduced a version of Hudson's (1987) estimator that improved it in two ways. First, he took the comparison of the identical sequences out of Hudson's definition of k and used instead the average number of pairwise differences, which he denoted by

$$\pi = \frac{2}{n(n - 1)} \sum_{\ell=1}^{n-1} \sum_{m=\ell+1}^{n} k_{\ell m}$$

As we have noted in (3.2) of Chapter 1, $\pi = \Delta_n$ is an unbiased estimator of θ. Corresponding to π, one can define

$$S_\pi^2 = \frac{2}{n(n - 1)} \sum_{\ell=1}^{n} \sum_{m=1}^{n} (k_{\ell m} - \pi)^2$$

Since $k_{\ell\ell} = 0$, $\bar{k} = \pi(n - 1)/n$ and

$$S_k^2 = \left(\frac{n - 1}{n}\right) S_\pi^2 + \left(\frac{n - 1}{n^2}\right) \pi^2$$

The second change was to replace Hudson's biased estimator of θ^2, which in the current notation can be written as π^2, by an unbiased one. To do this, Wakeley (1997) computed that

$$\text{var}\,(\pi) = \left[\frac{n+1}{3(n-1)}\right]\theta + f_\pi(R,n)\theta^2$$

where

$$f_\pi(R,n) = \frac{2}{n(n-1)R^2}\Big\{-2R - [2n(n+1) - 7 - R]I_1$$
$$+ [2n(n+1)(13+2R) - 55 - R]\frac{I_2}{\sqrt{97}}\Big\}$$

and

$$I_1 = \ln\left[\frac{R^2 + 13R + 18}{18}\right] \quad \text{and} \quad I_2 = \ln\left[\frac{(13 - \sqrt{97} + 2R)(13 + \sqrt{97})}{(13 + \sqrt{97} + 2C)(13 - \sqrt{97}}\right]$$

Using this, he formulated his improved estimator $\hat{R}_\pi$ as the solution of

$$S_\pi^2 = \left[\frac{2(n-2)}{3(n-1)}\right]\pi + g_\pi(\hat{R}_k,n)\left\{\frac{\pi^2 - [(n+1)/3(n-1)]\pi}{f_\pi(\hat{R}_k,n) + 1}\right\}$$

where

$$g_\pi(R,n) = \frac{(n-2)}{n(n-1)R^2}\Big\{-2R(n+1) - [n - 7 - R(n+1)]I_1$$
$$+ [49n - 55 + R(15n - 1)]\frac{I_2}{\sqrt{97}}\Big\}$$

Wakeley (1997) applied his new estimator to data from Schaeffer and Miller (1993) that consisted of 99 sequences of a 3.5 kb region containing the alcohol dehydrogenase gene of *Drosophila psuedoobscura*. Hudson's estimate $\hat{R}_k = 315$ compared with Wakeley's estimate $\hat{R}_\pi = 282$. Using simulations, Wakeley computed approximate 95% confidence intervals for the two estimators to be [185,484] and [172,453].

Griffiths and Marjoram (1996) have developed an estimator of R based on likelihood methods. Hey and Wakeley (1997) have introduced one based on the location of incongruent sites in the sequence. Wall (2000) has performed simulations to compare all of the estimators we have mentioned in this section.

2.3   Population Subdivision

The island model was introduced by Wright (1943). Here we will follow the formulation of Maruyama (1970), who had n subpopulations with N diploid individuals each. In constructing the population in generation $t + 1$ from generation t, individuals pick their parents at random from the same subpopulation with probability $1 - m$ and at random from one of the other $n-1$ subpopulations with probability m. In ecology this is called a metapopulation model. This structure with $n=6$ can be illustrated by the following picture.

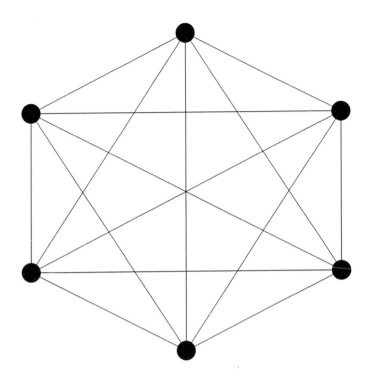

Let u be the mutation rate, $\theta = 4Nu$, and $M = 4Nm$. If we consider two lineages in the genealogical process and measure time in units of $2N$ generations, then the two lineages:

coalesce at rate 1 when they are in the same population,

experience mutations at rate $2u \cdot 2N = \theta$,

migrate at rate $2m \cdot 2N = M$.

Identity by descent

Let $p_s(\theta)$ and $p_d(\theta)$ be the probabilities that two lineages are identical by descent when they are picked from the same or different populations. By considering what happens at the first event:

$$p_s(\theta) \quad = \quad \frac{1}{1+\theta+M} \cdot 1 + \frac{M}{1+\theta+M} p_d(\theta)$$

$$p_d(\theta) \quad = \quad \frac{M/(n-1)}{\theta + M} p_s(\theta) + \frac{M(n-2)/(n-1)}{\theta + M} p_d(\theta)$$

The second equation implies that

$$p_d(\theta) = \frac{M/(n-1)}{\theta + M/(n-1)} p_s(\theta) = \frac{M}{(n-1)\theta + M} p_s(\theta)$$

Using this in the first equation, we have

$$p_s(\theta) = \frac{1}{1+\theta+M} + \frac{M}{1+\theta+M} \cdot \frac{M}{(n-1)\theta + M} p_s(\theta)$$

Noting $(1+\theta+M)((n-1)\theta + M) - M^2 = \theta(n-1) + \theta^2(n-1) + M\theta(n-1) + M + M\theta$ we have

$$p_s(\theta) \quad = \quad \frac{\theta(n-1) + M}{\theta^2(n-1) + \theta(n-1+Mn) + M}$$

$$p_d(\theta) \quad = \quad \frac{M}{\theta^2(n-1) + \theta(n-1+Mn) + M}$$

Setting $\gamma = M/(n-1)$ and $D = \theta^2 + \theta(1+n\gamma) + \gamma$ we have

$$(3.1) \qquad\qquad p_s(\theta) = \frac{\theta + \gamma}{D} \qquad p_d(\theta) = \frac{\gamma}{D}$$

Note that in the limit of fast migration, $\gamma \to \infty$

$$p_s(\theta) = p_d(\theta) = \frac{1}{n\theta + 1}$$

This may look different from the usual result for a homogeneously mixing population but since $n\theta = (4Nn)u$ this is the by now familiar formula for a population with total size Nn.

Mean coalescence time

Let T_s be the coalescence time for two (distinct) individuals chosen from the same population and $t_s = T_s/2N$. It is easy to see that

$$p_s(\theta) = Ee^{-2uT_s} = Ee^{-\theta t_s}$$

In words, $p_s(\theta)$ is the Laplace transform of t_s. Differentiating the last formula, we see that $-p_s'(\theta) = E(t_s e^{-\theta t_s})$ so $-p_s'(0) = Et_s$. To use this formula, we note that $D' = 2\theta + (1 + n\gamma)$ so

$$(3.2) \qquad\qquad -p_s'(\theta) = - \left\{ \frac{1}{D} - \frac{(\theta + \gamma)D'}{D^2} \right\}$$

Setting $\theta = 0$, which implies $D = \gamma$ and $D' = 1 + n\gamma$, we have

$$(3.3) \qquad\qquad Et_s = -p_s'(0) = - \left\{ \frac{1}{\gamma} - \frac{\gamma(1+n\gamma)}{\gamma^2} \right\} = n$$

Note that the mean of t_s does not depend on the migration rate. However, we can see from the Laplace transform, $p_s(\theta)$, that the distribution does.

Repeating the calculation for t_d, we have

$$(3.4) \qquad -p_d'(\theta) = -(-\gamma D'/D^2)$$

and it follows that

$$(3.5) \qquad Et_d = -p_d'(0) = \frac{\gamma(1 + n\gamma)}{\gamma^2} = n + \frac{1}{\gamma}$$

One can derive this result more simply by noting that two lineages that start in different populations will require an average of $(n-1)/M = 1/\gamma$ units of time to enter the same population so

$$Et_d = \frac{1}{\gamma} + Et_s$$

The average number of pairwise differences between two individuals sampled from the same population, Δ_s, has $E\Delta_s = \theta Et_s$. Likewise $E\Delta_d = \theta Et_d$. Combining this with (3.2) and (3.3) shows that

$$E\Delta_d - E\Delta_s = \frac{\theta}{\gamma} = \frac{\theta(n-1)}{M} = \frac{(n-1)u}{m}$$

Example 3.1. Slatkin (1987) used this to analyze data of Kreitman and Aguadé (1986a) for 87 samples of a 2.7 kilobase region encompassing the *Adh* locus in *Drosophila*. Sixty of the samples were from Raleigh, North Carolina and 27 from Putah Creek, California, near Davis. Slatkin argued that their restriction enzyme technique was sensitive enough to detect all insertions and deletions and approximately 20% of the base pair substitutions.

The average number of insertions and deletions was 2.1 between members of the Raleigh population and 1.93 for Putah Creek. The average number of base pair differences detected by their method between members of the Raleigh population was 3.6 and 3.61 for Putah Creek. Five times the second number plus the first gives 20.1 and 19.98, which we average to get 20.04. The average number of differences between populations computed by the same method was 20.71. The difference, which is 0.67, is our estimate of $(n-1)u/m$. As Slatkin says, "these data suggest that either $(n-1)u$ is very small or m is relatively large. The latter seems likely for *D. melanogaster*, a species that is commensal with humans and whose dispersal is likely to be via trucks on interstate highways."

Variances

By continuing the analysis above we can compute the variances of t_s, t_d, Δ_s, and Δ_d. To begin, we note that $p_s''(0) = Et_s^2$ and using (3.2)

$$p_s''(\theta) = \frac{-D'}{D^2} - \frac{D'}{D^2} - \frac{(\theta + \gamma)D''}{D^2} + 2\frac{(\theta + \gamma)(D')^2}{D^3}$$

Since $D = \theta^2 + \theta(1 + n\gamma) + \gamma$, $D' = 2\theta + 1 + n\gamma$, and $D'' = 2$ we have

$$
\begin{aligned}
p_s''(0) &= -\frac{2(1 + n\gamma)}{\gamma^2} - \frac{2\gamma}{\gamma^2} + \frac{2(1 + n\gamma)^2}{\gamma^2} \\
&= \frac{2}{\gamma^2}((n-1)\gamma + (n\gamma)^2)
\end{aligned}
$$

Since $Et_s = n$, it follows that

(3.6) $$\operatorname{var}(t_s) = n^2 + \frac{2n - 2}{\gamma}$$

The calculation for t_d is somewhat easier. Using (3.4) gives

$$
\begin{aligned}
p_d''(\theta) &= -\frac{\gamma D''}{D^2} + 2\frac{\gamma(D')^2}{D^3} \\
p_d''(0) &= -\frac{2\gamma}{\gamma^2} + \frac{2\gamma(1 + n\gamma)^2}{\gamma^3} = 2\left(n + \frac{1}{\gamma}\right)^2 - \frac{2}{\gamma}
\end{aligned}
$$

Since $Et_d = n + 1/\gamma$, it follows that

(3.7) $$\operatorname{var}(t_d) = \left(n + \frac{1}{\gamma}\right)^2 - \frac{2}{\gamma} = n^2 + \frac{2n - 2}{\gamma} + \frac{1}{\gamma^2}$$

To check this, note that two lineages that start in different populations take an exponentially distributed amount of time with mean $1/\gamma$ to come to the same population so

$$\operatorname{var}(t_d) = \frac{1}{\gamma^2} + \operatorname{var}(t_s)$$

Effective population size

Following Nei and Takahata (1993), we will now try to make sense out of our collection of formulas by introducing an effective population size. Let T_r be the coalescence time of two individuals sampled at random from the entire population and $t_r = T_r/2N$. Combining (3.3) and (3.5)

$$
\begin{aligned}
ET_r &= 2N\left[\frac{1}{n} \cdot n + \frac{n-1}{n} \cdot \left(n + \frac{1}{\gamma}\right)\right] \\
&= 2Nn\left[1 + \frac{(n-1)}{n^2\gamma}\right]
\end{aligned}
$$

Recalling $\gamma = M/(n-1) = 4nm/(n-1)$, we have

(3.8) $$ET_r = 2Nn\left[1 + \frac{(n-1)^2}{4Nmn^2}\right]$$

Since in a homogeneously mixing population of effective size N_e we have $ET_r = 2N_e$, this shows that from the viewpoint of the expected coalescence time, an island model has effective population size

(3.9)
$$N_e = Nn \left[1 + \frac{(n-1)^2}{4Nmn^2}\right]$$

One can see from this that the effective population size is always larger than the actual population size and can be much greater when $4Nm$ is small.

Since the nucleotide diversity $\pi = 2\mu ET_r$, it is clear that with this definition we have $\pi = 4N_e\mu$. However, as we will now see, this simple approach does not quite work for the homozygosity. Let F be the probability that two individuals chosen at random are identical by descent. Using (3.1) and $\gamma = M/(n-1)$, we have

$$F = \frac{1}{n}p_s(\theta) + \frac{n-1}{n}p_d(\theta) = \frac{M/(n-1) + \theta/n}{D}$$

Recalling that $D = \theta^2 + \theta(1+n\gamma) + \gamma$, we have

$$\frac{1}{F} = \frac{\theta^2 + \theta\left(1 + \frac{nM}{n-1}\right) + \frac{M}{n-1}}{\frac{\theta}{n} + \frac{M}{n-1}}$$

Breaking the numerator up as $\theta^2 + \theta n M/(n-1)$ plus $M/(n-1) + \theta/n$ plus $\theta - \theta/n$, we can write the above as

$$\theta n + 1 + \frac{\frac{n-1}{n}\theta}{\frac{\theta}{n} + \frac{M}{n-1}} = 1 + 4Nun + \frac{(n-1)^2 u}{(n-1)u + mn}$$

since $\theta = 4Nu$ and $M = 4Nm$. In a homogeneously mixing population of size N_e, $1/F = 1 + 4N_e u$, so we have

$$N_e = Nu \left[1 + \frac{(n-1)^2}{4Nn(n-1)u + 4Nmn^2}\right]$$

The new formula is not quite the old one, (3.9), unless $m \gg u$. The equality under this condition is not surprising: if migration is much faster than mutation then the coalescence time should have the lack of memory property of the exponential distribution and in this case the formula for the Laplace transform of the exponential distribution implies

$$Ee^{-2uT_r} = \frac{1}{1 + 2uET_r}$$

Fixation indices

To quantify the impact of population structure on genetic differentiation, Wright (1951) introduced a quantity that can be defined as follows (see Nei 1975, page 151)

(3.10)
$$F_{ST} = \frac{f_0 - \bar{f}}{1 - \bar{f}}$$

where f_0 is the probability that two genes sampled from the same subpopulation are identical by descent and $\bar{f}$ is that probability for two individuals sampled at random from the entire population.

The probability of identity of two genes is the probability that no mutation occurred before their coalescence time T so

$$f = \sum_{t=1}^{\infty}(1-\mu)^{2t}P(T=t) \approx \sum_{t=1}^{\infty}(1-2t\mu)P(T=t) = 1 - 2\mu ET$$

the middle approximation being valid if $\mu \ll ET$. Using this with the previous formula shows that

$$(3.11) \qquad\qquad F_{ST} \approx \frac{\bar{T} - \bar{T}_0}{\bar{T}}$$

where $\bar{T}_0$ is the average coalescence time of two genes drawn from the same population and $\bar{T}$ is the the average coalescence time for two genes sampled at random from the entire population. An advantage of (3.11) over (3.10) is that it does not depend on the mutation rate.

In the case of the finite island model, $\bar{T} = ET_r = 2NEt_r$, and $\bar{T}_0 = ET_s = 2NEt_s$, so using (3.8) and (3.3) we have

$$F_{ST} = \frac{(n-1)^2}{4Nmn^2} \bigg/ \left(1 + \frac{(n-1)^2}{4Nmn^2}\right)$$

and it follows that

$$(3.12) \qquad\qquad F_{ST} = \left(1 + 4Nm \cdot \frac{n^2}{(n-1)^2}\right)^{-1}$$

a formula first derived by Takahata (1983); see also (5) in Takahata and Nei (1984). Contradicting our previous convention, we will now follow the usage in a different part of the literature by defining $M = Nm$ to be the number of migrating gametes per generation. When the number of colonies is large we can replace $n^2/(n-1)^2$ by 1 and we have

$$(3.13) \qquad\qquad M = \frac{1}{4}\left(\frac{1}{F_{ST}} - 1\right)$$

Once we have a recipe for estimating F_{ST} from data, the last formula can be used to estimate the migration rate. When there are only two populations, $\bar{T} = (Et_s + Et_d)/2$ and $\bar{T}_0 = Et_s$, (3.11) becomes

$$\frac{Et_d - Et_s}{Et_s + Et_d}$$

and using (3.13) we have

$$M = \frac{1}{4}\left(\frac{Et_s + Et_d}{Et_d - Et_s} - 1\right) = \frac{Et_s}{2(Et_d - Et_s)}$$

Recalling that $E\Delta_i = \theta E t_i$, we can estimate M by

$$(3.14) \qquad \hat{M} = \frac{\hat{\Delta}_s}{2(\hat{\Delta}_d - \hat{\Delta}_s)}$$

where $\hat{\Delta}_s$ is the mean number of differences between two sequences sampled from the same population and $\hat{\Delta}_d$ is the mean number of differences between two sequences sampled from different populations.

This estimator is closely related to but slightly different than others that have been introduced. Weir and Cockerham's (1984) $\hat{\theta}$ and Lynch and Crease's (1990) N_{ST} estimate $(Et_d - Et_s)/Et_s$ so one has

$$\hat{M} = \frac{1}{2} \cdot \left(\frac{1}{\hat{\theta}} - 1 \right)$$

Hudson, Slatkin, and Maddison (1992) estimate F_{ST} by $\hat{F} = 1 - \hat{\Delta}_s/\hat{\Delta}_d$ so they again have

$$(3.15) \qquad \hat{M} = \frac{1}{2} \cdot \left(\frac{1}{\hat{F}} - 1 \right)$$

Example 3.2. To illustrate the estimation of F_{ST} and inferences about spatial structure, we will use data from Hamblin and Veuille (1999), who sequenced 809 bp of the *vermillion* locus in four African populations of *D. simulans*. Values of F_{ST} as computed by the formula of Hudson, Slatkin, and Maddison are given above the diagonal in the following table. Note that $F_{ST} \geq 0$ by definition but the comparison of Kenya and Tanzania produced a negative estimate.

	Kenya	Tanzania	Zimbabwe	Cameroon
Kenya		-0.033	0.178	0.107
		(0.854)	(0.001)	(0.006)
Tanzania	∞		0.122	0.077
			(0.007)	(0.014)
Zimbabwe	4.6	7.2		0.159
				(0.014)
Cameroon	8.3	12	5.3	

To determine the significance of these values, they used the method of Hudson, Boos, and Kaplan (1992). To explain the method, we consider the comparison of the 13 sequences from Kenya and the 10 from Zimbabwe. If the two populations were part of a homogeneously mixing whole, then the distribution of the computed value of F_{ST} does not change if we pick 13 of the 23 sequences at random (without replacement) to be the Kenya sample and call the remaining 10 the Zimbabwe sample. They repeated this procedure 1000 times. The number in parentheses below the estimate $\hat{F}$, 0.001 in this case, indicates the fraction of times the randomized data set gave a larger value of F_{ST}. In all cases except the Kenya and Tanzania comparison we can reject with confidence the assumption of homogeneous mixing. Using (3.15) now we can estimate the number of migrants per generation $\hat{M}$. The results are given below the diagonal. In the case of the Kenya-Tanzania comparison, the estimated $\hat{M}$ is negative, so we write ∞.

Example 3.3. Seielstad, Minch, and Cavalli-Sforza (1998) have recently made an interesting application of F_{ST} estimates. They collected data on Y chromsome single nucleotide polymorphisms and compared them with published studies of autosomal and mitochondrial DNA variation.

Genetic system	within populations	within continents	between continents	F_{ST}	M
mtDNA	0.814	0.061	0.125	0.186	4.38
autosomes	0.856	0.057	0.088	0.144	1.49
Y chromosome	0.355	0.118	0.527	0.645	0.55

These authors approximate F_{ST} by the variation among populations (i.e., 1 minus the within-population variability). To infer migration rates from this, we can use (3.13) for autosomes, but mtDNA and the Y chromosome are haploid and exist in only one of the two sexes so their effective population size is $1/4$ as large and we must use $F_{ST} = (1 + M)^{-1}$ instead of (3.13).

The results are given in the table. Comparing the inferred migration rate from mtDNA, which resides only in females, with that from the Y chromosome in males, we conclude that females migrate about eight times as often as males. At first, this may seem surprising since men travel more than women in many societies. However, the most important parameter from a genetic perspective is the distance between the birthplace of the parents and of the children. Marriages in agricultural economies where land is inherited by sons, and probably in early foraging economies as well, tend to be patrilocal; that is, the wife moves to join the husband. Thus women tend to be more mobile than men as far as transgenerational movements are concerned.

2.4   Spatial Structure: Stepping Stone Model

The stepping stone model was introduced by Kimura (1953), but the first mathematical analysis was done over a decade later by Kimura and Weiss (1964) and Weiss and Kimura (1965). After about another decade, this model was rediscovered in the probability literature by Clifford and Sudbury (1973) and Holley and Liggett (1975).

In the one-dimensional stepping stone model, space is represented as a sequence of colonies $0 \leq x < L$, each of which consists of N diploid or $2N$ haploid individuals. To avoid edge effects, we will suppose that the colonies form a ring. The next figure shows a picture of the situation with $L = 12$.

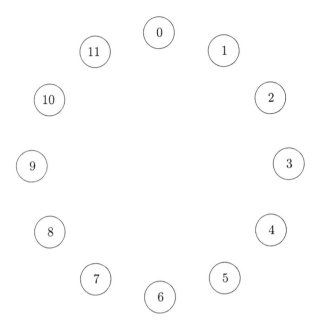

To implement this mathematically, we compute the displacement from colony x to y modulo L. That is, we add a (positive or negative) multiple of L to the difference $y - x$ to make the answer lie in $(-L, 2, L/2]$. For example if $L = 12$, $x = 10$, and $y = 1$ then $y - x = -9$ and $(y - x) \bmod 12 = -9 + 12 = 3$. In words, colony 1 is a distance 3 from colony 10 in the clockwise direction. For an example with a negative result, consider $x = 0$ and $y = 11$. In this case $(y - x) \bmod 12 = 11 - 12 = -1$. In words, colony 11 is a distance 1 from colony 0 in the counterclockwise direction. The choice of $(y - x) \bmod 12 \in \{-5, \ldots 6\}$ is different from the usual mathematical practice of defining $(y - x) \bmod 12$ to lie in $\{0, 1, \ldots 11\}$. The reader will see the reason for this change when we describe the dynamics of the model.

The population evolves in discrete time, with generation $n + 1$ obtained from generation n in the following way. Consider a given individual in colony x. With probability μ, this individual mutates to a new type and, with probability $(1 - \mu)p(x, y)$, assumes the type of an individual chosen at random (in generation n) from the colony at y. All such mutations and choices are assumed to be independent for all individuals at all colonies.

We assume that the transition probability $p(x, y)$ is given by

$$p(x, y) = (1 - \nu)I(x, y) + \nu q(y - x),$$

where $I(x, y)$ is 1 if $x = y$ and 0 otherwise, and the difference $y - x$ is computed and modulo L. Here ν is the migration probability and $q(z)$ is a probability distribution on the integers $\mathbf{Z}$ with $q(0) = 0$ that has the following properties.

(i) *symmetry.* $q(x) = q(-x)$.

(ii) *finite range.* $q(x) = 0$ if $|x| \geq K$.

(iii) *irreducibility.* It is possible to get from any colony x to any other colony y by a sequence of steps each of which has positive probability.

The most common example is the *nearest neighbor* model which has $q(1) = q(-1) = 1/2$. In words, when migration occurs, it occurs to the two neighboring colonies with equal probability. We will begin with the analysis of this simple case. For further simplicity, we will first consider the case of an infinite sequence of colonies indexed by the integers. Let $\psi(x, y)$ be the probability that two individuals, one chosen from colony x and one from colony y, are identical by descent in equilibrium. (When $x = y$ we suppose that two distinct individuals are chosen.) Clearly this probability only depends on the distance between the colonies, so we consider instead $\phi(x) = \psi(0, x)$.

Considering what happens in one generation and supposing that μ and ν are small enough so that we can ignore the probability of two events affecting the two individuals we are considering, we have that

(4.1) $\phi(x) = \nu\phi(x - 1) + (1 - 2\mu - 2\nu)\phi(x) + \nu\phi(x + 1)$ for $x \neq 0$

Rearranging, we have

$$0 = \phi(x - 1) - \left(2 + \frac{2\mu}{\nu}\right)\phi(x) + \phi(x + 1)   \text{ for } x \neq 0$$

Restricting our attention to $x \geq 1$ in the last equation, we have a second-order difference equation whose general solution is $A\lambda_1^x + B\lambda_2^x$, where the λ_i are the roots of

$$0 = 1 - \left(2 + \frac{2\mu}{\nu}\right)\lambda + \lambda^2$$

The quadratic formula tells us that the roots are

$$\lambda_i = \frac{2 + \frac{2\mu}{\nu} \pm \sqrt{\left(2 + \frac{2\mu}{\nu}\right)^2 - 4}}{2} = \frac{2 + \frac{2\mu}{\nu} \pm \sqrt{\frac{8\mu}{\nu} + \frac{4\mu^2}{\nu^2}}}{2}$$

If $\mu \ll \nu$ then $\lambda_i \approx 1 \pm \sqrt{2\mu/\nu}$.

Noting that $(\lambda - a)(\lambda - b) = \lambda^2 - (a + b)\lambda + ab$, we see that $\lambda_1\lambda_2 = 1$ and we have $\lambda_1 > 1 > \lambda_2$. From this we see that for $x \geq 0$, $\phi(x) = B\lambda_2^x$, for otherwise the probability $\phi(x)$ would become unbounded as $x \to \infty$. Using the symmetry $\phi(-x) = \phi(x)$, it follows that

$$\phi(x) = B\lambda_2^{|x|}$$

To determine the constant B we use the equation analogous to (4.1) for $x = 0$. Now $\phi(1) = \phi(-1)$ and the probability of coalescence of two lineages in the same colony on one step is $1/2N$, so if we ignore the occurrence of two events in one generation

$$\phi(0) = 2\nu\phi(1) + (1 - 2\mu - 2\nu - 1/2N)\phi(0) + 1/2N$$

Rearranging gives

(4.2) $$(2\mu + 2\nu + 1/2N)\phi(0) - 2\nu\phi(1) = 1/2N$$

Substituting in $\phi(x) = B\lambda_2^{|x|}$ and solving gives

$$B = \frac{1/2N}{2\mu + 2\nu(1 - \lambda_2) + 1/2N}$$

When $\mu \ll \nu$ we have $\lambda_2 \approx 1 - \sqrt{2\mu/\nu}$ so

(4.3) $$\phi(0) = B \approx \frac{1}{1 + 4N\sqrt{2\mu\nu}} \quad \text{and} \quad \phi(x) \approx B(1 - \sqrt{2\mu/\nu})^{|x|}$$

which agrees with formulas on page 89 of Malécot (1969).

We are now ready to tackle the more complicated case of a ring of L sites. Again we let $\phi(x) = \psi(0, x)$. If we define $\phi(L) = \phi(0)$, then by the reasoning that led to (4.1)

(4.4) $$\phi(x) = \nu\phi(x-1) + (1 - 2\mu - 2\nu)\phi(x) + \nu\phi(x+1) \quad \text{for } 0 < x < L$$

This is the same second order difference equation, so it has solutions $A\lambda_1^x + B\lambda_2^x$ for the same values of λ_1 and λ_2. The solution of interest has the symmetry property $\phi(x) = \phi(L - x)$ and in particular $\phi(0) = \phi(L)$, so

$$A + B = A\lambda_1^L + B\lambda_2^L \quad \text{and hence} \quad A(\lambda_1^L - 1) = B(1 - \lambda_2^L)$$

From this it follows that there is a constant C so that $A = C(1 - \lambda_2^L)$ and $B = C(\lambda_1^L - 1)$ and hence

(4.5) $$\phi(x) = C(1 - \lambda_2^L)\lambda_1^x + C(\lambda_1^L - 1)\lambda_2^x$$

To check our computations we note that using $\lambda_1\lambda_2 = 1$

$$\begin{aligned}
\phi(L - x) &= C(1 - \lambda_2^L)\lambda_1^{L-x} + C(\lambda_1^L - 1)\lambda_2^{L-x} \\
&= C(\lambda_1^L - 1)\lambda_1^{-x} + C(1 - \lambda_2^L)\lambda_2^{-x} \\
&= C(\lambda_1^L - 1)\lambda_2^x + C(1 - \lambda_2^L)\lambda_1^x = \phi(x)
\end{aligned}$$

To compute C we use (4.2) with the fact that $\phi(0) = C(\lambda_1^L - \lambda_2^L)$ and $\phi(1) = C(\lambda_1 - \lambda_2^{L-1} + \lambda_1^{L-1} - \lambda_2)$ to conclude

$$C = \frac{1/2N}{(2\mu + 1/2N)(\lambda_1^L - \lambda_2^L) + 2\nu(\lambda_1^L - \lambda_2^L - \lambda_1^{L-1} + \lambda_2^{L-1} - \lambda_1 + \lambda_2)}$$

If λ_1^L is large (and hence λ_2^L is small), then $\phi(x) \approx C\lambda_1^{L-x} + C\lambda_1^x$ and

$$C \approx \frac{1}{\lambda_1^L} \cdot \frac{1}{1 + 4N\mu + 4N\nu(\lambda_1 - 1)}$$

When $\mu \ll \nu$, we have $\lambda_1 \approx 1 + \sqrt{2\mu/\nu}$. If L is large and $x/L \leq 1/2 - \epsilon$, then $\lambda_1^{L-x} \gg \lambda_1^x$ so we have

$$\phi(x) \approx \frac{\lambda_2^x}{1 + 4N\sqrt{2\mu\nu}}$$

which agrees with our previous result for the stepping stone model on an infinite linear grid given in (4.3).

Recalling that $\lambda_1 \approx 1 + \sqrt{2\mu/\nu}$, we see that λ_1^L is large when $L\sqrt{\mu/\nu}$ is large or equivalently when $L^2/\nu \gg 1/\mu$. To interpret the last inequality, we note that the displacement kernel q has variance 1 and steps are taken with probability ν so it takes about L^2/ν steps to go a distance L. On the right-hand side, $1/\mu$ is the average amount of time it takes for a lineage to encounter a mutation, so when $L^2/\nu \gg 1/\mu$ it is very likely that a mutation will occur before the lineage has moved a distance L, and we expect very little difference between the circle and the line.

Our next goal is to show that if the opposite inequality $L^2/\nu \ll 1/\mu$ holds then the stepping stone model behaves like a homogeneously mixing population. The intuition behind this guess is that when $L^2/\nu \ll 1/\mu$ it is very unlikely that a mutation will occur before the lineage has moved a distance that is a large multiple of L and hence traveled around the circle many times, forgetting its starting point. To check this intuition with our formula, we note that (4.5) implies that

$$\begin{aligned}
\phi(x) &= C(1 - \lambda_2^L)\lambda_1^x + C(\lambda_1^L - 1)\lambda_2^x \\
&= C(\lambda_1^x - \lambda_2^x) + C(\lambda_1^{L-x} - \lambda_2^{L-x})
\end{aligned}$$

Using the formula for C now, we have

$$\phi(x) = \frac{\lambda_1^x - \lambda_2^x + \lambda_1^{L-x} - \lambda_2^{L-x}}{(1 + 4N\mu)(\lambda_1^L - \lambda_2^L) + 4N\nu(\lambda_1^L - \lambda_2^L - \lambda_1^{L-1} + \lambda_2^{L-1} - \lambda_1 + \lambda_2)}$$

Using the fact that

$$\frac{\lambda_1^k - \lambda_2^k}{\lambda_1 - \lambda_2} = \sum_{j=1}^{k} \lambda_1^{k-j}\lambda_2^{j-1} \approx k$$

when $L^2/\nu \ll 1/\mu$ and hence $\lambda_1^L \approx 1$ we have

$$\phi(x) \approx \frac{x + (L - x)}{(1 - 4N\mu)L + 4N\nu(L - (L-1) - 1)} = \frac{1}{1 + 4N\mu}$$

the result for a homogeneously mixing population.

The one-dimensional stepping stone model is appropriate for populations at the edge of a lake or along a coastline. However, for most applications, a two-dimensional version in which there is a rectangular grid of colonies indexed by (x_1, x_2) with $0 \leq x_1, x_2 < L$ is a better model. The next figure shows a picture of the case $L = 10$.

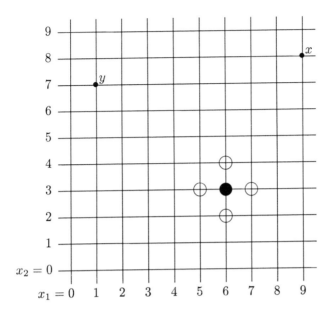

Here, for simplicity, we have not drawn the 100 circles that represent the colonies. The reader should think of the colonies as being at the intersections of the lines and indexed by the numbers that indicate the row and column. For example, the colony indicated by the solid dot is $(6, 3)$.

As in the case of the one-dimensional model, we will avoid edge effects by using modulo arithmetic to compute displacements. This time there are two coordinates, so we compute the difference componentwise. In the example above, $L = 10$ so the displacement from $(x_1, x_2) = (9, 8)$ to $(y_1, y_2) = (1, 7)$ is $(-8, -1) \bmod 10 = (2, -1)$. In words, points on the right edge are adjacent to those on the left, and those on the top edge are adjacent to those on the bottom. To visualize this, mentally cut the grid out of the page. Use tape to attach the right edge to the left to make a cylinder. Then tape the circle at the top edge to the one at the bottom to form a donut shape that mathematicians call a torus. The torus does not look much like our flat universe but it does have the advantage that the world is homogeneous, i.e., looks the same from every point.

The dynamics in two dimensions are almost exactly the same as in one dimension. The only difference is that there are now two coordinates. Again, the population evolves in discrete time, with generation $n+1$ obtained from generation n in the following way. Consider a given individual in colony (x_1, x_2). With probability μ, this individual mutates to a new type and, with probability $(1 - \mu)p((x_1, x_2), (y_1, y_2))$, assumes the type of an individual chosen at random (in generation n) from the colony at (y_1, y_2). All such mutations and choices are assumed to be independent for all individuals at all colonies.

We assume that the transition probability $p((x_1, x_2), (y_1, y_2))$ is given by

$$p((x_1, x_2), (y_1, y_2)) = (1 - \nu)I((x_1, x_2), (y_1, y_2)) + \nu q(y_1 - x_1, y_2 - x_2),$$

where $I(x, y)$ is 1 if $(x_1, x_2) = (y_1, y_2)$, and 0 otherwise, and the differences $y_i - x_i$ are computed and modulo L. $q(z_1, z_2)$ is a probability distribution on the points in two dimensions with integer coordinates $\mathbf{Z}^2$ with $q(0, 0) = 0$ that has the following properties.

(i) *symmetry.* $q(x_1, x_2) = q(-x_1, -x_2)$, $q(x_1, x_2) = q(x_2, x_1)$.

(ii) *finite range.* $q(x_1, x_2) = 0$ if $\max\{|x_1|, |x_2|\} \geq K$.

(iii) *irreducibility.* It is possible to get from any colony (x_1, x_2) to any other colony (y_1, y_2) by a sequence of steps each of which has positive probability.

The most common example is the *nearest neighbor* model which has $q(1, 0) = q(-1, 0) = q(0, 1) = q(0, -1) = 1/4$. In words, migration occurs to one of the four nearest neighboring colonies with equal probability. In the figure, the four nearest neighbors of the black dot are indicated by circles.

The first result is quite general and applies to stepping stone models in any dimension. In order to treat all of these cases at the same time and to simplify the notation in the two-dimensional case, we will write x for a generic colony. In one dimension, x is an integer. In two dimensions, x is shorthand for (x_1, x_2). Let $\psi(x, y)$ be the probability that two individuals, one chosen from the colony at x and one from the colony at y are identical by descent in equilibrium. (When $x = y$ we suppose that two distinct individuals are chosen.) The first step in computing ψ is the following result of Malécot (1969):

$$(4.6) \qquad \psi(x, y) = \frac{1 - \psi(0, 0)}{2N} \sum_{n=1}^{\infty} (1 - \mu)^{2n} p^{2n}(x, y)$$

Here $p^k(x, y)$ is the probability of going from x to y in k steps. Intuitively it is just the kth power of the matrix $p(x, y)$. Formally it is defined inductively by $p^1(x, y) = p(x, y)$ and for $k \geq 2$

$$p^k(x, y) = \sum_z p(x, z) p^{k-1}(z, y)$$

Proof of (4.6). The proof follows pages 77–81 of Malécot (1969) but corrects the mistake in his (3.4.2). Let $\psi_n(x, y)$ be the probability that two individuals, one chosen from x and one from y are identical by descent in generation n. When $x = y$ we suppose that two distinct individuals are chosen. By definition, $p(x, y)$ is the probability that an individual in colony x in generation $n+1$ is the offspring of one at y in generation n. Recalling that the number of chromsomes in a colony is $2N$ and considering what happens on one step, we see that

$$\psi_{n+1}(x,y) = (1-\mu)^2 \sum_{x',y'} \psi_n(x',y')p(x,x')p(y,y')$$

$$+ (1-\mu)^2 \sum_z \frac{1-\psi_n(z,z)}{2N} p(x,z)p(y,z)$$

where the second term compensates for the two individuals choosing the same parent. Setting $\psi_{n+1} = \psi_n = \psi$ to compute the equilibrium and iterating once, we have

$$\psi(x,y) = (1-\mu)^2 \sum_z \frac{1-\psi(z,z)}{2N} p(x,z)\, p(y,z)$$

$$+ (1-\mu)^2 \sum_{x',y'} p(x,x')p(y,y')$$

$$\left\{ (1-\mu)^2 \sum_z \frac{1-\psi(z,z)}{2N} p(x',z)p(y',z) \right.$$

$$\left. + (1-\mu)^2 \sum_{x'',y''} \psi(x'',y'')p(x',x'')p(y',y'') \right\}$$

Noting $\sum_{x'} p(x,x')p(x',z) = p^2(x,z)$, the above becomes

$$\psi(x,y) = (1-\mu)^2 \sum_z \frac{1-\psi(z,z)}{2N} p(x,z)p(y,z)$$

$$+ (1-\mu)^4 \sum_z \frac{1-\psi(z,z)}{2N} p^2(x,z)p^2(y,z)$$

$$+ (1-\mu)^4 \sum_{x'',y''} \psi(x'',y'')p^2(x,x'')p^2(y,y'')$$

Iterating n times, letting $n \to \infty$ and noting that the last term tends to 0 when $\mu > 0$, we have

$$\psi(x,y) = \sum_{n=1}^{\infty}(1-\mu)^{2n} \sum_z \frac{1-\psi(z,z)}{2N} p^n(x,z)p^n(y,z)$$

$$= \frac{1-\psi(0,0)}{2N} \sum_{n=1}^{\infty}(1-\mu)^{2n}p^{2n}(x,y)$$

where in the last step we have used $\psi(z,z) = \psi(0,0)$ and $p^n(y,z) = p^n(z,y)$. $\qquad\square$

For the rest of the section, we will restrict our attention to the two-dimensional case. By translation invariance, it is enough to consider $\phi(x) =$

$\psi(0, x)$. To compute ϕ, we introduce the Fourier transforms

$$\hat{\phi}(k) = \sum_x e^{ik \cdot x} \phi(x) \quad \text{and} \quad \hat{p}(k) = \sum_x e^{ik \cdot x} p(0, x)$$

where $k \cdot x = k_1 x_1 + k_2 x_2$ is the dot product of the vectors $k = (k_1, k_2)$ and $x = (x_1, x_2)$. Because of the symmetry properties in (i), the transforms $\hat{\phi}(k)$ and $\hat{p}(k)$ are real. Let $\Lambda(L) = \mathbf{Z}^2 \cap [0, L)^2$. As we will explain below, transforming (4.6) and using the inversion formula for Fourier transforms with the symmetry mentioned above, we obtain

$$(4.7) \quad \phi(x) = \frac{(1 - \mu)^2 (1 - \phi(0))}{2NL^2} \sum_{k \in 2\pi\Lambda(L)/L} \frac{\hat{p}^2(k) \cos(k_1 x_1) \cos(k_2 x_2)}{1 - (1 - \mu)^2 \hat{p}^2(k)}$$

where $0 = (0, 0)$ and $\hat{p}^2(k)$ is shorthand for $(\hat{p}(k))^2$. In words the sum is over all vectors $k = (k_1, k_2)$ of the form $(2\pi\ell_1/L, 2\pi\ell_2/L)$ where $(\ell_1, \ell_2) \in \Lambda(L)$. This result is a close relative of the $K = \infty$ special case of (3.7) in Maruyama (1971). To make the connection, note that in his formulation migrations in the two directions are independent so his $\xi_{k_1, k_2} = \hat{p}^2(k)$.

Proof of (4.7). Maruyama (1971) proved this by diagonalizing matrices. However, with a little Fourier analysis, the proof is quite simple. Transforming (4.6), we have

$$\hat{\phi}(k) = \frac{1 - \phi(0)}{2N} \sum_{n=1}^{\infty} (1 - \mu)^{2n} \hat{p}^{2n}(k) = \frac{1 - \phi(0)}{2N} \frac{(1 - \mu)^2 \hat{p}^2(k)}{1 - (1 - \mu)^2 \hat{p}^2(k)}$$

The inversion formula on $(\mathbf{Z} \bmod L)^2$ is

$$\phi(x) = \frac{1}{L^2} \sum_{k \in 2\pi\Lambda(L)/L} e^{-ik \cdot x} \hat{\phi}(k)$$

Using this on the previous formula we have

$$\phi(x) = \frac{(1 - \mu)^2 (1 - \phi(0))}{2NL^2} \sum_{k \in 2\pi\Lambda(L)/L} \frac{\hat{p}^2(k) e^{-ik \cdot x}}{1 - (1 - \mu)^2 \hat{p}^2(k)}$$

To get rid of the complex exponential we note that

$$e^{ik \cdot x} = (\cos(k_1 x_1) + i \sin(k_1 x_1)) \cdot (\cos(k_2 x_2) + i \sin(k_2 x_2))$$

and the symmetry properties of $\hat{p}^2(k)$ imply that the terms involving a sine will sum to 0.   □

At first, it may be disturbing that the unknown $1 - \phi(0)$ is on the right-hand side of (4.7). This problem is easily remedied. Setting $x = 0$ in (4.7), we have $\phi(0) = A(1 - \phi(0))$ where

$$(4.8) \quad A = \frac{(1 - \mu)^2}{2NL^2} \sum_{k \in 2\pi\Lambda(L)/L} \frac{\hat{p}^2(k)}{1 - (1 - \mu)^2 \hat{p}^2(k)}$$

and solving we have $\phi(0) = (1+1/A)^{-1}$. A significant simplification of (4.7) occurs if we average over all $x \in \Lambda(L)$. Since $\sum_{x \in \Lambda(L)} \cos(k_1 x_1) \cos(k_2 x_2) = 0$ except when $k = 0$, and in this case $\hat{p}(0) = 1$, we have

$$(4.9) \quad \bar{\phi} \equiv \frac{1}{L^2} \sum_{x \in \Lambda(L)} \phi(x) = \frac{(1-\mu)^2(1-\phi(0))}{2NL^2} \cdot \frac{1}{2\mu - \mu^2} \approx \frac{1-\phi(0)}{4NL^2\mu}$$

when μ is small.

The results in (4.7)–(4.9) are exact and valid for any L but are difficult to understand. Thus it is natural to suppose L is large and look for approximations. Motivated by our results in one dimension the first case to consider is: $1/\mu \ll L^2/v\sigma^2$. To explain this condition, we note that the time required for a mutation to occur in one family line is $1/\mu$ at which time the variance of the total displacement from its starting point is $v\sigma^2/\mu \ll L^2$, i.e., the lineage has moved a distance much smaller than L. In this case, we can replace the torus by the infinite two dimensional lattice. Using the Fourier inversion formula for $\mathbf{Z}^2$ and dropping the factor $(1-\mu)^2$, which is close to 1, we get

$$(\star) \quad \phi(x) \approx \frac{(1-\phi(0))}{2N} \int_{[-\pi,\pi]^2} \frac{\hat{p}^2(\kappa) \cos(\kappa_1 x_1) \cos(\kappa_2 x_2)}{1 - (1-\mu)^2 \hat{p}^2(\kappa)} \frac{d\kappa}{(2\pi)^2}$$

In this situation, Nagylaki (1974) has derived the asymptotics:

$$(4.10) \qquad \phi(0) \approx \left[1 - \frac{8\pi v\sigma^2 N}{\ln(2\mu)}\right]^{-1}$$

$$(4.11) \qquad \phi(x) \approx -\frac{2\phi(0)}{\ln(2\mu)}[K_0(\sqrt{2\mu}|\xi|) - K_0(|\xi|)]$$

where $|\xi| = (\xi_1^2 + \xi_2^2)^{1/2}$, $\xi_i = x_i/\sqrt{v\sigma^2}$, and K_0 is one of the many Bessel functions invented to solve problems in physics (see e.g., page 78 of Watson 1966). The exact definition of K_0 is unimportant for our purposes, but it is useful to know that

$$(4.12) \qquad K_0(x) \approx \begin{cases} \ln(1/x) & \text{when } x \text{ is small} \\ e^{-x}\sqrt{\pi/2x} & \text{when } x \text{ is large} \end{cases}$$

Formula (4.11) is often given without the second factor $-K_0(|\xi|)$ (see, e.g., Slatkin and Barton 1989, page 1353) but that term is very important when ξ is small. To see this, let $|\xi| \to 0$ in (4.11) and use the first formula in (4.12) to see that if we ignore the second term then we get the nonsensical result $\phi(x) \to \infty$. (Recall that $\phi(x)$ is a probability and hence must always be ≤ 1.)

Proofs of (4.10) and (4.11). Here we follow Nagylaki (1974). Letting $R(k) = \hat{p}^2(k)$ and reintroducing the complex exponential, we can write $(\star)$

as

$$\phi(x) \approx \frac{1 - \phi(0)}{2N} \int_{[-\pi,\pi]^2} \frac{e^{ik \cdot x} R(k)}{1 - (1 - \mu)^2 R(k)} \frac{d^2 k}{4\pi^2}$$

Noting that $R(k)$ is the Fourier transform of a distribution with mean 0 and covariance $2v^2 I$ where $v = \nu\sigma^2$, and letting $\ell_j = k_j v$ and $\ell^2 = \ell_1^2 + \ell_2^2$, leads to (see, e.g., (3.8) on page 103 of Durrett 1995)

$$R(k) \sim 1 - \ell^2 + O(\ell^3) \sim (1 + \ell^2)^{-1} + O(\ell^3)$$

Using these approximations and setting $\xi_i = x_i/v$, we have

$$(\star\star) \qquad \phi(x) \approx \frac{1 - \phi(0)}{2N} \frac{1}{2\pi v^2} \left[\frac{1}{2\pi} \int_{[-\pi/v,\pi/v]^2} \frac{e^{i\ell \cdot \xi} d^2\ell}{(1 + \ell^2)(2\mu + \ell^2)} \right]$$

If the migration rate ν is small and hence v is close to 0, the integral inside the brackets is

$$\approx \frac{1}{2\pi(1 - 2\mu)} \int \frac{e^{i\ell \cdot \xi}}{(2\mu + \ell^2)} - \frac{e^{i\ell \cdot \xi}}{(1 + \ell^2)} d^2\ell = \frac{K_0(\sqrt{2\mu}|\xi|) - K_0(|\xi|)}{1 - 2\mu}$$

the last bit of calculus coming from page 323 of Malécot (1967). In words, "the bidimensional Fourier transform of $(m^2 + x^2)^{-1}$ is $K_0(m|\xi|)$." Using (4.12) now shows

$$K_0(\sqrt{2\mu}|\xi|) - K_0(|\xi|) \to -\frac{1}{2} \ln(2\mu)$$

as $|\xi| \to 0$. Using the results from this paragraph in $(\star\star)$, we have

$$1 - \phi(0) \approx -\frac{8\pi v^2 N}{\ln(2\mu)} \phi(0)$$

and solving gives

$$\phi(0) \approx [1 - 8\pi v^2 N / \ln(2\mu)]^{-1}$$

Plugging the previous formula for $1 - \phi(0)$ into $(\star\star)$ gives

$$\phi(x) \approx -\frac{2}{\ln(2\mu)} \phi(0)[K_0(\sqrt{2\mu}|\xi|) - K_0(|\xi|)] \qquad \square$$

In one dimension, when $1/\mu \gg L^2/\nu\sigma^2$, the stepping stone model behaves like a homogeneously mixing population. Slatkin and Barton (1989) have asserted that this is also true in two dimensions. However, Cox and Durrett (2001) have recently shown that is not correct. Their results rely on earlier work of Cox and Griffeath (1986), Cox (1989), and Cox and Greven (1991). The proofs of these results (Theorems 4.1, 4.2, 4.4, and 4.5 below) are somewhat lengthy and more sophisticated than most of the rest of the material in the book, so they are stated here without their proofs, which may be found in the paper cited. To study the behavior of the stepping stone model, Cox and Durrett (2001) work backwards in time to define a coalescing random walk with killing. Individuals whose state is the result of a new mutation are killed since we no longer have to work backwards to determine their state. Other particles make a jump from colony x to colony y with probability $p(x, y)$ and land at a randomly chosen site within the colony.

Suppose for the moment that the mutation rate $\mu = 0$ and consider the genealogy of a sample of size two chosen at random from the population. As we work backwards, let T_0 be the amount of time required until the two lineages first reside in the same colony, and let t_0 be the total amount of time needed for the two lineages to coalesce to one. Let X_n be the difference in the locations of the two particles in generation n (computed modulo L). Since the two particles were chosen randomly from the torus, $\Lambda(L)$, the distribution of X_0 is the uniform distribution on $\Lambda(L)$, which we denote by π. Let P_π denote the distribution of the difference of two random walks starting from a pair of points chosen randomly on the torus. It is clear that random walkers starting from two randomly chosen locations on the torus will take at least L^2 units of time to hit. The next result shows that the actual amount of time required for T_0 is of order $L^2 \log L$.

Theorem 4.1. For any $t > 0$, as $L \to \infty$, uniformly for $\nu \in (0, 1]$,

$$P_\pi\left(T_0 > \frac{L^2 \log L}{2\pi\nu\sigma^2} t\right) \to e^{-t}$$

Sketch of proof. To explain the size of the answer, note that $P_\pi(X_n = 0) = 1/L^2$, and the local central limit theorem implies $P_0(X_n = 0) \sim (2\pi(2\nu\sigma^2)n)^{-1}$, so

$$1 = \sum_{n=0}^{L^2-1} P_\pi(X_n = 0) = \sum_{m=0}^{L^2-1} P_\pi(T_0 = m) \sum_{k=0}^{L^2-m} P_0(X_k = 0)$$

$$\approx P_\pi(T_0 \leq L^2) \frac{\log(L^2)}{2\pi(2\nu\sigma^2)}$$

Rearranging gives $P_\pi(T_0 \leq L^2) \approx 2\pi\sigma^2\nu/\log L$. To prove that the limit is exponential, Cox and Durrett (2001) show that X_n comes to equilibrium in time $o(L^2 \log L/\nu)$, so the limit distribution of $T_0/(L^2 \log L/\nu)$ must have the lack of memory property that characterizes the exponential. □

The typical distance between two points compared in Theorem 4.1 is of order L^2. When we look at closer distances the result changes. Let P_x denote the law of the difference of two walks when one starts in colony 0 and one in colony x. (If $x = 0$, we pick two distinct individuals from colony 0.)

Theorem 4.2. *Suppose* $x = x_L$ *satisfies* $\lim_{L \to \infty}(\log^+ |x|)/\log L = \beta \in [0, 1]$. *Then for any* $t > 0$, *as* $L \to \infty$, *uniformly for* $\nu \in (0, 1]$,

$$P_x\left(T_0 > \frac{L^2 \log L}{2\pi\nu\sigma^2} t\right) \to \beta e^{-t}$$

Sketch of proof. This generalizes a result in Cox and Greven (1991). The main idea behind Theorem 4.2 is that if $(\log^+ |x|)/\log L \to \beta$ then

$$P_x(T_0 \leq L^2/\nu) \to 1 - \beta.$$

When $T_0 > L^2/\nu$, it is also likely that $T_0 > L^2\sqrt{\log L}/\nu$ at which time the distribution of X_n has become uniform over the torus, and the longer time behavior is as in Theorem 4.1. □

Getting the two lineages to the same colony at time T_0 is only the first part of the coalescence time t_0. For the second part after T_0, we need only be concerned with the distribution of t_0 under P_0. We begin with a surprising formula of Strobeck (1987) which shows that $E_0 t_0$ is independent of the value of the migration rate $\nu > 0$ and of the dispersal kernel $q(x)$. The proof we give here is new and is a simple application of the cycle trick for Markov chains (see, for example, Theorem 5.4.3 in Durrett 1996).

Theorem 4.3. $E_0 t_0 = 2NL^2$.

Proof. When both lineages are in the same colony, they have probability $1/2N$ per generation to hit, so $E_0 t_0 = 2N E_0 T_0'$, where T_0' is the first time $t \geq 1$ that the two lines are in the same colony. (Recall that E_0 refers to picking two distinct individuals from the same colony.) The stationary distribution for the migration process is uniform, so it follows from the cycle trick representation of the stationary distribution that $E_0 T_0' = L^2$. □

Comparing Theorems 4.1 and 4.3, we see that there are two extreme possibilities:

$$ET_0 = O(L^2 \log L/\nu) \ll O(2NL^2) = Et_0 \quad \text{or} \quad ET_0 \gg Et_0$$

In the first case, the two lineages will come to the same colony in $o(NL^2)$ so the actual starting positions of the particles don't matter, and the limit distribution will have the lack of memory property.

Theorem 4.4. *If* $\lim_{L \to \infty} N\nu/\log L = \infty$, *then for any* $t > 0$, *as* $L \to \infty$,

$$\sup_{x \in \Lambda(L)} |P_x(t_0 > 2NL^2 t) - e^{-t}| \to 0$$

Conventional wisdom, see pages 125–126 of Kimura and Maruyama (1971), says that "marked local differentiation of gene frequencies can occur if $N\nu < 1$ where N is the effective size of each colony and ν is the rate at which each colony exchanges individuals with the four surrounding colonies." In the other direction, "if $N\nu > 1$ local differentiation is less pronounced and especially if $N\nu \geq 4$, the whole population tends to behave as a panmictic unit." As Theorem 4.4 and the next result show, $N\nu$ must be larger than $\log L$ in order for the system to behave as if it were homogeneously mixing.

Theorem 4.5. *If* $\lim_{L\to\infty} 2\pi\sigma^2 N\nu/\log L = \alpha \in [0, \infty)$ *then for any* $t > 0$ *as* $L \to \infty$,

$$P_\pi\left(t_0 > (1 + \alpha)\frac{L^2 \log L}{2\pi\nu\sigma^2}t\right) \to e^{-t}$$

If $x = x_L$ *satisfies* $\lim_{L\to\infty}(\log^+ |x|)/\log L = \beta \in [0, 1]$ *then, as* $L \to \infty$,

$$P_x\left(t_0 > (1 + \alpha)\frac{L^2 \log L}{2\pi\nu\sigma^2}t\right) \to \left(\beta + (1 - \beta)\frac{\alpha}{1 + \alpha}\right)e^{-t}$$

Our results in Theorems 4.4 and 4.5 about the coalescence time t_0 allow us to compute the distribution of any quantity that involves only pairwise comparison of DNA sequences. We will now consider three of these: (i) the probability that two randomly chosen individuals are identical by descent, (ii) the decay of genetic correlation with distance, and (iii) Wright's (1951) measure of population subdivision, F_{ST}.

Identity by descent

Two individuals will be identical by descent if (and only if) no mutation has occurred before t_0. If these individuals are picked at random from the population and we let h denote the probability that they are identical by descent, then

(4.13)
$$h = E_\pi(1 - \mu)^{2t_0}.$$

If t_0/c_L is close to 0 with probability $1 - \rho$ and a mean one exponential random variable with probability ρ, as is the case in all of the conclusions of Theorems 4.4 and 4.5, then

(4.14) $h \approx (1 - \rho) + \rho \displaystyle\int_0^\infty e^{2c_L \ln(1-\mu)t}e^{-t}\, dt = (1 - \rho) + \dfrac{\rho}{1 - 2c_L \ln(1 - \mu)}$

In the case of Theorem 4.4, $\rho = 1$ and $c_L = 2NL^2$. Using the approximation $\ln(1 - x) \approx -x$ for small x, and letting $N_T = NL^2$ denote the total number of individuals in the system, then

(4.15) $h \approx \dfrac{1}{1 - 4NL^2 \ln(1 - \mu)} \approx (1 + 4N_T\mu)^{-1}$

for small μ, the classic result for a homogeneously mixing population with N_T individuals. In contrast, if we let $L \to \infty$ with constant colony size N, then we end up in the $\alpha = 0$ case of the first result of Theorem 4.5. Again $\rho = 1$ but this time the normalizing constant is $c_L = L^2 \log L / (2\pi\sigma^2\nu)$ so using (4.14) we end up with

$$(4.16) \qquad h \approx \left(1 + \frac{(L^2 \log L)}{\pi\sigma^2\nu} \mu \right)^{-1}$$

Turning (4.15) around, we see that the value of h given in (4.16) is that of a homogeneously mixing population with effective population size

$$(4.17) \qquad N_e = \frac{L^2 \log L}{4\pi\sigma^2\nu}$$

For a numerical example consider a 50 by 50 grid of colonies of size 20 for a total of 50,000 individuals ($L = 50, N = 20$). Suppose there is migration with equal probability to each of the other 24 points in a 5×5 square centered at the point ($\sigma^2 = 50/24$), and let $\nu = 0.1$ to have the number of migrants per generation $N\nu = 2$. In this case the effective population size is

$$N_e \approx \frac{2500(3.91202)}{4(3.14159)(50/24)0.1} \approx 3,736$$

versus the actual population size $N_T = 50,000$.

It is interesting to contrast the last calculation with the island model in which there are s subpopulations with N individuals. In this case (3.9) shows that island model behaves like a homogeneously mixing population of size

$$N_e = Ns \left(1 + \frac{(s-1)^2}{4N\nu s^2} \right)$$

Note that the first factor Ns is the actual population size, while the factor in parentheses is larger than 1. Thus in contrast to the stepping stone model, in the island model the effective population size N_e is always larger than the actual population size.

Decay of correlation with distance

Pick one individual from the colony at 0 and one from the colony at x (and if $x = 0$ pick two distinct individuals from the colony at 0). Let $\phi(x)$ be the probability the two individuals are identical by descent. As Slatkin (1991) has observed, when the mutation rate is small, $1 - \phi(x) \approx 2\mu E_x t_0$. Noting that $E_x t_0 = E_x T_0 + E_0 t_0$, we have

$$(4.18) \qquad \phi(0) - \phi(x) \approx 2\mu E_x T_0$$

By Theorem 4.2, if $L \to \infty$ and $\log^+ |x| / \log L \to \beta$, then we should have

$$E_x T_0 \approx \beta \frac{L^2 \log L}{2\pi\sigma^2\nu}$$

Replacing β by $\log^+ |x|/\log L$ on the right-hand side and using (4.18), we see that, for small μ,

$$(4.19) \qquad \phi(0) - \phi(x) \approx 2\mu \, \frac{\log^+ |x|}{\log L} \cdot \frac{L^2 \log L}{2\pi\sigma^2\nu} = \mu \cdot \log^+ |x| \cdot \frac{L^2}{\pi\sigma^2\nu}$$

That is, the difference $\phi(0) - \phi(x)$ is proportional to $\log^+ |x|$.

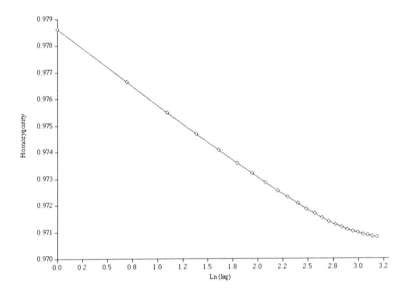

To get a check on the quality of this approximation, we may use the exact results of (4.5) to compute $\phi(m,0)$ for the case $L = 50$, $N = 20$, with nearest neighbor migration ($\sigma^2 = 0.5$) at rate $\nu = 0.05$, and with a mutation rate $\mu = 10^{-7}$. The first figure shows $\phi(m,0)$ plotted against $\log m$. Note that $\phi(m,0)$ does decrease roughly linearly with the logarithm of the distance between the colonies until the effect of wraparound on the torus kicks in. The heterozygosities $1-\phi(m,0)$ are quite small here, but they do range from 0.021 to 0.029, an increase of about 40% as we move across the system. This contradicts a claim of Slatkin and Barton (1989) who predict that the population should be effectively panmictic when $\sigma^2\nu/\mu >$ $> L^2$ since in that case $\frac{\sigma^2\nu}{\mu} = 250,000 \gg 2500 = L^2$ but there is significant spatial structure. To further investigate the values of μ for which a system is effectively panmictic we have considered the last example for various values of the mutation rate. The next figure plots $\phi(0)$ as determined by (4.7), (4.11), and (4.15) using squares, diamonds and circles. Let $\mu_0 = \nu\sigma^2/L^2 = 10^{-5}$ and $\mu_1 = \nu\sigma^2/(L^2 \log L) \approx (10^{-5})/3.91$. Note that, as our theory predicts, the large mutation approximation works well for $\mu \gg \mu_0$ while mean field theory works well for $\mu \ll \mu_1 \approx 2.5 \times 10^{-6}$.

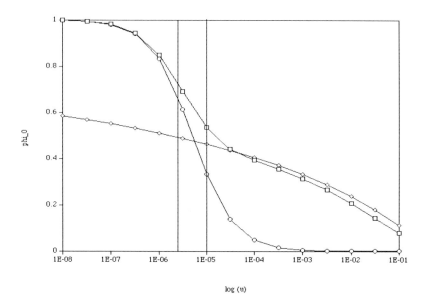

F_{ST}

In (3.10) we defined

$$(4.20) \qquad F_{ST} = \frac{\phi(0) - \bar{\phi}}{1 - \bar{\phi}}$$

where as above, $\phi(0)$ is the probability of identity by descent for two individuals sampled from the same colony, and $\bar{\phi}$ is the probability for two individuals sampled at random from the entire population. In (3.11) we showed

$$(4.21) \qquad F_{ST} \approx \frac{E_\pi t_0 - E_0 t_0}{E_\pi t_0} = \frac{E_\pi T_0}{E_\pi T_0 + E_0 t_0}$$

Using Theorems 4.1 and 4.3, it follows that if $2\pi\sigma^2 N\nu/\log L \to \alpha \in (0, \infty)$ then

$$(4.22) \qquad F_{ST} \approx \frac{\frac{L^2 \log L}{2\pi\nu\sigma^2}}{\frac{L^2 \log L}{2\pi\nu\sigma^2} + 2NL^2} \approx \frac{1}{1 + 2\alpha}$$

This says that F_{ST} is close to 0 if and only if $N\nu \gg \log L$. Crow and Aoki (1984) did a numerical study of F_{ST} for the nearest neighbor stepping stone model and found (see their page 6075) that F_{ST} is roughly proportional to $\log n$, where $n = L^2$ is the number of colonies. In the cases they considered, $\log L/(2\pi\nu\sigma^2) \ll 2N$, so the first term in the denominator of (4.22) can be ignored, and we have

$$F_{ST} \approx \frac{\log L}{4N\pi\nu\sigma^2} = \frac{1}{8N\pi\nu\sigma^2} \log(L^2)$$

confirming their prediction.

It is interesting to compare (4.22) with the corresponding formula for the island model given in (3.12)

$$F_{ST} = \frac{1}{1 + 4N\nu s^2/(s-1)^2}$$

When s is large we can suppress the factor $s^2/(s-1)^2$, so that $F_{ST} \approx (1 + 4N\nu)^{-1}$, and as noted in (3.13) one can estimate the scaled migration rate $M = N\nu$ by

(4.23)
$$\widehat{M} = \frac{1}{4}\left(\frac{1}{F_{ST}} - 1\right)$$

Suppose the population being sampled has a stepping stone structure, but one uses the island model formula (4.23). Using (4.22) in (4.23), and the assumption $2N\pi\sigma^2\nu/\log L \approx \alpha$, we find that

(4.24)
$$\widehat{M} \approx \frac{\alpha}{2} \approx N\nu\sigma^2 \cdot \frac{\pi}{\log L}$$

so the resulting estimate $\widehat{M}$ has a bias that depends on the size of the system. Here we have kept the σ^2 with $N\nu$ since in the stepping stone model the scaled migration rate $N\nu\sigma^2$ is what one can most simply estimate from observations. If we imagine the world to be a 50×50 grid ($L = 50$), then the correction factor $\pi/\log L$ is about 0.4, so there is a significant amount of bias from using an island model formula on a stepping stone population. This result has no impact on the work of Seielstad et al. (1998) discussed in the previous section since they used the ratio of estimates from mtDNA and Y chromosome data and when this is done the extra factor cancels out.

3
Natural Selection

In this chapter, we will consider various forms of selection and investigate their effects on the genealogy of a sample.

3.1 Directional Selection

In this section, we will consider the Moran model with two alleles with selection and no mutation. Let 1 and $1 - s$ be the relative fitnesses of the two alleles. Thinking of these as the probability that an offspring of that type is viable, we can formulate the transition rates of the Moran model with selection as

$$i \to i+1 \qquad \text{at rate } b_i = 2N - i \cdot \frac{i}{2N}$$

$$i \to i-1 \qquad \text{at rate } d_i = i \cdot \frac{2N - i}{2N} \cdot (1 - s)$$

Since there is no mutation, the A allele will either be lost or become fixed in the population. Let $g(i)$ be the probability that it becomes fixed when there are initially i copies. By considering what happens the first time the process leaves i, we see that

$$g(i) = \frac{b_i}{b_i + d_i} g(i+1) + \frac{d_i}{b_i + d_i} g(i-1)$$

Rearranging, we have

$$g(i+1) - g(i) = \frac{d_i}{b_i}(g(i) - g(i-1)) = (1-s)(g(i) - g(i-1))$$

Now $g(0) = 0$, so if we let $c = g(1)$ and iterate, it follows that

$$(\star) \qquad\qquad g(i+1) - g(i) = c(1-s)^i$$

If $s = 0$, $(\star)$ says $g(i+1) - g(i)$ is constant, i.e., $g(i)$ is linear. Since $g(0) = 0$ and $g(2N) = 1$, we must have

$$(1.1) \qquad\qquad g(i) = i/2N$$

Let us now consider the *rate of substitution* defined as the number of mutants reaching fixation per unit time. If neutral mutations occur at a rate of u per gene per generation, then the number of mutants arising at a locus in a diploid population of size N is $2Nu$ per generation. Since the probability of fixation for each of these mutations is $1/2N$ by (1.1), the rate at which new mutations is fixed in the population is u, independent of the population size. This result is due to Kimura (1968).

In the case $s \neq 0$, summing we have

$$g(j) = \sum_{i=0}^{j-1} c(1-s)^i = c\frac{1 - (1-s)^j}{s}$$

We must have $g(2N) = 1$ so $c = s/(1 - (1-s)^{2N})$ and it follows that

$$(1.2) \qquad\qquad g(j) = \frac{1 - (1-s)^j}{1 - (1-s)^{2N}}$$

When $j = 1$, the numerator is just s. If selection is strong, i.e., $2Ns$ is large then $(1-s)^{2N} \approx 0$ and the probability of fixation of a new mutant is just s.

When s is small, $(1-s) \approx e^{-s}$, so (1.2) can be written as

$$(1.3) \qquad\qquad g(j) \approx \frac{1 - e^{-js}}{1 - e^{-2Ns}}$$

The genealogical process for the Moran model is that of the Wright-Fisher model but run twice as fast. If we replace s by $2s$ to compensate for this and write $j = 2Np$, we get the classic result of Kimura (1962) that the probability of fixation for the Wright-Fisher model is

$$(1.4) \qquad\qquad \approx \frac{1 - e^{-4Nsp}}{1 - e^{-4Ns}}$$

It is instructive, and useful for later results, to give another derivation of (1.1) and (1.2). This begins with the observation that when $s = 0$, $b_i/(b_i + d_i) = 1/2$, so

$$i = \frac{b_i}{b_i + d_i}(i+1) + \frac{d_i}{b_i + d_i}(i-1)$$

From this we can see that when the process jumps, the average value of X_t stays the same, so EX_t is constant in time. Ultimately the process will be absorbed at $2N$ or at 0 but since the expected value is constant in time

$$x = 2N \cdot P_x(X_\infty = 2N) + 0 \cdot P_x(X_\infty = 0)$$

and solving we have $P_x(X_\infty = 2N) = x/2N$ in agreement with (1.1).

When $s \neq 0$, $b_i/(b_i + d_i) = 1/(2 - s)$. A little calculation shows that

$$(1-s)^{i+1}\frac{1}{2-s} + (1-s)^{i-1}\frac{1-s}{2-s} = (1-s)^i\frac{1-s}{2-s} + (1-s)^i\frac{1}{2-s} = (1-s)^i$$

so in this case the value of $(1 - s)^{X_t}$ stays constant in time. Reasoning as before,

$$(1-s)^x = (1-s)^{2N}P_x(X_\infty = 2N) + 1 \cdot [1 - P_x(X_\infty = 2N)]$$

and solving we have

$$P_x(X_\infty = 2N) = \frac{1 - (1-s)^x}{1 - (1-s)^{2N}}$$

in agreement with (1.2).

Our next goal is to compute the expected time to fixation given that fixation occurs. Kimura and Ohta (1969) did this using the diffusion approximation. However, it is possible to do their computation without leaving the discrete setting, so we will take that approach here. Let $\tau = \min\{t : X_t = 0 \text{ or } X_t = 2N\}$ be the fixation time. Let S_y be the amount of time spent at y before time τ. Clearly,

$$(1.5) \qquad E_x\tau = \sum_{y=1}^{2N-1} E_x S_y$$

Let N_y be the number of visits to y. Let $q(y) = (2 - s)(2N - y)y/2N$ be the rate at which the chain leaves y. Since each visit to y lasts for an exponential amount of time with mean $1/q(y)$ we have

$$(1.6) \qquad E_x S_y = \frac{1}{q(y)} E_x N_y$$

If we let $T_y = \min\{t : X_t = y\}$ be the first hitting time of y then

$$P_x(N_y \geq 1) = P_x(T_y < \infty)$$

Letting $T_y^+ = \min\{t : X_t = y \text{ and } X_s \neq y \text{ for some } s < t\}$ be the time of the first return to y, we have

$$P_x(N_y \geq k + 1 | N_y \geq k) = P_y(T_y^+ < \infty)$$

The last formula shows that, conditional on $N_y \geq 1$, N_y is geometric with success probability $P_y(T_y^+ = \infty)$. Combining this with the previous formula, we have

$$(1.7) \qquad E_x N_y = \frac{P_x(T_y < \infty)}{P_y(T_y^+ = \infty)}$$

We will begin with the case $s = 0$. Since the average value of X_t is constant in time,

$$(1.8) \qquad P_x(T_y < T_0) = \frac{x}{y} \quad \text{for } 0 \le x \le y$$

Similar reasoning shows that

$$x = y P_x(T_y < T_{2N}) + 2N[1 - P_x(T_y < T_{2N})]$$

and solving gives

$$(1.9) \qquad P_x(T_y < T_{2N}) = \frac{2N - x}{2N - y} \quad \text{for } y \le x \le 2N$$

When the process leaves y it goes to $y - 1$ or $y + 1$ with equal probability so

$$\begin{aligned} P_y(T_y^+ = \infty) &= \frac{1}{2} \cdot P_{y+1}(T_{2N} < T_y) + \frac{1}{2} \cdot P_{y-1}(T_0 < T_y) \\ &= \frac{1}{2} \cdot \frac{1}{2N - y} + \frac{1}{2} \cdot \frac{1}{y} = \frac{2N}{2y(2N - y)} \end{aligned}$$

Combining (1.7)–(1.9) gives

$$E_x N_y = \begin{cases} \frac{x}{y} \cdot \frac{2y(2N-y)}{2N} & 0 \le x \le y \\ \frac{2N-x}{2N-y} \cdot \frac{2y(2N-y)}{2N} & y \le x \le 2N \end{cases}$$

Since $q(y) = 2y(2N - y)/2N$, (1.6) gives us

$$(1.10) \qquad E_x S_y = \begin{cases} \frac{x}{y} & 0 \le x \le y \\ \frac{2N-x}{2N-y} & y \le x \le 2N \end{cases}$$

We are interested in the expected fixation time conditional that the chain reaches $2N$ before 0. If we let $h(x) = P_x(T_{2N} < T_0)$ and let $p_t(x, y)$ be the transition probability for the Moran model, then it follows from the definition of conditional probability and the Markov property that

$$\bar{p}_t(x, y) = \frac{P_x(X_t = y, T_{2N} < T_0)}{P_x(T_{2N} < T_0)} = p_t(x, y) \cdot \frac{h(y)}{h(x)}$$

Integrating from $t = 0$ to ∞ we see that the conditioned chain has

$$(1.11) \qquad \bar{E}_x S_y = \int_0^\infty \bar{p}_t(x, y)\, dt = \frac{h(y)}{h(x)} E_x S_y$$

(1.8) implies $h(z) = z/2N$, so using (1.10) we have

$$(1.12) \qquad \bar{E}_x S_y = \begin{cases} 1 & 0 \le x \le y \\ \frac{2N-x}{x} \cdot \frac{y}{2N-y} & y \le x \le 2N \end{cases}$$

By the reasoning that led to (1.5)

$$\bar{E}_x\tau = \sum_{y=1}^{2N-1} \bar{E}_x S_y = \sum_{y=x}^{2N-1} 1 + \frac{2N-x}{x} \cdot \sum_{y=1}^{x-1} \frac{y}{2N-y}$$

The first sum is $2N - x$. If we let $p = x/2N$ then

$$\sum_{y=1}^{x-1} \frac{y}{2N-y} = 2N \sum_{y=1}^{x-1} \frac{y/2N}{1-y/2N} \cdot \frac{1}{2N} \approx 2N \int_0^p \frac{u}{1-u}\, du$$

To evaluate the integral we note that it is

$$= \int_0^p -1 + \frac{1}{1-u}\, du = -p - \ln(1-p)$$

Combining the last three formulas

$$(1.13) \qquad \bar{E}_x\tau \approx 2N(1-p) + \frac{2N(1-p)}{p}(-p - \ln(1-p))$$

$$= -\frac{2N(1-p)}{p}\ln(1-p)$$

Recalling that the Moran model moves twice as fast as the Wright-Fisher model, this agrees with the classic result due to Kimura and Ohta (1969). As $p \to 0$, $-\ln(1-p)/p \to 1$ so

$$\bar{E}_x\tau \to 2N$$

Our next step is to investigate what happens when $s > 0$. In this case the average value of $(1-s)^{X_t}$ stays constant in time, so if $0 \le x \le y$

$$(1-s)^x = (1-s)^y P_x(T_y < T_0) + 1 \cdot [1 - P_x(T_y < T_0)]$$

and solving gives that for $0 \le x \le y$

$$(1.14) \quad P_x(T_y < T_0) = \frac{1-(1-s)^x}{1-(1-s)^y} \qquad P_x(T_0 < T_y) = \frac{(1-s)^x - (1-s)^y}{1 - (1-s)^y}$$

Likewise, if $y \le x \le 2N$

$$(1-s)^x = (1-s)^y P_x(T_y < T_{2N}) + (1-s)^{2N} \cdot [1 - P_x(T_y < T_{2N})]$$

and solving gives that if $y \le x \le 2N$ then

$$(1.15) \qquad P_x(T_y < T_{2N}) = \frac{(1-s)^x - (1-s)^{2N}}{(1-s)^y - (1-s)^{2N}}$$

$$P_x(T_{2N} < T_y) = \frac{(1-s)^y - (1-s)^x}{(1-s)^y - (1-s)^{2N}}$$

From (1.14) and (1.15), it follows that

$$(1.16) \qquad P_y(T_y^+ = \infty) = \frac{1}{2-s} P_{y+1}(T_{2N} < T_y) + \frac{1-s}{2-s} P_{y-1}(T_0 < T_y)$$

$$= \frac{1}{2-s} \cdot \frac{(1-s)^y - (1-s)^{y+1}}{(1-s)^y - (1-s)^{2N}}$$
$$+ \frac{1-s}{2-s} \cdot \frac{(1-s)^{y-1} - (1-s)^y}{1 - (1-s)^y}$$

If $s > 0$ is fixed and N is large, $(1-s)^{2N} \approx 0$, so using (1.16)

$$P_y(T_y^+ = \infty) \approx \frac{s}{2-s} + \frac{1-s}{2-s} \cdot \frac{s(1-s)^{y-1}}{1 - (1-s)^y}$$

It will turn out that most of the answer will come from large values of y. In this case, the last formula simplifies to

(1.17) $$P_y(T_y^+ = \infty) \approx \frac{s}{2-s}$$

If we take $x = 1$, then there is only one case to consider, so using (1.7) and (1.14) with the last formula, we have for large y

$$E_1 N_y \approx \frac{1 - (1-s)^1}{1 - (1-s)^y} \cdot \frac{2-s}{s}$$

Using $q(y) = (2-s)(2N-y)y/2N$ with (1.6) now we have

$$E_1 S_y \approx \frac{1 - (1-s)^1}{1 - (1-s)^y} \cdot \frac{2-s}{s} \cdot \frac{2N}{(2-s)y(2N-y)}$$

$h(x) = P_x(T_{2N} < T_0) = (1 - (1-s)^x)/(1 - (1-s)^{2N})$ so using (1.11)

$$\bar{E}_1 S_y \approx \frac{2N}{sy(2N-y)}$$

(1.17) and hence the last three formulas are only valid for large y. As the first part of the next computation will show, we can ignore the contribution from small y.

To evaluate the asymptotic behavior of $\sum_{y=1}^{2N-1} \bar{E}_1 S_y$ we will divide the sum into three parts. Let $M = 2N/(\ln N)$.

$$\sum_{y=1}^{M} \frac{2N}{y(2N-y)} \approx \sum_{y=1}^{M} \frac{1}{y} \approx \ln(2N/\ln N) = \ln N + \ln 2 - \ln\ln N \approx \ln N$$

At the other end, changing variables $z = 2N - y$ shows

$$\sum_{y=2N-M}^{2N-1} \frac{2N}{y(2N-y)} = \sum_{z=1}^{M} \frac{2N}{z(2N-z)}$$

In the middle,

$$\sum_{y=M+1}^{2N-M-1} \frac{2N}{y(2N-y)} = \sum_{y=M+1}^{2N-M-1} \frac{1}{\frac{y}{2N}\left(1 - \frac{y}{2N}\right)} \cdot \frac{1}{2N}$$
$$\approx \int_{1/\ln N}^{1-1/\ln N} \frac{1}{u(1-u)}\, du$$

To evaluate the integral, we note $1/u(1-u) = 1/u + 1/(1-u)$ so it is

$$= 2 \int_{1/\ln N}^{1-1/\ln N} \frac{1}{u} \, du = \ln(1 - 1/\ln N) + \ln \ln N$$

The first term tends to 0 as $N \to \infty$. The second is much smaller than $\ln N$, so combining our computations, we have

$$(1.18) \qquad E_1(\tau | T_{2N} < T_0) = \sum_{y=1}^{2N-1} \bar{E}_1 S_y \approx \frac{2}{s} \ln N$$

To obtain more insight into what is happening during the fixation of a favorable allele, we will now give a second derivation of (1.18). As above, we divide the process into three phases.

I. If $i/2N$ is small, then

$$i \to i + 1 \qquad \text{at rate } b_i \approx i$$
$$i \to i - 1 \qquad \text{at rate } d_i \approx (1 - s)i$$

This is a continuous time branching process in which each of the i particles gives birth at rate 1 and dies at rate $1 - s$. Letting Z_t be the number of particles at time t, it is easy to see from the description that

$$\frac{d}{dt} EZ_t = sEZ_t$$

so $EZ_t = Z_0 e^{st}$. A result from the theory of branching processes (see Athreya and Ney 1972) shows that as $t \to \infty$

$$(1.19) \qquad e^{-st} Z_t \to W$$

The limit W may be 0 and will be if the branching process dies out, that is, $Z_t = 0$ for some t. However, on the event that the process does not die out $\{Z_t > 0$ for all $t\}$, we have $W > 0$.

Let T_1 be the first time that there are $M = 2N/\ln N$ particles. There is nothing special about this precise value. Using (1.19), we see that $Z_t \approx e^{st} W$ so when the mutation survives

$$\frac{2N}{\ln N} \approx \exp(sT_1) W$$

and solving gives

$$T_1 \approx \frac{1}{s} \ln \left(\frac{2N}{W \ln N} \right) \approx \frac{1}{s} \ln(2N)$$

II. Let T_2 be the first time that there are $2N - M$ particles. As we will now show, during the second phase from T_1 to T_2 the process behaves like the solution of the logistic differential equation. Let X_t be the number of copies of the mutant allele at time t, and let $Y_t^N = X_t/2N$. Y_t makes transitions as follows:

$$i/2N \rightarrow (i+1)/2N \qquad \text{at rate } b_i = 2N - i \cdot \frac{i}{2N}$$

$$i/2N \rightarrow (i-1)/2N \qquad \text{at rate } d_i \approx (1-s)2N - i \cdot \frac{i}{2N}$$

When $Y_0^N = i/2N = y$, the infinitesimal mean

$$\frac{d}{dt}EY_t^N = b_i \cdot \frac{1}{2N} + d_i \cdot \left(-\frac{1}{2N}\right) = s\frac{2N-i}{2N} \cdot \frac{i}{2N} = sy(1-y)$$

while the infinitesimal variance

$$\frac{d}{dt}E(Y_t^N - y_0)^2 = (b_i + d_i) \cdot \frac{1}{(2N)^2} = (2-s)\frac{2N-i}{2N} \cdot \frac{i}{2N} \cdot \frac{1}{2N} \rightarrow 0$$

In this situation, results in Section 8.7 of Durrett (1996) show that as $N \rightarrow \infty$, Y_t^N converges to Y_t, the solution of the logistic differential equation

$$dY_t = sY_t(1 - Y_t)$$

It is straightforward to check that the solution of this equation is

$$Y_t = \frac{1}{1 + Ce^{-t}}$$

where $C = (1-Y_0)/Y_0$. In the case of interest, $Y_0 = 1/\ln(N)$, so $C \approx \ln(N)$ and $Y_t = 1 - 1/(\ln N)$ when

$$(\ln N)e^{-t} = \frac{\ln N}{\ln N - 1} - 1 = \frac{1}{\ln N - 1} \sim \frac{1}{\ln N}$$

Solving, we find that $T_2 - T_1 \approx 2\ln\ln N$.

III. To achieve fixation of the mutation after time T_2, each of the remaining $M = 2N/(\ln N)$ individuals must be replaced. The number of nonmutants j makes transitions

$$j \rightarrow j+1 \qquad \text{at rate } d_{2N-j} \approx (1-s)j$$
$$j \rightarrow j-1 \qquad \text{at rate } b_{2N-j} \approx j$$

That is, the number of nonmutants Z_t is a continuous time branching process in which each of the j particles gives birth at rate $(1-s)$ and dies at rate 1. By arguments in part I, $EZ_t = Z_0e^{-st}$ so it takes about $(1/s)\ln(2N)$ units of time to reach 0. □

Weak selection

Intermediate between no selection ($s = 0$) and strong selection (s fixed) is weak selection, where $2Ns$ tends to a limit as $N \rightarrow \infty$. Formulas (1.14)–(1.16) are valid for any $s > 0$. Combining the two fractions in (1.16) over a common denominator

$$P_y(T_y^+ = \infty) = \frac{[(1-s)^y - (1-s)^{y+1}] \cdot [1 - (1-s)^{2N}]}{(2-s) \cdot [(1-s)^y - (1-s)^{2N}] \cdot [1 - (1-s)^y]}$$

Dividing top and bottom by $(1-s)^y$, the above

$$= \frac{s \cdot [1 - (1-s)^{2N}]}{(2-s) \cdot [1 - (1-s)^{2N-y}] \cdot [1 - (1-s)^y]}$$

$$= \frac{s \cdot [1 - (1-s)^{2N}]}{(2-s) \cdot [(1-s)^y - (1-s)^{2N}] \cdot [(1-s)^{-y} - 1]}$$

Using (1.14) and (1.15) with (1.7) and our two expressions for $P_y(T_y^+ = \infty)$ we have

$$E_x N_y = \frac{[1 - (1-s)^x] \cdot (2-s) \cdot [1 - (1-s)^{2N-y}]}{s[1 - (1-s)^{2N}]} \qquad 0 \le x \le y$$

$$= \frac{[(1-s)^x - (1-s)^{2n}] \cdot (2-s) \cdot [(1-s)^{-y} - 1]}{s[1 - (1-s)^{2N}]} \qquad y \le x \le 2N$$

Using $q(y) = (2-s)(2N - y)y/2N$ now with (1.6) gives

$$E_x S_y = \frac{2N[1 - (1-s)^x] \cdot [1 - (1-s)^{2N-y}]}{s[1 - (1-s)^{2N}] \cdot (2N - y)y} \qquad 0 \le x \le y$$

$$= \frac{2N[(1-s)^x - (1-s)^{2N}] \cdot [(1-s)^{-y} - 1]}{s[1 - (1-s)^{2N}] \cdot (2N - y)y} \qquad y \le x \le 2N$$

By (1.14) $h(y)/h(x) = [1 - (1-s)^y]/[1 - (1-s)^x]$ so

$$\bar{E}_x S_y = \frac{2N[1 - (1-s)^y] \cdot [1 - (1-s)^{2N-y}]}{s[1 - (1-s)^{2N}] \cdot (2N - y)y} \qquad 0 \le x \le y$$

$$= \frac{2N(1-s)^x - (1-s)^{2N}}{1 - (1-s)^x}$$
$$\cdot \frac{[1 - (1-s)^y] \cdot [(1-s)^{-y} - 1]}{s[1 - (1-s)^{2N}] \cdot (2N - y)y} \qquad y \le x \le 2N$$

Up to this point, all of the calculations are valid for any $s > 0$. Letting $x = 2Np$, $y = 2Nq$, and assuming s is small so $(1-s) \approx e^{-s}$, the above is

$$\approx \frac{[1 - e^{-2Nqs}] \cdot [1 - e^{-2N(1-q)s}]}{s[1 - e^{-2Ns}] \cdot (1-q)q} \cdot \frac{1}{2N} \qquad 0 \le x \le y$$

$$\approx \frac{e^{-2Nps} - e^{-2Ns}}{1 - e^{-2Nps}} \cdot \frac{[1 - e^{-2Nqs}] \cdot [e^{2Nqs} - 1]}{s[1 - e^{-2Nps}] \cdot (1-q)q} \cdot \frac{1}{2N} \qquad y \le x \le 2N$$

From this it follows that

$$\sum_{y=1}^{N-1} \bar{E}_x S_y \approx \int_p^1 \frac{[1 - e^{-2Nqs}] \cdot [1 - e^{-2N(1-q)s}]}{s[1 - e^{-2Ns}] \cdot (1-q)q} \, dq$$

$$+ \quad \frac{e^{-2Nps} - e^{-2Ns}}{1 - e^{-2Nps}} \int_0^p \frac{[1 - e^{-2Nqs}] \cdot [e^{2Nqs} - 1]}{s[1 - e^{-2Ns}] \cdot (1 - q)q} \, dq$$

which agrees with results Kimura and Ohta (1969) derived from the diffusion approximation. Letting $2Ns = \sigma$, we have

$$\bar{E}_x \tau \approx 2N \int_p^1 \frac{[1 - e^{-\sigma q}] \cdot [1 - e^{-\sigma(1-q)}]}{\sigma[1 - e^{-\sigma}] \cdot (1 - q)q} \, dq$$

$$+ \quad 2N \frac{e^{-\sigma p} - e^{-\sigma}}{1 - e^{-\sigma p}} \int_0^p \frac{[1 - e^{-\sigma q}] \cdot [e^{\sigma q} - 1]}{\sigma[1 - e^{-\sigma}] \cdot (1 - q)q} \, dq$$

Since $1 - e^{-\sigma a} \le \sigma a$, the two integrals are finite. However they must be evaluated numerically. As a check on the last formula, we note $(e^{a\sigma} - 1)/\sigma \to a$ as $\sigma \to 0$ so

$$\bar{E}_x \tau \to 2N \int_p^1 1 \, dq + 2N \left(\frac{-p+1}{p} \right) \int_0^p \frac{q}{1-q} \, dq$$

which was the result for the neutral case given in (1.3).

Consider now the Moran model with selection and mutation. Generalizing from Section 1.2, we formulate the dynamics as follows:

(i) Each individual is replaced at rate 1. That is, individual x lives for an exponentially distributed amount with mean 1, and then is "replaced."

(ii) To replace individual x, we choose at random from the set of individuals (including x itself).

(iii) An a that is chosen mutates to A with probability u. An A that is chosen mutates to a with probability v.

(iv) The new, possibly mutated, letter replaces the old one at x with probability 1 if the new letter is an A but only with probability $(1 - s)$ if it is an a.

The probability that the choice in (ii) results in an A when there are i in the population is

$$p_i = \frac{i}{2N} \cdot (1 - v) + \frac{2N - i}{2N} \cdot u$$

With this notation in hand, we can write the transition rates for the Moran model as

$$i \to i + 1 \quad \text{at rate} \quad b_i = \frac{2N - i}{2N} \cdot p_i$$

$$i \to i - 1 \quad \text{at rate} \quad d_i = (1 - s) \frac{i}{2N} \cdot (1 - p_i)$$

In words, we can only gain an A if a site with a is chosen and the result of (ii) and (iii) produces an A. We can only lose an A if a site with A is chosen and the result of (ii) and (iii) produces an a that gets to replace the old letter in step (iv). Our next result generalizes (1.17) of Chapter 1.

(1.20) *Suppose the population size N is large and let $q = 2Nu$, $r = 2Nv$, and $\sigma = 2Ns$. Then the stationary distribution for the Moran model, when rescaled to lie on the unit interval $[0,1]$, is close to a distribution that has density*

$$f(x) = c_{q,r,\sigma} x^{q-1}(1-x)^{r-1}e^{x\sigma}$$

and $c_{q,r,\sigma}$ is a constant chosen to make $\int_0^1 f(x)\,dx = 1$.

Proof. The proof is simple since all of the work was done in the previous proof. Let b_k^* and d_k^* be the birth and death rates for the Moran model with mutation but no selection. (1.16) in Chapter 1 implies

$$\pi(i) = \pi(k)b_k \prod_{j=k+1}^{i-1} \frac{b_j}{d_j}\cdot\frac{1}{d_i} = (1-s)^{-(i-k)}\pi(k)b_k^* \prod_{j=k+1}^{i-1} \frac{b_j^*}{d_j^*}\cdot\frac{1}{d_i^*}$$

If we take $k = N$ as before and let $N \to \infty$ with $i/2N \to x$, then the first term tends to $e^{\sigma(x-1/2)}$. The previous proof takes care of the second term and the desired result follows.   □

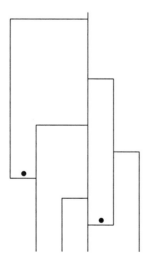

Krone and Neuhauser (1997) were the first to figure out how to study the genealogy of samples in models with selection. Departing from our usual approach in order to keep a closer contact with their work, we will consider a haploid population of N individuals that evolves according to the Moran model. We focus on one locus and limit the discussion to the case of two alleles A and a with relative fitnesses 1 and $1 - s$. Following Krone and Neuhauser, we consider only symmetric mutation: a's mutate to A's at rate u and A's mutate to a's at rate u.

We first construct the genealogy ignoring mutation. The details may look a little strange but the point of the construction is not to mimic reality but simply to develop a scheme that will simulate the Moran model with selection. As in the ordinary case with $s = 0$, when we work backwards in time each individual in the population is subject to replacement at a total rate 1. However, this time there are two types of events. At rate 1, we have a replacement event that chooses a parent at random and always replaces the individual by the parent. At rate s, we choose a parent at random but replace the individual by the parent only if the parent is A. Since we will not know until the end of the genealogical computation whether or not replacement should occur, we must follow the lineages of both the individual and the parent and the result is branching in the genealogy. The preceding picture gives a possible outcome for a sample of four individuals. Here dots mark the edges that can only be used by A's.

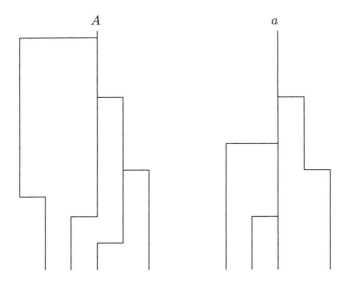

If we speed up time by N and let $\sigma = Ns$ this results in a process in which coalescence occurs at rate $j(j - 1)/2$ and mutations occur at rate σj when there are j lineages. The time at which the genealogy reaches one individual is denoted T_{UA}, where UA stands for ultimate ancestor. As the next two pictures show, depending on the state of the ultimate ancestor, it may or may not be the most recent common ancestor of the sample. Note also that the topology of the tree is different in the two cases.

The first thing to be proved is that the process ultimately will coalesce to one lineage. Since the process is a birth and death chain in which $b_i/d_i \to 0$, this is a fairly straightforward exercise. See Theorem 3.2 in Krone and Neuhauser (1997) for details. They have shown in addition that

$$E_n T_{UA} = 2 \left(1 - \frac{1}{n}\right) + 2 \sum_{m=1}^{n-1} \frac{1}{m(m+1)} \frac{e^\sigma}{\sigma^{m+1}} \int_0^\sigma t^{m+1} e^{-t} \, dt$$

When $\sigma = 0$, the second term is 0 and the answer reduces to that for the ordinary coalescent.

To compute the time of the most recent common ancestor, one must work backwards to T_{UA} and then forwards from that time to see what lineages in the genealogy are real. For this reason, exact computations are difficult. To get around this difficulty, Krone and Neuhauser (1997) computed expected values to first order in σ, which corresponds to considering lineages with 0 or 1 mutation. Theorem 4.19 in Krone and Neuhauser (1997) shows that if σ is small and $\theta = 2Nu$ then the probability that two individuals chosen at random are identical by descent is

$$\frac{1}{1+\theta} - \frac{\theta(5+2\theta)}{4(1+\theta)^2(3+\theta)(3+2\theta)}\sigma + O(\sigma^2)$$

Again, when $\sigma = 0$ this reduces to the classic answer for the ordinary coalescent. When $\theta = 1$, this becomes

$$\frac{1}{2} - \frac{7}{320}\sigma + O(\sigma^2)$$

The coefficient of σ is small in this case. Figure 9 of Krone and Neuhauser (1997) shows it is < 0.025 for all $\theta \in [0, \infty)$.

To get results for σ that are not small, one has to turn to simulation. When σ gets to be 5–10, this becomes difficult because there are a large number of lineages created before the ultimate ancestor occurs. Slade (2000ab) has recently developed some methods for trimming the tree in addition to proving some new theoretical results for the coalescent with selection.

3.2   Balancing Selection

We begin by considering the Wright-Fisher model with diploid individuals and a locus with two alleles: A_1 and A_2. Let w_{ij} be the relative fitness of $A_i A_j$ and assume that $w_{12} = w_{21}$. Let u be the probability of mutation from A_1 to A_2 and v be the probability of mutation from A_2 to A_1. If

$x = i/2N$ is the current frequency of allele A_1, then the frequency in the next generation is

$$\psi_i = \frac{1}{\bar{w}}\Big\{[w_{11}x^2 + w_{12}x(1-x)](1-u)$$
$$+ [w_{21}x(1-x) + w_{22}(1-x)^2]v\Big\}$$

where $\bar{w} = w_{11}x^2 + w_{12} \cdot 2x(1-x) + w_{22}(1-x)^2$ is the average fitness. The actual number of copies of A_1 in the next generation will be j with probability

$$p_{ij} = \binom{2N}{j}\psi_i^j(1-\psi_i)^{2N-j}$$

We concentrate here on the case with no mutation $u = v = 0$ and consider the large population limit so evolution of the frequency of A_1 given by

$$x' = \frac{1}{\bar{w}}[w_{11}x^2 + w_{12}x(1-x)]$$

Introducing $m_i = xw_{i1} + (1-x)w_{i2}$ as the marginal fitness of A_i we have $\bar{w} = xm_1 + (1-x)m_2$ and

$$x' = \frac{xm_1}{xm_1 + (1-x)m_2}$$

There are now several cases to consider

(i) *Directional selection.* $w_{11} > w_{12} > w_{22}$. In this case, $m_1 > m_2$ so if $x \in (0,1)$

$$\frac{x'}{x} = \frac{m_1}{xm_1 + (1-x)m_2} > 1$$

and if we let x_n be the frequency in generation n, then $x_n \to 1$ whenever $x_0 > 0$.

Obviously, when $w_{11} < w_{12} < w_{22}$ we have the same outcome in the other direction. This leaves us with two cases.

(ii) *Underdominance.* $w_{11} > w_{12} < w_{22}$. Heterozygotes are less fit.

(iii) *Overdominance.* $w_{11} < w_{12} > w_{22}$. Heterozygotes are more fit.

As we will now show, there is a fixed point $\bar{x}$ in each case. The fixed point is repelling in the first case and attracting in the second. To have a fixed point, we must have

$$\frac{m_1}{xm_1 + (1-x)m_2} = 1$$

or $m_1 = m_2$. Setting $xw_{11} + (1-x)w_{12} = xw_{12} + (1-x)w_{22}$ and solving gives

$$(2.1) \qquad \bar{x} = \frac{w_{22} - w_{12}}{(w_{22} - w_{12}) + (w_{11} - w_{12})}$$

In case (ii), $w_{22} - w_{12} > 0$ and $w_{11} - w_{12} > 0$, while in case (iii), $w_{22} - w_{12} < 0$ and $w_{11} - w_{12} < 0$. Therefore, in either case $\bar{x} \in (0,1)$.

To determine whether the fixed points are attracting or repelling we note that

$$\begin{aligned} m_1 &= w_{12} + x(w_{11} - w_{12}) \\ m_2 &= w_{22} + x(w_{12} - w_{22}) \end{aligned}$$

In case (ii), m_1 is increasing and m_2 is decreasing so

$$\text{if } x > \bar{x} \text{ then } m_1 > m_2 \text{ and } x' > x$$
$$\text{if } x < \bar{x} \text{ then } m_1 < m_2 \text{ and } x' < x$$

This implies that if $x_0 > \bar{x}$ then $x_n \to 1$, while if $x_0 < \bar{x}$ then $x_n \to 0$.

In case (iii), m_1 is decreasing and m_2 is increasing so

$$\text{if } x > \bar{x} \text{ then } m_1 < m_2 \text{ and } x' < x$$
$$\text{if } x < \bar{x} \text{ then } m_1 > m_2 \text{ and } x' > x$$

This is not quite enough to conclude that convergence to $\bar{x}$ for x' might overshoot the fixed point $\bar{x}$ and we could have a periodic orbit with period 2. To rule this out, we begin with the observation that the mean fitness $\bar{w} = w_{11}x^2 + w_{12} \cdot 2x(1-x) + w_{22}(1-x)^2$ has

$$\frac{d\bar{w}}{dx} = 2w_{11}x + w_{12}(2-4x) - 2w_{22}(1-x) = 0$$

when $x = (w_{22} - w_{12})/(w_{22} - 2w_{12} + w_{11}) = \bar{x}$ and $d^2\bar{w}/dx^2 = 2(w_{11} - 2w_{12} + w_{22}) < 0$ in case (iii), indicating a maximum. Some tedious algebra (see (1.39) in Ewens 1979) shows that the change in mean fitness

$$\begin{aligned} \bar{w}' - \bar{w} &= 2x(1-x)\{w_{11}x + w_{12}(1-2x) - w_{22}(1-x)\}^2 \\ &\quad \cdot \{w_{11}x^2 + [w_{12} + (w_{11} + w_{22})/2]x(1-x) + w_{22}(1-x)^2\}\bar{w}^{-2} \end{aligned}$$

This is > 0 for $x \neq \bar{x}$ and the desired result follows.

In the case of overdominance, the selective advantage of the heterozygote maintains both alleles at positive frequencies, so this case is called *balancing selection*. In what follows, we will be interested in the case in which

$$w_{11} = 1 - s_1 \qquad w_{12} = 1 \qquad w_{22} = 1 - s_2$$

In this case, (2.1) shows that the fixed point is

$$(2.2) \qquad \bar{x} = s_2/(s_1 + s_2)$$

We will also suppose that there is mutation from A_1 to A_2 with probability u per generation and from A_2 to A_1 with probability v. If we assume that mutation occurs after selection has acted, then

$$(2.3) \qquad x' = \frac{x m_1 (1 - u) + (1 - x) m_2 v}{x m_1 + (1 - x) m_2}$$

The corresponding equation for the fixed point is a cubic and hence cannot be solved explicitly. Following Ewens (1979) page 13, "We have in mind mainly the case where selective differences are of order 1% while the mutation rates are of order 10^{-5} or 10^{-6}. It is clear that under this assumption that if selection and mutation are taken into account there will exist a new stable equilibrium differing trivially (2.2). We thus do not consider this case further."

Kaplan, Darden, and Hudson (1988) were the first to study genealogies in models with balancing selection. The details are somewhat involved algebraically but the theme here and in the next two sections is that this form of selection can be treated as if it were population subdivision. Let $f_{A_j}(A_k, t)$ denote the probability that a randomly chosen gene from generation t is of allelic type A_k and its parental gene from generation $t - 1$ is of allelic type A_j. From (2.3) it follows that if X_t is the frequency of A_1 in generation t then

$$
\begin{aligned}
f_{A_1}(A_1, t) &= \frac{1 - u}{\bar{w}_{t-1}} X_{t-1} m_1 (t - 1) \\
f_{A_1}(A_2, t) &= \frac{u}{\bar{w}_{t-1}} X_{t-1} m_1 (t - 1) \\
f_{A_2}(A_2, t) &= \frac{1 - v}{\bar{w}_{t-1}} (1 - X_{t-1}) m_2 (t - 1) \\
f_{A_2}(A_1, t) &= \frac{v}{\bar{w}_{t-1}} (1 - X_{t-1}) m_2 (t - 1)
\end{aligned}
$$

where $\bar{w}_{t-1} = X_{t-1}^2 w_{11} + 2 X_{t-1}(1 - X_{t-1}) w_{12} + (1 - X_{t-1})^2 w_{22}$ is the mean fitness in generation $t - 1$ and

$$
\begin{aligned}
m_1(t - 1) &= X_{t-1} w_{11} + (1 - X_{t-1}) w_{12} \\
m_2(t - 1) &= X_{t-1} w_{12} + (1 - X_{t-1}) w_{22}
\end{aligned}
$$

are the two marginal fitnesses.

Suppose that n genes are chosen at random from the 0th generation and let $Q(0) = (i, j)$ if the sample contains i A_1 alleles and j A_2 alleles. For $t < 0$, let $Q(t)$ denote the number of A_1 and A_2 ancestral genes of the sample in generation t. To compute the transition probability of $Q(t)$, we let $f(A_i, t) = f_{A_1}(A_i, t) + f_{A_2}(A_i, t)$ be the probability of picking a gene of allelic type A_i regardless of the type of the parental gene. The probability that a sampled A_2 allele from generation t has an A_1 parental gene equals

$$\frac{f_{A_1}(A_2, t)}{f(A_2, t)} = \frac{u X_{t-1} m_1 (t - 1)}{u X_{t-1} m_1 (t - 1) + (1 - v)(1 - X_{t-1}) m_2 (t - 1)}$$

If we assume the allele frequencies are in equilibrium then $X_{t-1} \approx \bar{x}$ and $m_1(t-1) \approx m_2(t-1)$, so assuming $u = \beta_1/2N$ and $v = \beta_2/2N$ are small,

$$\frac{f_{A_1}(A_2,t)}{f(A_2,t)} \approx \frac{\bar{x}\frac{\beta_1}{2N}}{\bar{x}\frac{\beta_1}{2N} + (1-\bar{x})\left(1 - \frac{\beta_2}{2N}\right)} \approx \frac{\beta_1\bar{x}}{1-\bar{x}} \cdot \frac{1}{2N}$$

Ignoring the possibility of two mutations on one step,

$$P(Q(t-1) = (i+1, j-1)|Q(t) = (i,j)) = \frac{j\beta_1\bar{x}}{1-\bar{x}} \cdot \frac{1}{2N}$$

A similar argument shows that

$$P(Q(t-1) = (i-1, j+1)|Q(t) = (i,j)) = \frac{i\beta_2(1-\bar{x})}{\bar{x}} \cdot \frac{1}{2N}$$

In the cases of interest, u and v are small, so most individuals pick their parents from the same subpopulation. Ignoring the possibility of two coalescences or a coalescence and a mutation on one step we have

$$P(Q(t-1) = (i-1, j)|Q(t) = (i,j)) = \binom{i}{2}\frac{1}{2N\bar{x}}$$

$$P(Q(t-1) = (i, j-1)|Q(t) = (i,j)) = \binom{j}{2}\frac{1}{2N(1-\bar{x})}$$

As advertised above, this is the same as a two-island model with populations of sizes $2N\bar{x}$ and $2N(1-\bar{x})$ and migration probabilities $\beta_2(1-\bar{x})/2N$ and $\beta_1\bar{x}/2N(1-\bar{x})$ per individual per generation for the two populations.

As Hudson and Kaplan (1988) observed, it is not hard to generalize the setup above to include recombination. If one is investigating the genealogy of a neutral locus B that is separated from A by recombination with probability r per generation, this adds a term of the form

$$\frac{1}{\bar{w}_{t-1}} r X_{t-1}(1 - X_{t-1}) w_{12}$$

to $f_{A_1}(A_2,t)$ and subtracts it from $f_{A_2}(A_2,t)$, so repeating the calculations above shows that if $r = R/2N$ is small

$$P(Q(t-1) = (i+1, j-1)|Q(t) = (i,j)) = \frac{j\bar{x}(\beta_1 + R(1-\bar{x}))}{1-\bar{x}} \cdot \frac{1}{2N}$$

$$P(Q(t-1) = (i-1, j+1)|Q(t) = (i,j)) = \frac{i(1-\bar{x})(\beta_2 + R\bar{x})}{\bar{x}} \cdot \frac{1}{2N}$$

Consider now a sample of size two of the B locus. Our first goal is to compute $M_{i,j}$, the mean coalescence time for two lineages when i starts linked to the A_1 allele and j starts linked to the A_2 allele. To simplify notation, we will let

$$\alpha_1 = \frac{(1-\bar{x})(\beta_2 + R\bar{x})}{\bar{x}} \qquad \alpha_2 = \frac{\bar{x}(\beta_1 + R(1-\bar{x}))}{1-\bar{x}}$$

$$\gamma_1 = 1/\bar{x} \qquad \gamma_2 = 1/(1-\bar{x})$$

Here α_i is the migration rate out of subpopulation i and γ_i is the coalescence rate within it. By considering what happens on the first event, it is easy to see that

$$M_{2,0} = \frac{1}{2\alpha_1 + \gamma_1} + \frac{2\alpha_1}{2\alpha_1 + \gamma_1}M_{1,1}$$

$$M_{0,2} = \frac{1}{2\alpha_2 + \gamma_2} + \frac{2\alpha_2}{2\alpha_2 + \gamma_2}M_{1,1}$$

$$M_{1,1} = \frac{1}{\alpha_1 + \alpha_2} + \frac{\alpha_1}{\alpha_1 + \alpha_2}M_{0,2} + \frac{\alpha_2}{\alpha_1 + \alpha_2}M_{2,0}$$

Plugging the first two equations into the third one, we have

$$(\alpha_1 + \alpha_2)M_{1,1} = 1 + \frac{\alpha_1}{2\alpha_2 + \gamma_2} + \frac{\alpha_1(2\alpha_2)}{2\alpha_2 + \gamma_2}M_{1,1}$$
$$+ \frac{\alpha_2}{2\alpha_1 + \gamma_1} + \frac{\alpha_2(2\alpha_1)}{2\alpha_1 + \gamma_1}M_{1,1}$$

Solving gives

$$M_{1,1} = \frac{1 + \frac{\alpha_1}{2\alpha_2 + \gamma_2} + \frac{\alpha_2}{2\alpha_1 + \gamma_1}}{\frac{\alpha_1\gamma_2}{2\alpha_2 + \gamma_2} + \frac{\alpha_2\gamma_1}{2\alpha_1 + \gamma_1}}$$

and then $M_{0,2}$ and $M_{2,0}$ can be computed from the preceding equations. To check this formula, we note that if $\gamma_1, \gamma_2 \gg \alpha_1, \alpha_2$ then

$$M_{1,1} \approx \frac{1}{\alpha_1 + \alpha_2}$$

In words, the two lineages wait an amount of time with mean $1/(\alpha_1 + \alpha_2)$ to come to the same population and then coalescence comes soon after that event.

In the other direction, if $\gamma_1, \gamma_2 \ll \alpha_1, \alpha_2$ then

$$M_{1,1} \approx \frac{1 + \frac{\alpha_1}{2\alpha_2} + \frac{\alpha_2}{2\alpha_1}}{\frac{\alpha_1\gamma_2}{2\alpha_2} + \frac{\alpha_2\gamma_1}{2\alpha_1}}$$

This may not look intuitive but there is an easy explanation. Migration is much faster than coalescence, so observing that in equilibrium lineages are in the first population with probability $\alpha_2/(\alpha_1 + \alpha_2)$ and in the second with probability $\alpha_1/(\alpha_1 + \alpha_2)$, then the probability of coalescence on one step is approximately

$$\left(\frac{\alpha_2}{\alpha_1 + \alpha_2}\right)^2 \gamma_1 + \left(\frac{\alpha_1}{\alpha_1 + \alpha_2}\right)^2 \gamma_2 = \frac{\alpha_2^2\gamma_1 + \alpha_1^2\gamma_2}{(\alpha_1 + \alpha_2)^2}$$

Inverting this to get the mean coalescence time and then multiplying top and bottom by $1/2\alpha_1\alpha_2$, the mean is then

$$\frac{(\alpha_1 + \alpha_2)^2}{\alpha_2^2\gamma_1 + \alpha_1^2\gamma_2} = \frac{1 + \frac{\alpha_1}{2\alpha_2} + \frac{\alpha_2}{2\alpha_1}}{\frac{\alpha_1\gamma_2}{2\alpha_2} + \frac{\alpha_2\gamma_1}{2\alpha_1}}$$

The same logic can be used to compute $h(i,j)$, the probability that two lineages are identical by descent when i starts in population 1 and j in population 2. Let u be the mutation rate and let $\theta = 4Nu$. By considering what happens at the first event,

$$(2\alpha_1 + \gamma_1 + \theta)h(2,0) = 2\alpha_1 h(1,1) + \gamma_1$$
$$(2\alpha_2 + \gamma_2 + \theta)h(0,2) = 2\alpha_2 h(1,1) + \gamma_2$$
$$(\alpha_1 + \alpha_2 + \theta)h(1,1) = \alpha_1 h(0,2) + \alpha_2 h(2,0)$$

Plugging the first two equations into the third one

$$(\alpha_1 + \alpha_2 + \theta)\, h(1,1) = \frac{\alpha_1(2\alpha_2)}{2\alpha_2 + \gamma_2 + \theta}h(1,1) + \frac{\alpha_1\gamma_2}{2\alpha_2 + \gamma_2 + \theta}$$
$$+ \frac{\alpha_2(2\alpha_1)}{2\alpha_1 + \gamma_1 + \theta}h(1,1) + \frac{\alpha_2\gamma_1}{2\alpha_1 + \gamma_1 + \theta}$$

which can be solved for $h(1,1)$.

Example 2.1. Hudson and Kaplan (1988) used this to study Kreitman's (1983) data on the *Adh* locus. To examine the distribution of polymorphic sites along the chromosome, a "sliding window" method was used. Three different quantities were computed to characterize the variability in the window centered at each nucleotide site k: $\pi_{FS}(k)$, $\pi_{FF}(k)$, and $\pi_{KK}(k)$, the average number of pairwise differences between Fast and Slow sequences, between Fast sequences, and between Slow sequences. The region sequenced contained protein coding sequences as well as introns and other noncoding sequences. To take at least partial account of the different levels of constraints in these regions, the size of the window was varied so as to keep the number of possible silent changes in the window constant. The window size chosen corresponds to 50 base pairs in noncoding regions.

If each nucleotide is treated as an individual locus and if it is assumed that the allelic frequencies at position 2 of codon 192 are maintained by strong balancing selection, then the theory above can be used to calculate the expectation of $\pi_{FS}(k)$, $\pi_{SS}(k)$, and $\pi_{FF}(k)$. These calculations require that values be assigned to β_1, β_2, and $\bar{x}$, and that for each site i we must compute θ_i and R_i, the recombination rate between i and the location i_0 of the balanced polymorphism. Here and in what follows, we means Hudson and Kaplan (1988). That is, our discussion uses the estimates in their paper.

At sites where m of the three possible mutations is a silent change (does not change the amino acid), then we assume that the rate $\theta_i = m\theta_0/3$. The heterozygosity per nucleotide at silent sites, π, has been estimated to be 0.006 for a region that is 13 kb long that includes the *Adh* locus, so we set $\theta_0 = 0.006$. The mutations that change lysine to threonine and threonine back to lysine are the second-position transversions $A \to C$ and $C \to A$. Since $\theta_0 = 4Nu$, then a plausible value for $\beta_1 = \beta_2 = \theta_0/6 = 0.001$, since these are $2N$ times the mutation rates. Since $\bar{x}$, the frequency of the Slow variant varies with geographic location (Oakeshott et al. 1982) it is not clear what value to assign to it. A more realistic model must take spatial structure into account, but here we simply set $\bar{x} = 0.7$, a value for a sample of *D. melanogaster* from Raleigh, North Carolina discussed in Kreitman and Aguadé (1986a).

Finally, we set $R_i = R_0|i - i_0|$. Recombination per base pair has been estimated for several regions of the *D. melanogaster* genome to be approximately 10^{-8} per generation in females (Chovnick, Gelbart, and McCarron 1977). There is no recombination in males. The neutral mutation rate has been estimated to be approximately 5×10^{-9} per year in many organisms. If we assume that *D. melanogaster* has 4 generations per year, then the ratio of the recombination rate to the neutral mutation rate per generation is approximately

$$\frac{10^{-8}/2}{(5 \times 10^{-9})/4} = 4$$

This implies that R_0 is approximately 4 times $\theta_0/2$, or 0.012.

With all of the parameters estimated, we can compute the expected values of $\pi_{FS}(k)$, $\pi_{SS}(k)$, and $\pi_{FF}(k)$ by using the formulas for $h(1,1)$, $h(2,0)$, and $h(0,2)$ above. The three graphs on pages 836 and 837 of Hudson and Kaplan (1988) show the results. In order to fit the FS data, the recombination rate needed to be lowered by a factor of 6 from what was expected. Even after that was done, the fit was not good for the SS data, which showed a surprising amount of polymorphism in the SS near the locus under selection.

In his survey paper, Hudson (1991) redid the analysis using the divergence between *D. melanogaster* and *D. simulans* to estimate the mutation rate on a locus-by-locus basis. Now the recombination value that produces this fit is only a factor of 2 smaller than the a priori estimate.

3.3   Background Selection

B. Charlesworth, Morgan and D. Charlesworth (1993) suggested an explanation for the observation of reduced variability in regions of low recombination: selection against linked deleterious alleles maintained by recurrent mutation ("background selection"). Following D. Charlesworth, B. Charlesworth, and Morgan (1995) and Hudson and Kaplan (1994, 1995, 1996), we will use a coalescent-based approach.

To begin, we assume that the locus A is linked to one other locus at which deleterious mutations occur at rate u per individual per generation and that there is no recombination between the two loci. All deleterious mutations are assumed to have the same effect: $1 - sh$ in the heterozygous state and $1 - h$ in the homozygous state. However, individual mutations will have low frequencies so we will ignore the latter possibility. Interaction between mutations is assumed to be multiplicative so that an individual heterozygous for i such mutations has fitness $(1 - sh)^i$.

Following Kimura and Maruyama (1966) and Hey (1991), we formulate the dynamics of the process and the corresponding coalescent as follows. Let f_i be the frequency of gametes with i mutations, $m_k = \exp(-u/2)(u/2)^k/k!$ be the probability that a gamete experiences k new mutations, and $w_j = (1 - sh)^j$ be the relative fitness of a gamete with j mutations. The proportion of descendent gametes with j mutations produced by parental gametes with i mutations is

$$p_{ij} = \frac{w_{ij}}{W} \quad \text{where} \quad w_{ij} = f_i w_i m_{j-i} \quad \text{and} \quad W = \sum_{ij} w_{ij}$$

Our first step is to check that the Poisson $f_i = e^{-u/2sh}(u/2sh)^i/i!$ is a stationary distribution for the process. To do this, we let $v = u/2$ and note that

$$\sum_{i=0}^{j} w_{ij} = \sum_{i=0}^{j} e^{-v/sh} \frac{(v/sh)^i}{i!}(1-sh)^i e^{-v} \frac{v^{j-i}}{(j-i)!}$$

$$= e^{-v(1+1/sh)} \frac{1}{j!} \sum_{i=0}^{j} \frac{j!}{i!(j-i)!}((v/sh)-v)^i v^{j-i}$$

$$= e^{-v(1+1/sh)} \frac{(v/sh)^j}{j!}$$

Summing over j now, we have

$$W = \sum_{j=0}^{\infty} e^{-v(1+1/sh)} \frac{(v/sh)^j}{j!} = e^{-v}$$

so $\sum_{i=0}^{j} p_{ij} = \sum_{i=0}^{j} w_{ij}/W = e^{-v/sh}(v/sh)^j/j!$.

By Bayes' theorem, the probability that a gamete with j mutations derives from one with i mutations is

$$q_{ji} = \frac{p_{ij}}{\sum_{i=0}^{j} p_{ij}} = \frac{e^{-v/sh} \frac{(v/sh)^i}{i!}(1-sh)^i \frac{v^{j-i}}{(j-i)!}}{e^{-v/sh} \frac{(v/sh)^j}{j!}} = \frac{j!}{i!(j-i)!}(1-sh)^i(sh)^{j-i}$$

In words, q_{ji} is a binomial distribution. To understand the amount of time such a chain will take to reach the 0 state from j, visualize the initial state as j white balls and that loss of mutation, with probability sh on each trial, results in a ball being painted green. This implies that the expected time to go from 1 to 0 has a geometric distribution with mean $1/sh$. Ignoring the possibility that two balls get painted on one turn, the total time to go from j to 0 then has mean

$$\leq \frac{1}{jsh} + \frac{1}{(j-1)sh} + \cdots + \frac{1}{2sh} + \frac{1}{sh} \approx \frac{\log(j+1)}{sh}$$

If $sh = 0.02$, as has been suggested by Crow and Simmons (1983), then on the average only 50 generations are needed for a sampled class 1 chromosome to get to class 0. Consider now a sample of size two. Ignoring the time to get to class 0 and the possibility that the two lineages coalesce before getting to class 0, the coalescent process occurs as for the neutral model, with a population size of $2Ne^{-u/2sh}$ instead of $2N$. If neutral mutations occur at rate μ per nucleotide per generation ,then the nucleotide diversity is $\pi_0 = 4N\mu$ under the neutral theory and reduced by background selection to

$$(3.1) \qquad \pi = 4N\mu e^{-u/2sh} = \pi_0 e^{-u/2sh}$$

a result first derived by Charlesworth, Morgan, and Charlesworth (1983); see their equation (3). For large sample sizes, the argument above is the same and suggests that the shape of the gene tree will be just like the shape of the neutral tree except that the effective population size is changed to $N_e = Ne^{-u/2sh}$. As a consequence, the frequency spectrum will be the same as under the neutral model, while the expected number of segregating sites will become

$$(3.2) \qquad ES = \left(\frac{\pi}{\pi_0}\right) \theta \sum_{j=1}^{n-1} \frac{1}{j}$$

Hudson and Kaplan (1994) have done simulations to show that background selection has very little effect on Tajima's D statistic.

We suppose now that there is recombination with probability R per generation between the selected locus and the neutral locus A. At recombination events, the selected locus is replaced by an independent copy drawn from the population and hence has a Poisson mean $u/2sh$ number of mutations. In the absence of recombination, the number of mutations decreases according to the binomial distribution with a fraction $(1 - sh)$ of the points retained. From this, we see that if the last recombination event happened k generations ago, an event of probability $R(1 - R)^k$ the number of deleterious mutations will have a Poisson distribution with mean $(1 - sh)^k u/2sh$. Thus, in equilibrium the number of deleterious mutations is a geometric mixture of Poisson distributions.

Eventually our analysis will involve a lot of deleterious loci with small mutation probabilities. To prepare for this, we need to consider what happens when u is small. In this case, there will always be 0 or 1 mutation, so supposing R and sh are small, the probability of one mutation by the argument above is

$$\sum_{k=0}^{\infty} R(1 - R)^k \frac{u}{2sh}(1 - sh)^k = \frac{uR}{2sh(R + sh + Rsh)} \approx \frac{uR}{2sh(R + sh)}$$

Actually, in many cases R will not be small but if, say, $R = 1$ and $sh = 0.02$, then $R + sh + Rsh = 1.04$ while $R + sh = 1.02$, so the approximation is still reasonable.

Consider now a sample of size 2 at the A locus, and let $\mu(k)$ be the equilibrium probability that a lineage in the coalescent has k deleterious mutations. If we suppose that particle movement is more rapid than coalescence, then the probability of coalescence on one step is

$$(3.3) \qquad\qquad \Lambda = \sum_k \frac{\mu(k)^2}{2N_k}$$

where $N_k = Ne^{-u/2sh}(u/2sh)^k/k!$ is the number of individuals in the population with k mutations. When u is small, we only have two classes to worry about: 0 and 1 mutation. In this case, $2N$ times the sum reduces to

$$\lambda = \frac{\left(\frac{uR}{2sh(R+sh)}\right)^2}{u/2sh} + \frac{\left(1 - \frac{uR}{2sh(R+sh)}\right)^2}{1 - u/2sh}$$

When u/sh is small, the above is

$$\approx \frac{uR^2}{2sh(R+sh)^2} + \left(1 - \frac{2uR}{2sh(R+sh)}\right) \cdot (1 + u/2sh)$$

$$\approx 1 + \frac{uR^2 - 2uR(R+sh) + u(R+sh)^2}{2sh(R+sh)^2} = 1 + \frac{ush}{2(R+sh)^2}$$

From this we see that when time is measured in units of $2N$ generations, the time to coalescence is roughly exponential with mean

$$(3.4) \qquad\qquad \lambda^{-1} \approx 1 - ush/2(R+sh)^2$$

Suppose now that the neutral locus A is followed by two selected loci B_1 and B_2 with the probability of a recombination between A and B_1 being R_1 and between B_1 and B_2 being $R_2 - R_1$. Let u_1 and u_2 be the mutation rates at the two loci. Combining the two loci into one locus with mutation rate $u = u_1 + u_2$ and then randomly allocating the mutations between the two loci with probabilities $p_i = u_i/(u_1 + u_2)$, it is easy to see that in the equilibrium of the process going forward, the number of deleterious mutations at the two loci are independent. To argue that this also holds for the process working backwards in time, we note that this is true when a recombination occurs between A and B_1 and all subsequent operations: thinning the number of mutations using the binomial or a recombination between B_1 and B_2 preserves this property.

The last argument is valid for any number of selected loci. We are now ready to divide up our segment of DNA into a lot of little pieces B_i and take a limit as the number of pieces goes to infinity. Let u_i be the mutation rate at B_i and let R_i be the recombination rate between A and B_i. Consider now a sample of size 2 at the A locus. When there are m loci the classes are denoted by vectors $\vec{k} = (k_1, k_2, \ldots, k_m)$ but the argument that leads to (3.3) stays the same. Let $\mu(\vec{k})$ be the equilibrium probability that a lineage in the coalescent has k_i deleterious mutations at locus i. If we suppose that particle movement is more rapid than coalescence, then the probability of coalescence on one step is approximately

$$\Lambda = \sum_{\vec{k}} \frac{\mu(\vec{k})^2}{2N_{\vec{k}}}$$

where $N_{\vec{k}} = N \prod_{i=1}^{m} e^{-u_i/2sh}(u_i/2sh)^{k_i}/k_i!$ is the number of individuals in the population with k mutations.

Since μ is itself a product, it is easy to see that $2N$ times the sum reduces to

$$\lambda = \prod_{i=1}^{m} \frac{\left(\frac{u_i R_i}{2sh(R_i+sh)}\right)^2}{u_i/2sh} + \frac{\left(1 - \frac{u_i R_i}{2sh(R_i+sh)}\right)^2}{1 - u_i/2sh}$$

$$\approx \prod_{i=1}^{m} 1 + \frac{u_i sh}{2(R_i + sh)^2} \approx \exp\left(\sum_{i=1}^{m} \frac{u_i sh}{2(R_i + sh)^2}\right)$$

To pass to the limit let x be the distance from the neutral locus measured in kb and suppose that $u_i = \int_{B_i} u(x)\, dx$. In this case

$$\lambda \approx \exp\left(\int_a^b \frac{u(x)sh}{2(sh + R(x))^2}\, dx\right)$$

where a and b are the endpoints of the region under consideration. Since the coalescence time is roughly exponential with mean λ^{-1}, this means

Theorem. The nucleotide diversity π compared to the predictions of the neutral theory, π_0, satisfies

$$(3.5) \qquad \frac{\pi}{\pi_0} \approx \exp\left(-\int_a^b \frac{u(x)sh}{2(sh + R(x))^2}\, dx\right)$$

Example 3.1. If we suppose $u(x) \equiv u$, $R(x) = r|x|$, $a = -L$, and $b = L$, then the expression above reduces to

$$\frac{\pi}{\pi_0} \approx \exp\left(-2\int_0^L \frac{ush}{2(sh + rx)^2}\, dx\right)$$

$$= \exp\left(\frac{2}{r}\left[\frac{ush}{2(sh + rL)} - \frac{u}{2}\right]\right) = \exp\left(-\frac{2uL}{2sh + 2rL}\right)$$

Writing $U = 2uL$ for the total deleterious mutation rate in the region and $R = 2rL$ for the total recombination rate, the above can be written as

$$(3.6) \qquad \frac{\pi}{\pi_0} \approx \exp\left(-\frac{U}{2sh + R}\right)$$

When $R = 0$, this reduces to the result in (3.1). Note that as we should expect, recombination lessens the impact of deleterious mutations.

(3.5) gives the effect of deleterious mutations on the variability at 0 but it is straightforward to extend this to calculate the effect at other places. Suppose we have a chromosome of length L and let $M(x)$ be the distance from 0 to x measured in Morgans. In this case, the reduction in variability at y is given by

$$(3.7) \qquad \frac{\pi}{\pi_0} \approx \exp\left(-\int_0^L \frac{u(x)sh}{2(sh + |M(x) - M(y)|)^2}\,dx\right)$$

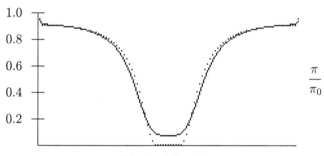

Physical Position

Example 3.2. Following Nordborg, Charlesworth, and Charlesworth (1996), we will now consider the case $M(x) = (x + \sin x)/12$ for $0 \le x \le 2\pi$. To explain their choice of this function we note that $M'(x) = (1 + \cos x)/12 = 0$ when $x = \pi$ so recombination is reduced near the centromere. The preceding plot shows what happens when $U = 0.1$ and $sh = 0.0003$ (dotted line) or $sh = 0.003$ (solid line). Note that near the centromere the weaker selection causes a greater reduction in variability. The graphs turn up sharply toward the ends because at the telomeres contributions only come from one side.

Example 3.3. Hudson and Kaplan (1995) applied (3.2) to predict levels of variation on the third chromosome of *D. melanogaster*. The total diploid deleterious mutation rate has been estimated from mutation accumulation studies to be 1.0 or larger (Crow and Simmons 1983, Keightley 1994). Since there are approximately 5000 cytological bands in the *Drosophila* genome, they estimated u, the deleterious mutation rate per generation per band, to be $1.0/5000 = 2 \times 10^{-4}$. To estimate recombination as a function of distance, Hudson and Kaplan used information in Flybase to determine map distance as a function of physical position for 107 locations on the third chromosome.

The map gives the values of $M(x)$ at a discrete sequence of points x_i. From these they estimated the reduction in variability at x_k by $\pi/\pi_0 = e^{-G}$, where

$$G = \sum_i \frac{ush}{2} \cdot \frac{|x_{i+1} - x_i|}{(sh + |M(x_{i+1}) - M(x_k)|/2)(sh + |M(x_i) - M(x_k)|/2)}$$

To compare with (3.7), we first note that the $1/2$ in the denominator is to account for the fact that there is no recombination in male *Drosophila*. Ignoring this 2, we can then derive their approximation as follows. Suppose without loss of generality that $M(x_k) \le M(x_i) < M(x_{i+1})$. If we suppose that $M(x)$ is linear on $[x_i, x_{i+1}]$, then ignoring the constant factor $ush/2$ the contribution to the integral in (3.7) from this interval is

$$\int_0^1 \frac{(x_{i+1} - x_i)\,dv}{[sh + v(M(x_{i+1}) - M(x_k)) + (1-v)(M(x_i) - M(x_k))]^2}$$

$$= -\frac{(x_{i+1} - x_i)/(M(x_{i+1}) - M(x_i))}{[sh + v(M(x_{i+1}) - M(x_k)) + (1-v)(M(x_i) - M(x_k))]}\Bigg|_0^1$$

$$= -\frac{(x_{i+1} - x_i)/(M(x_{i+1}) - M(x_i))}{[sh + (M(x_{i+1}) - M(x_k))]}$$

$$+ \frac{(x_{i+1} - x_i)/(M(x_{i+1}) - M(x_i))}{[sh + (M(x_i) - M(x_k))]}$$

$$= \frac{|x_{i+1} - x_i|}{(sh + |M(x_{i+1}) - M(x_k)|)(sh + |M(x_i) - M(x_k)|)}$$

Hudson and Kaplan compared the levels of variability at 17 loci on the third chromosome with predictions based on three different values of sh: 0.03, 0.02, and 0.005. The value of π_0 used, namely 0.014, was chosen to produce a good fit to the data as judged by eye. The fit given on page 1611 of Hudson and Kaplan (1995) is not very sensitive to the value of sh except near the centromere and is remarkably good except at the tips of the chromosomes.

Example 3.4. Another example of this type of analysis occurs in Hamblin and Aquadro's (1996) study of *Gld*. To estimate $M(x)$ they used information about the following loci in *D. simulans*. Here x_i is the band number, $M(x_i)$ is the distance from the tip measured in Morgans, and nd means not determined.

Locus	x_i	$M(x_i)$	Locus	x_i	$M(x_i)$
jv	175	0	Rh3	1089	nd
idh	285	0.064	Aldox	1299	0.754
Est-6	432	0.252	rosy	1403	nd
Pgm	567	0.381	Men	1413	0.877
ri	780	0.580	boss	1850	nd
Gld	996	0.590	Ald	1865	1.246
e	1059	0.600	ca	1990	1.300
H	1071	0.610	Acph-1	2000	1.340

The first step in making predictions from these data is to extend the definition of M to be linear in between the places where it is known.

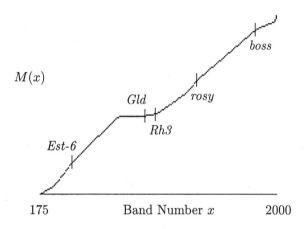

Taking $sh = 0.02$, $u = 0.0002$, and choosing $\pi_0 = 0.11$ as Hamblin and Aquadro (1996) did gives the following prediction for π. The circles give the observed levels of variability at *Est-6*, *Gld*, *Rh3*, *rosy*, and *boss*. We do not know the confidence intervals associated with the estimates of π but the general pattern seems consistent with the background selection model.

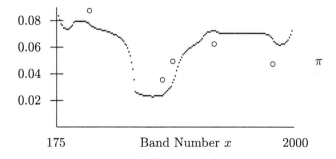

3.4   Hitchhiking

When a selectively favorable mutation occurs in a population and is subsequently fixed, the process will alter the frequency of alleles at closely linked loci. Alleles present on the chromosome on which the original mutation occurred will tend to increase in frequency, and other alleles will decrease in frequency. This is referred to as "hitchhiking" because an allele can get a lift in frequency from selection acting on a neighboring allele.

Following Maynard-Smith and Haigh (1974), we consider haploid individuals and begin by considering the behavior of the selected locus when alleles B and b have relative fitnesses $1 + s$ and 1. If we assume a very large population in which individuals of type B produce $1 + s$ times as many offspring as those of type b, then the fraction of individuals of type B in generation n, p_n, satisfies

$$(4.1) \qquad p_{n+1} = \frac{(1+s)p_n}{(1+s)p_n + (1-p_n)} = \frac{1+s}{1+sp_n} p_n$$

In n generations, B's will produce $(1+s)^n$ times as many offspring as b's will, so the general solution of the equation is

$$(4.2) \qquad p_n = \frac{(1+s)^n p_0}{1 - p_0 + (1+s)^n p_0}$$

Readers not convinced by the verbal argument can check that with this choice of p_n

$$\frac{(1+s)p_n}{1+sp_n} = \frac{(1+s)^{n+1}p_0}{1 - p_0 + (1+s)^n p_0 + s(1+s)^n p_0} = p_{n+1}$$

We will have $p_n \approx 1$ in (4.2) when $(1+s)^n p_0 = C$ and C is large, that is, $n = \ln(C/p_0)/\ln(1+s)$. If $p_0 = 1/2N$ and s is small, this condition is $n = (\ln 2NC)/s$ in accord with our previous result in (1.18) on the duration of a selective sweep.

Consider now a second neutral locus with alleles A and a. Introducing Q_n and R_n to denote the conditional probabilities $P(A|B)$ and $P(A|b)$ in generation n we have

Genotype	AB	aB	Ab	ab
Fitness	$1+s$	$1+s$	1	1
Frequency	$p_n Q_n$	$p_n(1-Q_n)$	$(1-p_n)R_n$	$(1-p_n)(1-R_n)$

The main result of Maynard-Smith and Haigh (1974) is

Theorem.

$$(4.3) \qquad Q_\infty = R_0(1-p_0) \sum_{n=0}^{\infty} \frac{(1-r)^n r}{1 - p_0 + p_0(1+s)^{n+1}}$$

To interpret this equation, we note that the initial frequency of the A allele is $R_0(1 - p_0)$ while its frequency after the sweep is Q_∞. Thus, the sum on the right-hand side gives the factor by which it has been reduced. To gain some insight into the sum, let X be a random variable with the shifted geometric distribution $P(X = n + 1) = (1 - r)^n r$ for $n \geq 0$ and note that the sum is

$$E\left(\frac{1}{1 - p_0 + p_0(1 + s)^X}\right)$$

The smaller r is, the larger X is and the smaller the expected value is, in accord with our intuition that when the recombination rate is smaller there is a greater impact on the allele frequencies.

Proof of (4.3). Let r be the probability of a recombination between the A and B loci per generation. Our first goal is to show

$$(4.4) \qquad Q_n - R_n = (1 - r)^n(Q_0 - R_0)$$

Even though it will take a lot of algebra to derive this, the answer is intuitive. A recombination event makes the two loci independent so the difference between the two conditional probabilities is $(1 - r)^n$ times the original difference.

To begin the proof of (4.3), we must compute Q_{n+1}. By considering the possible parent pairs we see that the probability of generating an AB offspring in generation $n + 1$ is

parents	number of offspring
AB,AB	$(1 + s)p_nQ_n \cdot (1 + s)p_nQ_n$
AB,aB	$(1 + s)p_nQ_n \cdot (1 + s)p_n(1 - Q_n)$
AB,Ab	$(1 + s)p_nQ_n \cdot (1 - p_n)R_n$
AB,ab	$(1 + s)p_nQ_n \cdot (1 - p_n)(1 - R_n) \cdot (1 - r)$
Ab,aB	$(1 - p_n)R_n \cdot (1 + s)p_n(1 - Q_n) \cdot r$

To explain the calculation, note that in the first case the offspring will always be AB. In the second and third, recombination has no effect. The offspring is AB $1/2$ of the time but there is a factor of 2 coming from the fact that the parents in the second case could be AB,aB or aB,AB. This $(1/2) \cdot 2$ occurs in the fourth and fifth cases as well. In the fourth, recombination must be avoided, while in the fifth it must occur to obtain the desired outcome. Adding up the first three rows with the part of the fourth that comes from the 1 in the $1 - r$ and then putting the rest in the second term, we have

$$(1+s)p_nQ_n \cdot ((1+s)p_n + 1 - p_n) + r(1+s)p_n(1-p_n)[R_n(1-Q_n) - Q_n(1-R_n)]$$

Dividing by the total number of offspring $(1 + p_n s)^2$, it follows that

$$p_{n+1}Q_{n+1} = \frac{(1 + s)p_nQ_n(1 + sp_n) + r(1 + s)p_n(1 - p_n)(R_n - Q_n)}{(1 + sp_n)^2}$$

Rearranging gives

(a) $$(1 + sp_n)^2 p_{n+1} Q_{n+1} =$$
$$[(1 + s)p_n \{Q_n(1 + sp_n) + r(1 - p_n)(R_n - Q_n)\}$$

(4.1) implies that

$$(1 + sp_n)^2 p_{n+1} = (1 + s)p_n(1 + sp_n)$$

Substituting this on the left-hand side of (a) and then dividing by $(1+s)p_n$, we have

(b) $$(1 + sp_n)Q_{n+1} = Q_n(1 + sp_n) + r(1 - p_n)(R_n - Q_n)$$

Considering Ab, we have

parents	number of offspring
Ab,Ab	$(1 - p_n)R_n \cdot (1 - p_n)R_n$
Ab,ab	$(1 - p_n)R_n \cdot (1 - p_n)(1 - R_n)$
Ab,AB	$(1 - p_n)R_n \cdot (1 + s)p_n Q_n$
Ab,aB	$(1 - p_n)R_n \cdot (1 + s)p_n(1 - Q_n) \cdot (1 - r)$
AB,ab	$(1 + s)p_n Q_n \cdot (1 - p_n)(1 - R_n) \cdot r$

Adding things up as before, we get

(c) $$(1 + sp_n)^2(1 - p_{n+1})R_{n+1} = (1 - p_n)R_n(1 + sp_n)$$
$$+r(1 + s)p_n(1 - p_n)(Q_n - R_n)$$

(4.1) implies that

$$(1+sp_n)^2(1-p_{n+1}) = (1+sp_n)^2 \cdot \frac{(1 + sp_n) - (1 + s)p_n}{1 + sp_n} = (1+sp_n)(1-p_n)$$

Substituting this on the left-hand side of (c) and then dividing by $(1 - p_n)$, we have

(d) $$(1 + sp_n)R_{n+1} = R_n(1 + sp_n) + r(1 + s)p_n(Q_n - R_n)$$

Subtracting (d) from (b) and then dividing by $(1 + sp_n)$ we have

$$Q_{n+1} - R_{n+1} = Q_n - R_n - \frac{r(1 - p_n) + r(1 + s)}{(1 + sp_n)}(Q_n - R_n)$$
$$= (1 - r)(Q_n - R_n)$$

proving (4.3).

If we assume that initially there is only one aB and no AB, then $Q_0 = 0$ and

(e) $$Q_n - R_n = -R_0(1 - r)^n$$

Using (b) and (e), we have

$$Q_{n+1} - Q_n = \frac{r(1 - p_n)}{1 + sp_n}R_0(1 - r)^n$$

Using (4.2) twice, we have

$$1 - p_n = \frac{1 - p_0}{1 - p_0 + p_0(1+s)^n} \qquad 1 + sp_n = \frac{1 - p_0 + p_0(1+s)^{n+1}}{1 - p_0 + p_0(1+s)^n}$$

Inserting this into the previous equation and summing, we have (4.3). $\square$

There is a different approach to this question, pioneered by Ohta and Kimura (1975) that leads to more insight. We assume that a favorable mutation B arises in the population at time $t = 0$ and is subsequently in the process of replacing allele b. As we have described in Section 2.1, the number of B's has a first phase in which it behaves like a supercritical branching process, a second in which the fraction of B's approximates the solution of the logistic differential equation, and a third in which the number of b's behaves like a subcritical branching process.

Kaplan, Hudson, and Langley (1989) incorporated these three phases into their simulation study of the impact of hitchhiking on the number of segregating sites. However, here we will simplify things by using the logistic differential equation

$$(f) \qquad\qquad \frac{dY_t}{dt} = sY_t(1 - Y_t)$$

to model the entire sweep. The solution to (f) is

$$(g) \qquad\qquad Y_t = \frac{Y_0}{Y_0 + (1 - Y_0)e^{-st}}$$

When $Y_0 = \epsilon$ the solution reaches $1/2$ at the time τ when $\epsilon = (1 - \epsilon)e^{-s\tau}$; that is, when

$$\left(\frac{1 - \epsilon}{\epsilon}\right) e^{-s\tau} = 1$$

or $\tau = (1/s)\ln((1/\epsilon) - 1)$. The solution in (g) has the symmetry property

$$(h) \qquad\qquad Y_{\tau+s} = 1 - Y_{\tau-s}$$

so it will reach $1 - \epsilon$ at time 2τ. The next graph gives a picture of Y_t when $\epsilon = 1/200$ and $s = 0.02$. In this case $\tau = 264.67$.

We conceptually divide the population into two parts: chromosomes with the advantageous mutant B and those with the disadvantageous allele b. Let $v(t)$ be the frequency of allele A in the B population and $w(t)$ be the frequency of allele A in the b population after t generations. Recombinations between chromosomes from the two populations occur at rate $rY_t(1 - Y_t)$ so we have

$$\frac{dv}{dt} = r(1 - Y_t)(w(t) - v(t))$$

$$\frac{dw}{dt} = rY_t(v(t) - w(t))$$

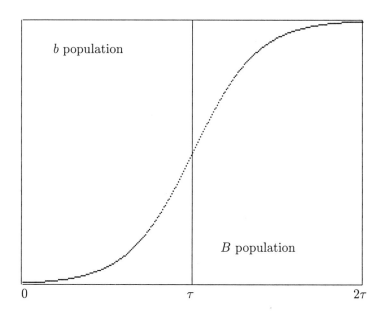

Subtracting the second equation from the first gives

$$\frac{d}{dt}(v(t) - w(t)) = -r(v(t) - w(t))$$

so we have

(i) $\qquad\qquad v(t) - w(t) = e^{-rt}(v(0) - w(0))$

which is the analogue of (4.4). Using (i) and (g) in our pair of differential equations gives

$$v(2\tau) = v(0) + r(w(0) - v(0)) \int_0^{2\tau} \frac{(1 - Y_0)e^{-st-rt}}{Y_0 + (1 - Y_0)e^{-st}} \, dt$$

$$w(2\tau) = w(0) + r(v(0) - w(0)) \int_0^{2\tau} \frac{Y_0 e^{-rt}}{Y_0 + (1 - Y_0)e^{-st}} \, dt$$

When $v(0) = 0$ and $w(0) = R_0$, the first equation becomes

(4.5) $\qquad v(2\tau) = R_0(1 - Y_0) \int_0^{2\tau} \frac{re^{-rt}}{(1 - Y_0) + Y_0 e^{st}} \, dt$

which is a close relative of the expression in (4.3). Using (i), we see that when $v(0) = 0$ and $w(0) = R_0$

$$w(2\tau) - v(2\tau) = e^{-2r\tau} R_0 = R_0 \left(\frac{\epsilon}{1 - \epsilon}\right)^{2r/s}$$

Depending on the size of r/s, this may or may not be close to 0.

Let $v_1(t)$ be the solution with $R_0 = 1$. A little thought reveals that $v_1(t)$ is the probability that the first locus of an individual in the B population comes from the b population at time 0. To get an approximation to $v_1(2\tau)$, note that the probability that a lineage will cross from the B population to the b population during the sweep is

$$(4.6) \qquad \approx r \int_0^{2\tau} 1 - Y_t \, dt = r\tau = \frac{r}{s} \ln(2N - 1)$$

since the symmetry property (h) implies

$$\int_0^\tau 1 - Y_{\tau-s} + 1 - Y_{\tau+s} \, ds = \int_0^\tau 1 \, ds$$

To judge the quality of the approximation, we consider the situation with a population size of $N = 10,000$ and selection coefficient $s = 0.01$ for various values of recombination r. The first two columns give the exact value from (4.3) and the approximation from (4.6). One can get a better approximation by noting that (4.6) counts the expected number of crossings, which has a Poisson distribution, so the probability of at least one is

$$(4.7) \qquad 1 - \exp(-(r/s)\ln(2N - 1))$$

r	(4.3)	(4.6)	(4.7)
0.0001	0.088216	0.099035	0.094289
0.0002	0.168381	0.198070	0.179687
0.0003	0.241252	0.297105	0.257034
0.0004	0.307515	0.396140	0.327087
0.0005	0.367785	0.495174	0.390535
0.0006	0.422622	0.594209	0.448001
0.0007	0.472532	0.693244	0.500048
0.0008	0.517969	0.792279	0.547188
0.0009	0.559349	0.891314	0.589883
0.0010	0.597043	0.990349	0.628553

As Kaplan, Hudson, and Langley (1989) observed in their equation (16), the heterozygosity after the sweep H_∞ is related to that before the sweep H_0 by

$$(4.8) \qquad \frac{H_\infty}{H_0} = p_{22}$$

where p_{22} is the probability that two lineages sampled from the B population at time 2τ are distinct at time 0. Since the time of the sweep is much smaller than the population size, two lineages will coalesce only if they both end up in the B population at time t. That is,

$$(4.9) \qquad p_{22} = 1 - (1 - v_1(2\tau))^2 = v_1(2\tau)(2 - v_1(2\tau))$$

which is equation (14a) of Stephan, Wiehe, and Lenz (1992).

Up to this point, we have only examined the evolutionary effect of one selective sweep. We will now consider recurring selected substitutions that occur according to a Poisson process at rate ν per nucleotide per generation. If the physical distance of a selected substitution from the neutral region is m bp, then its recombinational distance is ρm, where ρ is the recombination rate per base pair per generation. Writing $p_{22}(r, s, N)$ to display its dependence on the population parameters, we can see that the selective sweeps cause coalescence at an additional rate (per $2N$ generations) of

$$(4.10) \quad \mu = 2N \cdot 2\nu \int_0^\infty 1 - p_{22}(\rho x, s, N)\, dx = 4N \frac{\nu}{\rho} \int_0^\infty 1 - p_{22}(y, s, N)\, dy$$

so the time to coalescence has an exponential distribution with rate $1 + \mu$. A coalescence caused by a sweep forces the state of the neutral allele to be equal in the two sampled individuals, so the heterozygosity under repeated sweeps is $1/(1 + \mu)$ times that under the neutral theory. In symbols

$$(4.11) \qquad\qquad H = \frac{H_{neu}}{1 + \mu}$$

This is equation (21) of Stephan, Wiehe and Lenz (1992).

Stephan, Wiehe, and Lenz (1992) developed an approximation of p_{22}, see their (17), which allowed Wiehe and Stephan (1993) to conclude that

$$2 \int_0^\infty 1 - p_{22}(y, s, N)\, dy \approx sI$$

where $I \approx 0.075$ is a constant. Using this in (4.10) we have $\mu \approx I\alpha\nu/\rho$ where $\alpha = 2Ns$. Inserting this result into (4.11) we have

$$H \approx H_{neu} \cdot \frac{\rho}{\rho + \nu\alpha I}$$

From this it follows that

$$\frac{1}{H} = \frac{1}{H_{neu}} + \frac{\nu\alpha I}{H_{neu}} \cdot \frac{1}{\rho} = \beta_1 + \beta_2 \cdot \frac{1}{\rho}$$

Wiehe and Stephan (1993) used this relationship to fit data on 17 *Drosophila* loci from Begun and Aquadro (1992). Taking H to be the nucleotide diversity π, they found $\beta_1 = 125.54$ and $\beta_2 = 5.04 \times 10^{-7}$, which corresponds to $H_{neu} = 0.008$.

To interpret the parameters, we note that if we assume the per nucleotide mutation rate is 1×10^{-9}, then since $0.008 = H_{neu} = 4N_e\mu$, N_e is estimated to be 2×10^6. Assuming an average selective effect of 0.01, then $\alpha = 2N_e s = 4 \times 10^4$ and

$$\nu = \frac{\beta_2 H_{neu}}{I\alpha} = \frac{(5.04 \times 10^{-7}) \cdot 0.008}{0.075 \cdot 4 \times 10^4} = 1.34 \times 10^{-12}$$

Comparing this to the mutation rate 10^{-9}, we see that $1/(1.34 \times 10^{-3})$, or 1 out of every 746 mutations, are driven to fixation by selection. Aquadro,

Begun, and Kindahl (1994) repeated these calculations for 15 gene regions of the third chromosome of *Drosophila* with almost the same result.

The scheme described above can be used to understand the impact of selective sweeps on the genealogy of samples of size $n > 2$. If we let (I_t, J_t) be the number of lineages in the B and b populations respectively at time $2\tau - 4Nt$ and let $R = 4Nr$, then transitions occur at the following rates

transition	rate
$(i, j) \to (i - 1, j)$	$i(i - 1)/Y(2\tau - 4Nt)$
$(i, j) \to (i, j - 1)$	$j(j - 1)/(1 - Y(2\tau - 4Nt))$
$(i, j) \to (i - 1, j + 1)$	$iR(1 - Y(2\tau - 4Nt))$
$(i, j) \to (i + 1, j - 1)$	$jRY(2\tau - 4Nt)$

Since the chain is two-dimensional and temporally inhomogeneous, it is difficult to obtain exact results; however, we can develop the following approximation for large N.

(4.12) *Suppose there are k lineages at time 2τ. Let p be the probability in (4.6) and let $\sigma = (2/s) \ln \ln(2N)$. Each lineage flips a coin with probability p of heads to see if it crosses over to the b population. The lineages that do not cross over all coalesce between times 0 and σ. None of the ones that cross over coalesce.*

Proof. At times $t \geq \sigma$, $Y(t) \geq (\ln N)^2/2N$. The probability of a coalescence in the B population between time σ and 2τ is at most

$$\frac{2\tau}{4N} \cdot \frac{k(k - 1)}{(\ln(2N))^2/2N} \sim \frac{r}{s} \cdot \frac{k(k - 1)}{\ln(2N)} \to 0$$

In the other direction, the number of recombinations in the B population between times 0 and σ is at most

$$kr \int_0^\sigma 1 - Y_s \, ds$$

which is a small fraction of the total integral that goes into defining p. The last two calculations show that in the B population we can ignore recombinations during $[0, \sigma]$ and coalescence in $[\sigma, 2\tau]$. Similar calculations show that we can ignore recombinations in the B population in $[2\tau - \sigma, 2\tau]$ and coalescence in the b population in $[0, 2\tau - \sigma]$. Combining these facts gives the desired result. □

The error probabilities involved in (4.12) are rather large, $O(1/\ln(2N))$, so for exact results one must use numerical methods to compute the transition probability of (I_t, J_t). Braverman et al. (1995) used this technique to investigate the effect of selective sweeps on Tajima's D statistic.

4
Statistical Tests

In this chapter we will develop statistical tests designed to detect departures from "neutral evolution" where genealogies are described by the ordinary coalescent. There are two basic types of departures:

The End Comes Too Slowly. An example of this situation is

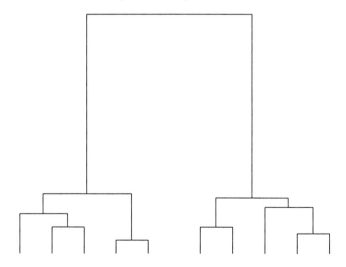

In this case, most of the mutations will have density 1/2. In less extreme situations, there will simply be an excess of mutations at intermediate frequencies. In Section 2.3, we saw that this can be caused by population subdivision. In Section 3.2, we saw that balancing selection can also cause this pattern.

The End Comes Too Quickly. An example of this situation is a *star-shaped* genealogy:

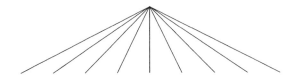

In this case, all of the mutations are singletons. In less extreme situations, there will simply be an excess of rare mutations. In Section 2.1, we saw that this can be caused by exponential growth in the population. In Section 3.1, we saw that a selective sweep can also cause this pattern.

4.1 Tajima's D Statistic

Once one has two ways of estimating the same thing, one can construct a hypothesis test by taking their difference. Tajima (1989) noticed that using the estimate Δ_n of $\theta = 4Nu$ based on pairwise differences and the estimate $\hat{\theta}$ based on the number of segregating sites from Section 1.4, one can define

$$d = \Delta_n - \hat{\theta}$$

with $Ed = 0$.

Our next step is to normalize the statistic d by dividing by its standard deviation in order to make the variance of d equal to 1. The main motivation for doing this is to try to make the distribution of the statistic independent of the unknown mutation rate θ. Recalling $\hat{\theta} = S_n/a_1$ and $a_1 = \sum_{i=1}^{n-1} 1/i$, we have

$$(1.1) \qquad \operatorname{var}(d) = \operatorname{var}(\Delta_n) - \frac{2}{a_1}\operatorname{cov}(S, \Delta_n) + \frac{1}{a_1^2}\operatorname{var}(S_n)$$

If we let $a_2 = \sum_{i=1}^{n-1} 1/i^2$, then (4.9) in Chapter 1 implies that

$$(1.2) \qquad \operatorname{var}(S_n) = a_1\theta + a_2\theta^2$$

From (4.6) in Chapter 1, we have $\operatorname{var}(\Delta_n) = b_1\theta + b_2\theta^2$, where

$$(1.3) \qquad b_1 = \frac{n+1}{3(n-1)} \quad \text{and} \quad b_2 = \frac{2(n^2+n+3)}{9n(n-1)}$$

Our next step is to compute the missing term

(1.4)
$$\mathrm{cov}\,(S_n, \Delta_n) = \theta + \left(\frac{1}{2} + \frac{1}{n}\right)\theta^2$$

Proof. We will proceed by induction on n. When $n = 2$, $S_2 = \Delta_2$ so

$$\mathrm{cov}\,(S_2, \Delta_2) = \mathrm{var}\,(S_2) = \theta + \theta^2$$

by (1.2), which agrees with the formula in (1.4).

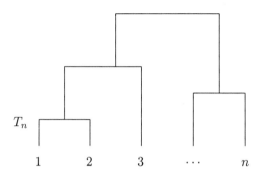

To do the inductive step, let T_n be the time of the first coalescence event and suppose that this event involves individuals 1 and 2. Let n_i be the number of mutations that occur on lineage i before time T_n, and let $s_n = \sum_{j=1}^{n} n_j$ be the total number of segregating sites created by time T_n. The total number of segregating sites for the sample of size n has

$$S_n = s_n + S_{n-1}$$

where S_{n-1} is the number that occur to the sample of size $n-1$ after time T_n. Since a pair of randomly chosen individuals has probability $1/\binom{n}{2}$ to be $\{1, 2\}$, we have

(a)
$$\mathrm{cov}\,(S_n, \Delta_n) = \frac{1}{\binom{n}{2}}\mathrm{cov}\,(S_n, n_1 + n_2) + \left(1 - \frac{1}{\binom{n}{2}}\right)\mathrm{cov}\,(S_n, \Delta_{ij})$$

where $\{i, j\} \neq \{1, 2\}$. To evaluate the first term, we note that

$$\mathrm{cov}\,(S_n, n_1 + n_2) = \mathrm{cov}\,(s_n, n_1 + n_2) = \mathrm{var}\,(n_1 + n_2) + \sum_{j=3}^{n}\mathrm{cov}\,(n_1 + n_2, n_j)$$

For the second term, we let Δ_{ij}^{n-1} be the number of pairwise difference on the i and j lineages after time T_n and note that what happens before T_n is uncorrelated with what happens after T_n so

$$\mathrm{cov}\,(S_n, \Delta_{ij}) = \mathrm{cov}\,(S_{n-1}, \Delta_{ij}^{n-1}) + \mathrm{cov}\,(s_n, n_i + n_j)$$

To evaluate the second term we note that symmetry implies

$$\text{cov}(s_n, n_i + n_j) = \text{cov}(s_n, n_1 + n_2)$$

Combining the last three equations with (a), we have $\text{cov}(S_n, \Delta_n) =$

(b) $\left(1 - \dfrac{1}{\binom{n}{2}}\right) \text{cov}(S_{n-1}, \Delta_{n-1}) + \text{var}(n_1 + n_2) + 2(n - 2)\text{cov}(n_1, n_2)$

It remains to compute $\text{var}(n_1 + n_2)$ and $\text{cov}(n_1, n_2)$. We can do this by generalizing (d)–(h) of the proof of (4.6) in Chapter 1. To compute the mean of n_i, note that in units of $2N$ generations the time of the first coalescence T_n has an exponential distribution with mean $1/\binom{n}{2}$, and that mutations occur at rate $2N\mu = \theta/2$, so if we condition on the time T_n then the number of mutations is Poisson with mean $T_n\theta/2$.

(c) $$E(n_i | T_n) = T_n\, \theta/2$$

and hence

(d) $$E n_i = \frac{\theta}{2} E T_n = \frac{\theta}{2} \cdot \frac{1}{\binom{n}{2}}$$

To compute the variance of n_i we recall that if Z has a Poisson distribution with mean λ, then $E Z^2 = \lambda + \lambda^2$ so

$$E(n_i^2 | T_2) = T_n\, \theta/2 + (T_n\, \theta/2)^2$$

Recalling that if X has an exponential distribution with mean μ then $E X^2 = 2\mu^2$, we have

(e) $$E(n_i^2) = \frac{\theta}{2} \cdot \frac{1}{\binom{n}{2}} + \frac{\theta^2}{4} \cdot \frac{2}{\binom{n}{2}^2}$$

Combining (d) and (e), it follows that

(f) $$\text{var}(n_i) = E(n_i^2) - (E n_i)^2 = \frac{\theta}{2} \cdot \frac{1}{\binom{n}{2}} + \frac{\theta^2}{4} \cdot \frac{1}{\binom{n}{2}^2}$$

Since n_1 and n_2 are conditionally independent given T_n we have

$$E(n_1\, n_2 | T_n) = \left(\frac{T_n\, \theta}{2}\right)^2$$

and hence

(g) $$E(n_1\, n_2) = \frac{\theta^2}{4} \cdot \frac{2}{\binom{n}{2}^2}$$

From this and (d), it follows that

(h) $$\text{cov}(n_1, n_2) = \frac{\theta^2}{4} \cdot \frac{1}{\binom{n}{2}^2}$$

so using (f) and (h) we have

$$(i) \quad \mathrm{var}\,(n_1 + n_2) = 2\,\mathrm{var}\,(n_1) + 2\,\mathrm{cov}\,(n_1, n_2) = \theta \cdot \frac{1}{\binom{n}{2}} + \theta^2 \cdot \frac{1}{\binom{n}{2}^2}$$

Combining (h), (i), (b), and the induction hypothesis,

$$\mathrm{cov}\,(S_n, \Delta_n) = \left(1 - \frac{1}{\binom{n}{2}}\right)\left(\theta + \left(\frac{1}{2} + \frac{1}{n-1}\right)\theta^2\right)$$

$$+ \theta \frac{1}{\binom{n}{2}} + \theta^2 \frac{1}{\binom{n}{2}^2} + 2(n-2)\frac{\theta^2}{4}\frac{1}{\binom{n}{2}^2}$$

The coefficient of θ on the right-hand side is 1. Combining the last two terms, we see that the coefficient of θ^2 is

$$\left(1 - \frac{2}{n(n-1)}\right)\left(\frac{1}{2} + \frac{1}{n-1}\right) + \frac{2n}{4} \cdot \frac{4}{n^2(n-1)^2}$$

Multiplying out the first term and simplifying the second gives

$$\frac{1}{2} - \frac{1}{n(n-1)} + \frac{1}{n-1} - \frac{2}{n(n-1)^2} + \frac{2}{n(n-1)^2} = \frac{1}{2} + \frac{1}{n}$$

completing the proof.   □

Combining (1.1)–(1.4), it follows that

$$\mathrm{var}\,(d) = c_1\theta + c_2\theta^2$$

where

$$c_1 = b_1 - \frac{1}{a_1} \quad \text{and} \quad c_2 = b_2 - \frac{n+2}{a_1 n} + \frac{a_2}{a_1^2}$$

To estimate θ in this expression, we will use $\hat{\theta} = S_n/a_1$. To deal with θ^2, we note that

$$E S_n^2 - E S_n = \mathrm{var}\,(S_n) - E S_n + (E S_n)^2 = (a_2 + a_1^2)\theta^2$$

so θ^2 can be estimated by $S_n(S_n - 1)/(a_2 + a_1^2)$ and the variance of d by

$$\widehat{\mathrm{var}}\,(d) = e_1 S_n + e_2 S_n(S_n - 1)$$

where $e_1 = c_1/a_1$ and $e_2 = c_2/(a_1^2 + a_2)$. This computation suggests the definition of a new statistic

$$D = d/\sqrt{\widehat{\mathrm{var}}\,(d)} = \frac{\Delta_n - S_n/a_1}{\sqrt{e_1 S_n + e_2 S_n(S_n - 1)}}$$

which is normalized to have variance ≈ 1.

There are no analytical results for the distribution of D, so to develop a hypothesis test Tajima had to use simulation. He first generated the genealogical relationship between the individuals but not the coalescence times by at each stage picking a pair of particles to coalesce. (4.10) in Chapter 1 shows that the number of mutations s_j that occur when there are j lineages has a shifted geometric distribution. Once Tajima decided on the number of mutations s_j, he sent each one to one of the j lineages chosen at random. For more details, see pages 588–589 of Tajima (1989). On the basis of these simulations, Tajima argued that D had approximately a beta distribution with parameters that he calculated from the minimum and maximum possible values of D. Using his approximating beta distribution, he then calculated the percentiles of the D statistic that are given in the table on his page 592.

Example 1.1. We begin by considering the mtDNA example of Aquadro and Greenberg (1983). In Examples 4.1 and 4.2 of Chapter 1, we computed that the estimates of θ based on Δ_7 and $S_7 = 44$ are 14.66 and 17.95. Using a small computer program, one can compute

$$
\begin{aligned}
a_1 &= 2.450000 & a_2 &= 1.491389 \\
b_1 &= 0.444444 & b_2 &= 0.312169 \\
c_1 &= 0.036281 & c_2 &= 0.035849 \\
e_1 &= 0.014809 & e_2 &= 0.004784
\end{aligned}
$$

and $\sqrt{\widehat{\operatorname{var}(d)}} = 3.114888$, so

$$
D = \frac{14.66 - 17.95}{3.114888} = -1.0562
$$

The negative value of D is consistent with the idea that an expansion of the human population might have produced an excess of rare alleles. However, from Table 2 on page 592 of Tajima (1989), we see that the 90% confidence interval for D in the case $n = 7$ is $(-1.498, 1.728)$, so this value of D is not significant.

Example 1.2. Duchene muscular dystrophy is a common inherited disease with an incidence worldwide of 1 in 3500 births. The Dmd locus is about 2.4 megabase long and consists of 79 exons that code for a 3685 amino acid protein called dystrophin. Dmd is on the X chromosome in a genomic region that experiences high rates of recombination. Fine scale mapping of the region reveals overall recombination frequencies of 12% across 2 Mb of DNA roughly six times the average value of 1 cM/Mb across the human genome. Nachman and Crowell (2000) studied parts of introns 7 and 44 in a worldwide sample of 41 alleles. In intron 7, they sequenced 2389 bp and observed the results given in the next table. The last two rows give the sequence from a single male common chimpanzee (*Pan troglodytes*) and a single male orangutan (*Pongo pygmaeus*).

Ignoring the insertion-deletion polymorphisms, there are 9 segregating sites, i.e., $S_{41} = 9$. $\sum_{i=1}^{40} 1/i = 4.278543$ so our estimate of θ based on the number of segregating sites is 2.103520. To compute the number of pairwise differences we note that in seven cases the mutant is a singleton, i.e., a $40 - 1$ split in the data, while in the other two cases the splits are $35 - 6$ and $36 - 5$. From this we see that the estimate of θ based on pairwise differences is

$$\Delta_{41} = \frac{7 \cdot 40 \cdot 1 + 35 \cdot 6 + 36 \cdot 5}{\binom{41}{2}} = \frac{670}{820} = 0.817073$$

Dividing by 2389 bp gives an estimate of the nucleotide diversity of $\pi = 0.0342\%$, considerably smaller than the value of 0.11% found by Li and Sadler (1991) at fourfold degenerate sites.

no.	0 1 4 5	0 2 2 5	0 2 6 8	0 5 1 0	0 5 5 1	0 6 8 8	1 2 9 9	0 4 8 1	0 5 4 0	0 6 3 4	0 7 1 1	0 9 2 5
30	A	T	A	A	-	T	T	A	-	T	G	G
1	.	G	G	.	G	.	.	T	A	.	.	.
1	.	.	G	.	G	.	.	T	A	C	.	.
1	.	.	G	.	G	.	.	T	A	.	.	.
1	.	.	G	.	G	X	.	T	A	.	.	.
1	.	.	.	.	.	.	.	T	A	.	.	.
1	.	.	G	.	.	.	.	.	.	.	.	A
1	.	.	.	.	.	.	.	.	.	.	A	.
1	.	.	.	.	.	.	C	.	.	.	.	.
1	G	.	.	.	.	.	.	.	.	.	.	.
1	.	.	G	.	.	.	.	.	.	.	.	.
1	.	.	.	G	.	.	.	.	.	.	.	.
Pan	.	.	G	.	G	.	.	C	.	.	.	.
Pongo	.	.	G	.	G	.	C	T	.	.	A	.

X = deletion of $TTAAG$

Using a small computer program, one can compute

$$a_1 = 4.278543 \qquad a_2 = 1.620244$$
$$b_1 = 0.350000 \qquad b_2 = 0.233740$$
$$c_1 = 0.116276 \qquad c_2 = 0.077123$$
$$e_1 = 0.027176 \qquad e_2 = 0.003870$$

and $\sqrt{\widehat{\text{var}}(d)} = 0.723368$, so

$$D = \frac{0.817073 - 2.103520}{0.723368} = -1.778413$$

The negative value of D is consistent with the idea that a recent selective sweep near intron 7 may have reduced variability there. From Table 2 on page 592 of Tajima (1989), we see that the 95% confidence interval is $(-1.803, 2.034)$ so the value of D is just barely not significant. It is interesting to note that Table 4 of Nachman and Crowell (2000) reports $p < 0.05$ based on their computed value of $D = -1.79$.

Example 1.3. Przeworski, Hudson, and DiRienzo (2000) have collected the results of a number of uses of Tajima's D statistic. Here n is the number of chromosomes in the sample, π is the estimate of the nucleotide diversity, and θ_W is Watterson's estimate of θ, S/a_n scaled by dividing by the number of nucleotides sequenced to make its units, like those of π, to be percentages.

Region	chr.	n	bp	S	π	θ_W	D
β-globin	11	349	2670	19	0.157	0.110	1.06
PDHA1	X	35	4200	24	0.178	0.139	0.97
Dys44	X	250	7622	34	0.093	0.073	0.74
LPL	8	142	9700	79	0.166	0.149	0.36
ACE	17	22	24,000	74	0.091	0.085	0.32
MC1R	16	242	951	6	0.114	0.104	0.19
DMD44	X	41	3000	19	0.141	0.148	-0.15
APOE	19	192	5491	22	0.053	0.069	-0.62
ZFX	X	336	1089	10	0.082	0.144	-0.94
Xq13.3	X	70	10,163	33	0.033	0.067	-1.62

Most of the values of π are consistent with Li and Sadler's 0.11%. However, those of Xq13.3 (0.033) and APOE (0.053) are somewhat lower, while those of PDHA1 (0.178) and LPL (0.166) are somewhat higher. In no case is the value of Tajima's D significantly different from 0. Note that six values are positive while four are negative. In particular, these values do not show the signature of a population expansion.

Example 1.4. The last conclusion fits with Hey's (1997) observation that mitochondrial and nuclear genes present conflicting portraits of human history. His study focused on four loci:

		n	bp	π	D
mtDNA	COII	6	684	0.34	-1.397
mtDNA	control region	189	764	1.75	-1.755
nuclear	β-globin	60	3000	0.18	1.491
nuclear	PDHA1	8	1769	0.113	1.406

For each of the mtDNA data sets, there is an excess of low-frequency polymorphisms and D is negative, consistent with patterns expected in an expanding population. However, the positive values from nuclear genes suggest that human populations were relatively large and not subject to bottlenecks during the time that human ancestors evolved to modern form.

As Hey explains, natural selection at either nuclear or mitochondrial genes could be responsible for the observed differences. For example, balancing selection at nuclear genes will increase the levels of intermediate-frequency polymorphisms. In mtDNA, there is no recombination, so natural selection cannot act as effectively to eliminate deleterious mutations. These mutations are expected to create a background selection effect simultaneously knocking down the effective population size and shifting the site frequency distribution toward an excess of the high-low pattern, as observed.

4.2   Fu and Li's D

Fu and Li (1993) defined a branch of a genealogy to be external if it directly connects to an external node. Other branches are called internal.

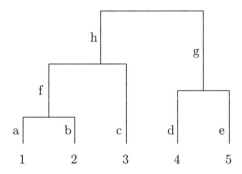

In the picture, a, b, c, d, and e are external branches, while f, g, and h are internal branches. In general, if we have a genealogy of n individuals then there are n external branches and $n - 2$ internal branches.

Following the notation in Fu and Li (1993), let η_e and η_i be the number of mutations that take place on external and internal branches. To compute the expected values of η_e and η_i, we begin by letting

$$
\begin{aligned}
J_n &= \text{the total length of all branches} \\
I_n &= \text{the total length of internal branches} \\
L_n &= \text{the total length of external branches}
\end{aligned}
$$

To remove the population size from our calculations we will suppose that all of these quantities are written in units of $2N_e$ generations. Letting $\theta = 4N_e\mu$ be the rescaled mutation rate, it follows that

(2.1) $E(\eta_e|L_n) = (\theta/2)L_n$ $E(\eta_i|I_n) = (\theta/2)I_n$

Returning to the two pictures at the beginning of the chapter, in the star-shaped phylogeny all branches are external, while in the slow coalescence example L_n is small compared to I_n. Thus, Fu and Li hope to identify departures from neutral evolution by comparing the size of η_e and η_i.

The first step in formulating a test statistic is to compute the expected values of L_n and I_n, and hence using (2.1) the expected values of η_e and η_i. Let $\ell_{n,k}$ be the length of the external branch ending at the kth individual in the sample, let K be uniformly distributed on $\{1, 2, \ldots, n\}$, and let $\ell_n = \ell_{n,K}$ denote the length of a randomly chosen external branch. Clearly

$$(2.2) \qquad EL_n = \sum_{k=1}^{n} E\ell_{n,k} = nE\ell_n$$

Let t_n be exponential with rate $\binom{n}{2}$. The genealogy of a sample of size n can be generated from that of a sample of size $n-1$ by adding two external branches of length t_n to the end of a randomly chosen external branch and extending the other $n-2$ external branches by t_n. If we do this, then

$$(\star) \qquad \ell_n = \begin{cases} t_n & \text{with probability } 2/n \\ \ell_{n-1} + t_n & \text{with probability } (n-2)/n \end{cases}$$

From this, it follows that

$$E\ell_n = Et_n + \frac{n-2}{n}E\ell_{n-1}$$

To solve this recursion, we recall $Et_n = 2/n(n-1)$, let $g_n = n(n-1)\ell_n$, and multiply the last equation by $n(n-1)$ to get

$$Eg_n = 2 + Eg_{n-1}$$

Since $\ell_2 = t_2$ has $E\ell_2 = 1$, $Eg_2 = 2$. Using this with the recursion we see that $Eg_n = 2(n-1)$ and $E\ell_n = 2/n$. Using (2.2) and (2.1) now we have

$$(2.3) \qquad EL_n = 2 \qquad E\eta_e = \theta$$

In words, the expected number of external mutations is independent of the sample size.

To compute the other expected values, we note that (4.7) in Chapter 1 implies

$$(2.4) \qquad EJ_n = 2a_n \qquad \text{where } a_n = \sum_{i=1}^{n-1} \frac{1}{i}$$

Subtracting (2.3) from this and using (2.1), we have

$$(2.5) \qquad EI_n = 2a_n - 2 \qquad E\eta_i = \theta(a_n - 1)$$

Comparing (2.5) and (2.3) shows that

$$d = \eta_i - (a_n - 1)\eta_e$$

has $Ed = 0$.

As in the case of Tajima's D, our test statistic will be the standardized variable

$$D = \frac{d}{\sqrt{\text{var}\,(d)}}$$

Thus, our next task is to compute $\text{var}(\eta_i - (a_n - 1)\eta_e)$. This calculation is a little tedious, so the reader should feel free to skip ahead to the answer given in (2.6). One reason for giving the details is to correct an error in Fu and Li (1993). See (k) and (ℓ) below. This should not be viewed as an indictment of these two authors. Many times I found errors in my own computation by comparing my formulas to theirs.

To begin, we note that the derivation of (4.7) in Chapter 1 shows that

$$J_n = \sum_{j=2}^{n} j\xi_j$$

where the ξ_j are independent exponentials with rate $\binom{j}{2}$. Elementary probability tells us that the variance of ξ_j is $4/j^2(j-1)^2$. Using the facts that $\text{var}(cX) = c^2 \text{var}(X)$ and the variance of a sum of independent random variables is the sum of the variances, we have

(a)
$$\text{var}(J_n) = \sum_{j=2}^{n} \frac{4}{(j-1)^2} = 4b_n$$

To compute the variance of L_n, we begin with the observation that (2.2) implies

(b)
$$E(L_n^2) = nE(\ell_n^2) + n(n-1)E(\ell_n\ell_n')$$

where ℓ_n and ℓ_n' are two different randomly chosen external branches. To compute the first term on the right-hand side, we note that $(\star)$ implies

$$
\begin{aligned}
E\ell_n^2 &= \frac{2}{n}Et_n^2 + \frac{n-2}{n}E(t_n + \ell_{n-1})^2 \\
&= Et_n^2 + \frac{2(n-2)}{n}Et_n \cdot E\ell_{n-1} + \frac{n-2}{n}E\ell_{n-1}^2
\end{aligned}
$$

Recalling that $Et_n = 2/n(n-1)$, $Et_n^2 = 2\cdot4/n^2(n-1)^2$, $E\ell_{n-1} = 2/(n-1)$, introducing $g_n = n(n-1)\ell_n^2$, and multiplying the previous equation by $n(n-1)$, we have

$$Eg_n = \frac{8}{n(n-1)} + \frac{2(n-2)}{n}\cdot 2 \cdot \frac{2}{n-1} + Eg_{n-1}$$

The above simplifies to

$$Eg_n = \frac{8}{n} + Eg_{n-1}$$

Noting that $Eg_2 = 2E\ell_2^2 = Et_2^2 = 4 = \frac{8}{2}$, we have

$$Eg_n = 8\sum_{k=2}^{n}\frac{1}{k} = 8(a_{n+1} - 1)$$

and it follows that

$$(c) \qquad E\ell_n^2 = \frac{8(a_{n+1} - 1)}{n(n-1)}$$

Turning to $E(\ell_n \ell_n')$ and using $(\star)$, we see that

$\ell_n \ell_n' =$	with probability
t_n^2	$2/n(n-1)$
$(\ell_{n-1} + t_n)t_n$	$2(n-2)/n(n-1)$
$t_n(\ell_{n-1}' + t_n)$	$2(n-2)/n(n-1)$
$(\ell_{n-1} + t_n)(\ell_{n-1}' + t_n)$	$(n-2)(n-3)/n(n-1)$

Collecting like terms, we have

$$E(\ell_n \ell_n') = Et_n^2 + \frac{(n-2)}{n(n-1)}(4 + 2(n-3))Et_n E\ell_{n-1}$$
$$+ \frac{(n-2)(n-3)}{n(n-1)}E\ell_{n-1}\ell_{n-1}'$$

Recalling that $Et_n = 2/n(n-1)$, $Et_n^2 = 2 \cdot 4/n^2(n-1)^2$, and $E\ell_{n-1} = 2/(n-1)$, we have

$$E(\ell_n \ell_n') = \frac{8}{n^2(n-1)^2} + \frac{2(n-2)}{n^2(n-1)^2} \cdot 4 + \frac{(n-2)(n-3)}{n(n-1)}E\ell_{n-1}\ell_{n-1}'$$

Introducing $g_n = n(n-1)\ell_n \ell_n'/4$, we have

$$Eg_n = \frac{2}{n} + \frac{n-3}{n-1}Eg_{n-1}$$

This implies $Eg_3 = 2/3$. Iterating gives

$$
\begin{aligned}
Eg_n &= \frac{2}{n} + \frac{n-3}{n-1}Eg_{n-1} \\
&= \frac{2}{n} + \frac{n-3}{n-1}\left(\frac{2}{n-1} + \frac{n-4}{n-2}Eg_{n-2}\right) \\
&= \frac{2}{n} + \frac{2(n-3)}{(n-1)^2} + \frac{(n-3)(n-4)}{(n-1)(n-2)} \cdot \frac{2}{n-2} + \frac{(n-4)(n-5)}{(n-1)(n-2)} \cdot Eg_{n-3}
\end{aligned}
$$

To see the pattern we iterate once more and rewrite the first two terms

$$\frac{(n-1)(n-2)}{(n-1)(n-2)} \cdot \frac{2}{n} + \frac{(n-2)(n-3)}{(n-1)(n-2)} \cdot \frac{2}{n-1} + \frac{(n-3)(n-4)}{(n-1)(n-2)} \cdot \frac{2}{n-2}$$
$$+ \frac{(n-4)(n-5)}{(n-1)(n-2)} \cdot \frac{2}{n-3} + \frac{(n-5)(n-6)}{(n-1)(n-2)} \cdot Eg_{n-4}$$

When we finally reach $Eg_3 = 2/3$, its coefficient is $2 \cdot 1/(n-1)(n-2)$. Using this and noting that the first two terms of the sum below are 0, we can rewrite the above as

$$= \frac{1}{(n-1)(n-2)} \sum_{k=1}^{n} (k-1)(k-2) \cdot \frac{2}{k}$$

$$= \frac{2}{(n-1)(n-2)} \sum_{k=1}^{n} k - 3 + \frac{2}{k}$$

Using the fact that $\sum_{k=1}^{n} k = n(n+1)/2$ and $\sum_{k=1}^{n} 1/k = a_{n+1}$, we have

(d) $\qquad E(\ell_n \ell'_n) = \frac{8}{n(n-1)^2(n-2)} \left(\frac{n(n+1)}{2} - 3n + 2a_{n+1} \right)$

Using (d) and (c) in (b), we have

$$EL_n^2 = \frac{8(a_{n+1} - 1)}{n-1} + \frac{8}{(n-1)(n-2)} \left(\frac{n(n+1)}{2} - 3n + 2a_{n+1} \right)$$

Using (2.3) now and doing some algebra gives

$$\begin{aligned} \text{var}\,(L_n) &= EL_n^2 - (EL_n)^2 \\ &= \frac{8(a_{n+1} - 1)}{n-1} + \frac{4}{(n-1)(n-2)} (n^2 - 5n + 4a_{n+1}) - 4 \end{aligned}$$

Combining things over a common denominator of $(n-1)(n-2)$ we have

$$\frac{8(n-2)a_{n+1} - 8(n-2) + 4n^2 - 20n + 16a_{n+1} - 4(n^2 - 3n + 2)}{(n-1)(n-2)}$$

$$= \frac{8na_{n+1} - 16n + 8}{(n-1)(n-2)}$$

Using $a_{n+1} = a_n + (1/n)$ now, we have

(e) $\qquad \text{var}\,(L_n) = \frac{8na_n - 16n + 16}{(n-1)(n-2)}$

With this in hand, we are ready to compute the variance of η_e. The conditional distribution of η_e given L_n is Poisson with mean $(\theta/2)L_n$. From this and formulas for the moments of the Poisson distribution, we have $E(\eta_e|L_n) = (\theta/2)L_n$ and

$$E(\eta_e^2|L_n) = (\theta/2)L_n + (\theta/2)^2 L_n^2$$

Taking the expected value, we have

$$\text{var}\,(\eta_e) = E(\eta_e^2) - (E\eta_e)^2 = (\theta/2)EL_n + (\theta/2)^2\,\text{var}\,(L_n)$$

Using (2.3) and (e) now, we have

(f) $\qquad \text{var}\,(\eta_e) = \theta + c_n\theta^2 \quad \text{where} \quad c_n = \frac{2na_n - 4(n-1)}{(n-1)(n-2)}$

From (4.9) in Chapter 1, the number of segregating sites $S_n = \eta_e + \eta_i$ has

(g) $\qquad\qquad\qquad \text{var}\,(S_n) = \theta a_n + \theta^2 b_n$

where $b_n = \sum_{i=1}^{n-1} 1/i^2$. Using $\eta_i = S_n - \eta_e$, elementary probability tells us that

$$(h) \qquad \text{var}(\eta_i) = \text{var}(S_n) - 2\,\text{cov}(\eta_i, \eta_e) - \text{var}(\eta_e)$$

To complete the computation of $\text{var}(d) = \text{var}(\eta_i - (a_n - 1)\eta_e)$, it suffices to compute $\text{cov}(\eta_i, \eta_e)$. Conditioning on the values of I_n and L_n, we have

$$
\begin{aligned}
\text{cov}(\eta_i, \eta_e) &= E(\eta_i \eta_e) - E(\eta_i)E(\eta_e) \\
&= (\theta/2)^2 E(I_n L_n) - (\theta/2)EI_n \cdot (\theta/2)EL_n \\
&= (\theta/2)^2 \text{cov}(I_n, L_n)
\end{aligned}
$$

To compute $\text{cov}(I_n, L_n) = E(I_n L_n) - EI_n \cdot EL_n$, we note that $I_n = J_n - L_n$ so

$$E(I_n L_n) - EI_n EL_n = E(J_n L_n) - EL_n^2 - EJ_n EL_n + (EL_n)^2$$

Combining the last two formulas, we have

$$(i) \qquad \text{cov}(\eta_i, \eta_e) = \left(\frac{\theta}{2}\right)^2 \cdot (E(J_n L_n) - EJ_n EL_n - \text{var}(L_n))$$

In view of (2.3), (2.4), and (e), it remains to evaluate $E(J_n L_n)$. To do this, we return to our recursion:

$$J_n = J_{n-1} + nt_n \qquad L_n = L_{n-1} - \ell_{n-1} + nt_n$$

for $n \geq 3$. Multiplying the last two expressions we have

$$
\begin{aligned}
E(J_n L_n) &= E(J_{n-1}(L_{n-1} - \ell_{n-1})) + nEt_n E(L_{n-1} - \ell_{n-1}) \\
&\quad + nEJ_{n-1}Et_n + n^2 E(t_n^2)
\end{aligned}
$$

Since ℓ_{n-1} is one of the $n-1$ external branches chosen at random, we have $E(L_{n-1} - \ell_{n-1}) = \frac{n-2}{n-1}EL_{n-1}$, and

$$E(J_{n-1}(L_{n-1} - \ell_{n-1})|J_{n-1}, L_{n-1}) = \frac{n-2}{n-1}J_{n-1}L_{n-1}$$

Taking expected values and using $Et_n = 2/n(n-1)$, $Et_n^2 = 4/n^2(n-1)^2$, with $EJ_{n-1} = 2a_{n-1}$ and $EL_{n-1} = 2$, which come from (2.3) and (2.4), gives

$$
\begin{aligned}
E(J_n L_n) &= \frac{n-2}{n-1}E(J_{n-1}L_{n-1}) + \frac{2}{n-1} \cdot \frac{n-2}{n-1} \cdot 2 \\
&\quad + n \cdot 2a_{n-1} \cdot \frac{2}{n(n-1)} + n^2 \cdot \frac{4}{n^2(n-1)^2}
\end{aligned}
$$

Letting $g_n = (n-1)J_n L_n$ and multiplying the last equation by $(n-1)$, we have

$$(j) \qquad Eg_n = Eg_{n-1} + 4a_{n-1} + \frac{4(n-2)+4}{n-1} = Eg_{n-1} + 4(a_{n-1}+1)$$

When $n = 2$, $g_2 = E(J_2 L_2) = E(J_2^2) = 4 \cdot 2$. Using this with the recursion in (j), we have

$$Eg_n = 8 + 4 \sum_{k=2}^{n-1} (a_k + 1) = 4n + 4 \sum_{k=2}^{n-1} \sum_{j=1}^{k-1} \frac{1}{j}$$

Interchanging the order of the double sum gives

$$4 \sum_{j=1}^{n-2} \frac{1}{j} \sum_{k=j+1}^{n-1} 1 = 4 \sum_{j=1}^{n-2} \frac{n-1-j}{j} = 4(n-1)a_{n-1} - 4(n-2)$$

Combining the last two formulas gives $Eg_n = 4(n-1)a_{n-1} + 8$. Using $a_{n-1} = a_n - 1/(n-1)$, we have

(k) $$E(J_n L_n) = \frac{4((n-1)a_n + 1)}{n-1}$$

In contrast, formula (37) of Fu and Li (1993) says

(ℓ) $$E(J_n L_n) = \frac{4na_n}{n-1}$$

To translate this into our notation, observe that their $M = 4N_e$ (see their page 694) while our times are in units of $2N_e$ generations. This discrepancy arises from the fact that Fu and Li's recursion is not (j) but is

$$Eg_n = Eg_{n-1} + 4(a_n + 1)$$

To suppress the difference between our result and Fu and Li's we will let $e_n = E(J_n L_n)/4$. Using this in (i) with (e), (f) gives

(m) $$\operatorname{cov}(\eta_i, \eta_e) = \left(\frac{\theta}{2}\right)^2 \cdot (4e_n - 4a_n - 4c_n)$$

It remains to put the pieces together. Recalling that $d = \eta_i - (a_n - 1)\eta_e$, we have

$$\operatorname{var}(d) = \operatorname{var}(\eta_i) - (a_n - 1)2\operatorname{cov}(\eta_i, \eta_e) + (a_n - 1)^2 \operatorname{var}(\eta_e)$$

(h) tells us that $\operatorname{var}(\eta_i) = \operatorname{var}(S_n) - 2\operatorname{cov}(\eta_i, \eta_e) - \operatorname{var}(\eta_e)$ so we have

$$\operatorname{var}(d) = \operatorname{var}(S_n) - 2a_n \operatorname{cov}(\eta_i, \eta_e) + (a_n^2 - 2a_n)\operatorname{var}(\eta_e)$$

Using (g), (m), and (f) now gives

$$\begin{aligned}
\operatorname{var}(d) &= \theta a_n + \theta^2 b_n - 2a_n \theta^2(e_n - a_n - c_n) + (a_n^2 - 2a_n)(\theta + c_n \theta^2) \\
&= a_n(a_n - 1)\theta + \theta^2 [b_n + a_n(a_n - 2)c_n - 2a_n(e_n - a_n - c_n)]
\end{aligned}$$

Neatening things up a little, we have

(2.6) $$\operatorname{var}(d) = a_n(a_n - 1)\theta + \theta^2 [b_n + a_n^2 c_n - 2a_n(e_n - a_n)]$$

If we use Fu and Li's formula for e_n given in $(ℓ)$, $e_n - a_n = a_n/(n-1)$ and this reduces to their formula (31).

As in the case of Tajima's D, θ and θ^2 have to be estimated. Using the approach in Section 4.1 but writing it in the new notation, we let $\eta = \eta_e + \eta_i$ be the number of segregating sites and estimate θ by η/a_n, θ^2 by $\eta(\eta-1)/(a_n^2+b_n)$. Plugging these estimates into (2.6) and using Fu and Li's formula for e_n, we have that

$$D_{FL} = \frac{\eta - a_n\eta_e}{\sqrt{u_D\eta + v_D\eta^2}}$$

where v_D is given in Fu and Li's Table 1 and $u_D = a_n - 1 - v_D$. Since Fu and Li's formula for e_n is not correct, $\text{var}(D_{FL})$ is not exactly one. Fortunately, for the applications that have been made of this test, this is not important. Even though Fu and Li's normalization is not quite correct, one can use D_{FL} and the values in their Table 2 to perform their test. In connection with that table we should note that even if the normalization were correct, then the distribution of the test statistic would depend on θ. According to page 699 of Fu and Li (1993), the actual percentage points cannot be larger than the nominal levels given as long as the actual θ falls into the interval $[2, 20]$.

Example 2.1. Hamblin and Aquadro (1996) studied DNA sequence variation at the *glucose dehydrogenase (Gld)* locus in *Drosophila simulans*. The *Gld* locus is near the centromere of chromosome 3 in a region of low recombination. Hamblin and Aquadro sequenced 970 nucleotides from exon 4 from 11 *D. simulans* chromosomes sampled from a population in Raleigh, N.C. These 11 sequences and that of one *D. melanogaster* individual are given in the table above. As usual, dots in columns 2–11 indicate that the sequence agrees with individual 1. Here, the *D. melanogaster* sequence serves as an "outgroup."

These two *Drosophila* species diverged about 2.5 million years ago, which is about 25 million generations. Since a typical estimate of the *Drosophila* effective population size is one million, it seems likely that the most recent common ancestor of the 11 *D. simulans* individuals will occur before coalescence with the *D. melanogaster* lineage. Thus, the *D. melanogaster* sequence gives us information about the state of the most recent common ancestor of the *D. simulans* individuals and allows us to conclude which nucleotides represent mutations. Note that in all cases but position 5413, the nucleotide in *D. melanogaster* agrees with one of the *D. simulans* individuals. In this case, the state of the most recent common ancestor is ambiguous, but it is clear from the data that the mutation is internal.

	mel	1	2	3	4	5	6	7	8	9	10	11
4609	C	T	.	.	.	.	.	.	C	C	C	C
4612	C	C	.	.	.	.	.	.	.	.	T	T
4690	T	G	.	T	T	T	T	T	T	T	T	T
4723	T	T	.	.	.	C	C	C	C	C	.	.
4759	A	A	.	.	.	T	T	T	T	T	.	.
4783	C	G	.	.	.	C	C	C	.	.	.	.
4861	C	C	.	.	.	.	.	.	.	.	A	A
4996	C	C	.	.	.	.	.	.	A	A	.	.
4999	G	G	.	.	.	.	.	.	A	A	.	.
5014	T	T	.	.	.	.	.	.	C	C	C	C
5137	G	A	.	G	.	.	G	.	G	.	.	.
5158	A	G	.	.	.	.	.	.	.	.	A	A
5176	A	A	.	.	.	G	.	G	.	G	.	.
5197	G	A	.	.	.	.	.	.	C	C	G	G
5200	T	T	.	.	.	.	.	.	.	.	A	A
5350	C	C	.	.	.	.	.	T	T	.	T	T
5362	C	C	.	.	.	.	.	T	T	.	T	T
5392	C	C	.	.	.	T	T	T	T	T	T	T
5413	C	G	.	.	.	A	A	A	.	.	.	.
5425	T	T	.	.	.	.	.	.	C	C	.	.
5455	G	G	.	A	A	.	.	.	.	.	A	A
5425	T	T	.	.	.	.	.	.	C	C	.	.
5461	A	A	.	.	.	.	.	.	.	.	T	T
5510	C	C	.	.	.	.	.	.	A	A	.	.
5158	G	C	.	G	G	G	G	G	.	.	G	G
5554	G	G	.	.	.	.	.	.	.	.	A	A

There are 26 segregating sites, but since there are two mutations at 5197, the total number of mutations $\eta = 27$. This represents a deviation from the infinite sites model but in light of the calculations at the beginning of Section 1.4 is not an unexpected one. $27/\sqrt{970} = 0.866918$, so by (4.1) in Chapter 1, the probability that all 27 mutations will land at different sites is approximately

$$\exp(-(0.866918)^2/2) = 0.6868$$

However, as we will now see, it is very unusual for there to be only one external mutation at 5486. A little computation shows $a_{11} = 2.929$. Table 2 of Fu and Li gives $v_D = 0.214$, so $u_D = a_{11} - 1 - v_D = 1.929 - 0.214 = 1.715$. The value of Fu and Li's statistic is thus

$$D_{FL} = \frac{27 - 1 \cdot 2.929}{\sqrt{(1.715)(27) + (0.214)(27)^2}} = 1.69$$

When $n = 11$, a 95% confidence interval for D_{FL} is $(-2.18, 1.57)$. Thus, there is a significant deficiency of external mutations.

To perform Tajima's test on these data, we ignore the column with three mutations so that there are 25 segregating sites. The remaining columns show the following statistics

split	1 − 10	2 − 9	3 − 8	4 − 7	5 − 6
number	1	11	4	7	2

Using this and the fact that $\binom{11}{2} = 55$, we can compute that

$$\Delta_{11} = \frac{1 \cdot 10 + 11 \cdot 18 + 4 \cdot 24 + 7 \cdot 28 + 2 \cdot 30}{55} = \frac{560}{55} = 10.181818$$

Dividing Δ_{11} by the 970 bp gives an estimate of π of 0.0105, which is consistent with the estimates for *Adh*, *Amy*, and *rosy* discussed in Section 1.4. In contrast the estimate of θ based on the 25 segregating sites is $25/2.928968 = 8.535429$. Computing as in the previous section, we find

$$a_1 = 2.928968 \qquad a_2 = 1.549768$$
$$b_1 = 0.400000 \qquad b_2 = 0.272727$$
$$c_1 = 0.058583 \qquad c_2 = 0.049884$$
$$e_1 = 0.020001 \qquad e_2 = 0.004925$$

and $\sqrt{\widehat{\text{var}}(d)} = 1.858779$, so Tajima's D is

$$D_T = \frac{10.1818181 - 8.535429}{1.858779} = 0.885737$$

Consulting Tajima's table we see that a 90% confidence interval for D_T is $(-1.572, 1.710)$, so this value of D_T is far from significant.

When there is no outgroup available, the number of singletons may overestimate the number of mutations on external branches. To illustrate this, consider the following genealogy:

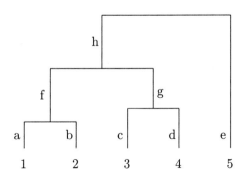

The mutations on h lead to singletons, even though h is an internal branch. Obviously, this problem can occur only if the last coalescence event in the phylogeny merges one lineage with the other $n - 1$. Formula (1.9a) in Chapter 1 shows that if $n > 2$, then this event has probability $2/(n - 1)$.

Let κ be the number of external branches leading to the root of the tree. In most cases $\kappa = 0$, but if $\kappa = 1$ let ξ_1 be the number of mutations on the internal branch leading to the root. Clearly, the number of singleton mutations, η_s, has

$$\eta_s = \eta_e + \kappa \xi_1$$

When $\kappa = 1$, the length of the internal branch leading to the root, when measured in units of $2N_e$ generations, has an exponential distribution with mean 1, so it follows from (2.3) that

$$E\eta_s = \theta + \frac{2}{n-1} \cdot \theta/2 = \frac{n\theta}{n-1}$$

The total number of mutations, η, has $E\eta = a_n\theta$ so

$$d^* = \frac{n}{n-1}\eta - a_n\eta_s$$

has $Ed^* = 0$.

As in the case of the two previous D's, our test statistic will be the standardized variable

$$D^* = d^*/\sqrt{\operatorname{var}(d*)}$$

Computations similar to the ones for D in this section show that

$$\operatorname{var}(d^*) = u'_n\theta + v'_n\theta^2$$

so we refer the reader to Appendix C of Fu and Li (1993) for details. Replacing θ and θ^2 by their estimates leads to

$$D^* = \frac{\eta(n/n-1) - a_n\eta_s}{\sqrt{u_{D*}\eta + v_{D*}\eta^2}}$$

where u_{D*} and v_{D*} are given in Fu and Li's Table 1.

Example 2.2. For an example of the use of D^*, we return to the Dmd example of the previous section. In this case $n = 41$, $\eta = 9$, and $\eta_s = 7$, so consulting Table 1 in Fu and Li, we have $a_{41} = 4.279$, $u_{D*} = 3.112$, $v_{D*} = 0.223$ so

$$D^* = \frac{9(41/40) - 4.278543 \cdot 7}{\sqrt{3.112(9) + 0.223(9)^2}} = -3.054$$

Table 2 of Fu and Li tells us that a 95% confidence interval for D^* is $(-2.50, 1.42)$, so we can reject the hypothesis of neutral evolution in this case.

In the case of the *Dmd* data, there is not one outgroup but two, so we can also perform the test with the D statistic. Each outgroup indicates that one singleton is actually an internal mutation, but curiously for the *Pan* sequence this is position 1299, while for the *Pongo* sequence this is position 0711. In either case then, we have $\eta = 9$ and $\eta_e = 6$. Fu and Li's Table 1 gives $v_D = 0.148$ and $a_{41} = 4.279$, so $u_D = a_{41} - 1 - v_D = 3.131$. The value of Fu and Li's statistic is thus

$$D_{FL} = \frac{9 - 4.279 \cdot 6}{\sqrt{3.131(9) + 0.148(9)^2}} = -2.631$$

This is closer to 0 but still outside the 95% confidence interval. If we resolve the conflict between the two outgroups by declaring that all mutations are external, then the D statistic becomes

$$D_{FL} = \frac{9 - 4.279 \cdot 6}{\sqrt{3.131(9) + 0.148(9)^2}} = -3.307$$

in contrast to the value of -3.21 reported in Nachman and Crowell (2000).

Example 2.3. Kaessmann, Heissig, von Haeseler, and Pääbo (1999) sequenced roughly 10 kb of noncoding DNA in a region of the X chromosome at map position $Xq13.3$. This part of the chromosome displays a rate of recombination of approximately 0.16 cM/Mb, approximately 1/8 of the average on the X chromosome (1.3 cM/Mb). A worldwide sample of $n = 69$ individuals identified $\eta = 33$ polymorphic positions. The data are given on page 79 of their paper. Nineteen of the mutations were singletons in the sample but in one case, the singleton nucleotide was the same as that in the gorilla and chimpanzee, so we have $\eta_e = 18$. Consulting Table 1 in Fu and Li we have $a_{69} = 4.804$ and $v_D = 0.119$ so $u_D = a_{69} - 1 - v_D = 3.685$. The value of Fu and Li's statistic is thus

$$D_{FL} = \frac{33 - 4.804 \cdot 18}{\sqrt{3.685(33) + 0.119(33)^2}} = -3.374$$

The 98% confidence interval in Fu and Li's Table 2 is $(-2.85, 1.78)$ when $n = 70$, so there is a significant departure from neutrality.

Kaessmann, Wiebe, and Pääbo (1999) followed up on this study by sequencing the region in 30 chimpanzees. Kaessmann, Wiebe, Weiss, and Pääbo (2001) added sequences for 11 gorillas and 14 orangutans. The combined results of these studies can be summarized in the following table:

	n	S	θ_w	D^*	p
humans	70	33	6.8	-3.35	< 0.02
chimpanzees	30	84	21.2	-2.03	> 0.05
gorillas	11	41	14.0	0.78	> 0.10
orangutans	14	77	24.2	0.44	> 0.10

Here n is the sample size, S is the number of segregating sites, $\theta_w = S/a_n$ is Watterson's estimate of θ, D^* is Fu and Li's statistics, and p is the probability of getting a value this far from 0 by chance.

The authors make two inferences from these data. The first, based on θ_w, is that humans differ from great apes in having a lower level of genetic variability, a conclusion consistent with earlier studies of mtDNA. The second, based on D^*, is that humans show a signal of population expansion that does not appear in apes. The value for chimpanzees is negative but not significantly so since the 95% confidence interval for a sample of size 30 is $(-2.53, 1.39)$. In contrast, the values for gorillas and orangutans are positive. A population expansion is, of course, just one of the possible explanations. Almost all of the samples are from individuals in different countries, so population subdivision may account for the excess of external mutations.

Fu and Li's and Tajima's D statistics are both based on the number of sites that show the various possible split patterns, i.e., in how many cases is one nucleotide occurs in k individual and the other in $n - k$. It is natural to ask if there are other ways of processing this data to obtain useful statistics. Fu (1996, 1997) has proposed other statistics. We refer the reader to his papers for details.

Simonsen, Churchill, and Aquadro (1995) developed new methods for constructing critical values of Tajima's D and Fu and Li's D^* and used simulations to determine the power of these tests. They found that Tajima's test was in general more powerful against the alternative hypotheses of selective sweep, population bottleneck, and population subdivision. However, Tajima's test can detect a selective sweep or bottleneck only if it has occurred within a specific interval of time in the recent past or population subdivision only when it has persisted for a long time. Recently, Wall and Przeworski (2000) have examined the power of Tajima's D and Fu and Li's D^* to detect population expansion in order to obtain insight into the question: When did the human population size start increasing?

4.3   The HKA Test

To motivate the test invented by Hudson, Kreitman, and Aguadé (1987), we begin with the somewhat surprising result due to Birky and Walsh (1988) that linkage to either advantageous or deleterious mutations does not affect the rate at which neutral mutations become fixed in the population. Let the frequency of a neutral allele A at a neutral locus be x. The frequency of the remaining alleles (collectively referred to as a) will then be $1 - x$. Suppose this locus is completely linked to another locus at which selected mutants arise. Let A^* (or a^*) denote the specific copy of A (or a) to which the newly arising selected mutant is linked. With probability x the linkage is to A, and the starting frequencies are

$$p(A^*) = 1/2N \quad p(A) = x - 1/2N \quad p(a) = 1 - x$$

With probability $1 - x$, the linkage is to a and the starting frequencies are

$$p(A) = x \quad p(a^*) = 1/2N \quad p(a) = 1 - x - 1/2N$$

Breaking things into the two cases,

$$
\begin{aligned}
P(A \text{ fixed}) \quad = \quad & x[P(A^* \text{ fixed}) + P(A \text{ fixed}|A^* \text{ lost})] \\
& + (1 - x)P(A \text{ fixed}|a^* \text{ lost})
\end{aligned}
$$

If the selected allele is lost, the probabilities of fixation for the neutral alleles are their relative frequencies, $p(a)/(p(A) + p(a))$, so:

$$P(A \text{ fixed}|A^* \text{ lost}) \quad = \quad \frac{x - 1/2N}{1 - 1/2N} = \frac{2Nx - 1}{2N - 1}$$

$$P(A \text{ fixed}|a^* \text{ lost}) \quad = \quad \frac{x}{1 - 1/2N} = \frac{2Nx}{2N - 1}$$

Letting f be the fixation probability for the selected locus and combining the last three equations, we have

$$
\begin{aligned}
P(A \text{ fixed}) \quad = \quad & xf + x(1 - f)\frac{2Nx - 1}{2N - 1} + (1 - x)(1 - f)\frac{2Nx}{2N - 1} \\
= \quad & xf + (1 - f)\frac{2Nx - x}{2N - 1} = x
\end{aligned}
$$

Thus, the fixation probability, and hence the rate of evolution of a neutral allele, is not changed by occurrence of a linked mutation under selection.

Suppose now that we have a sample from one species and one sequence from another. The ratio of the number of segregating sites in one species to the amount of divergence between the two species is determined by the time since divergence of the two species, the effective population size, and the size of the sample, but does not depend on the mutation rate at the locus. Hence, these ratios should be similar for different loci, and sufficiently large differences provide evidence for nonneutral evolution.

Having explained the motivation behind the HKA test, we turn now to the mechanics. Consider data collected from two species, referred to as species A and species B, and from $L \geq 2$ regions of the genome referred to as locus 1 through locus L. Assume that a random sample of n_A gametes from species A have been sequenced at all L loci and n_B gametes from species B have been sequenced at the same loci. Let S_i^A denote the number of sites that are polymorphic at locus i in the sample from species A. Similarly, let S_i^B denote the number of sites that are polymorphic at locus i in the sample from species B. Let D_i denote the number of differences between a random gamete from species A and a random gamete from species B. The $3L$ observations S_i^A, S_i^B, and D_i constitute the data with which the test devised by Hudson, Kreitman, and Aguadé (1987) is carried out.

It is assumed that each locus evolves according to the standard Wright-Fisher infinite sites model: (1) generations are discrete, (2) all mutations are selectively neutral, (3) the number of sites at each locus is very large, so that each mutation occurs at a previously unmutated site, (4) in each generation, mutations occur independently in each gamete and at each locus, (5) at locus i, the number of mutations per gamete in each generation is Poisson distributed with mean u_i, and (6) no recombination occurs within the loci. In addition, we assume that (7) all loci are unlinked, (8) species A and B are at stationarity at the time of sampling with population sizes $2N$ and $2Nf$ respectively, and (9) the two species were derived T' generations ago from a single ancestral population with size $2N(1+f)/2$ gametes.

Letting $\theta_i = 4Nu_i$ and $C(n) = \sum_{j=1}^{n-1} 1/j$, it follows from (4.8) in Chapter 1 that

$$E(S_i^A) = \theta_i C(n_A) \quad E(S_i^B) = f\theta_i C(n_B)$$

Using (4.9) in Chapter 1 and letting $C_2(n) = \sum_{j=1}^{n-1} 1/j^2$, we have

$$\begin{aligned} \mathrm{var}\,(S_i^A) &= E(S_i^A) + \theta_i^2 C_2(n_A) \\ \mathrm{var}\,(S_i^B) &= E(S_i^B) + (f\theta_i)^2 C_2(n_B) \end{aligned}$$

To compute the expected value of D_i, we note that it is $2u_i$ times the expected coalescence time of two individuals: one chosen at random from A and one from B. Those two lineages must stay apart for T' units of time and then coalescence occurs as in a single population of size $2N(1+f)/2$. Measured in units of $2N$ generations, the second phase takes an exponentially distributed amount of time with mean $(1+f)/2$, so letting $T = T'/2N$

$$ED_i = \theta_i(T + (1+f)/2)$$

To compute the variance, we note that in the first phase, the number of mutations is Poisson with mean $2u_iT' = \theta_iT$. By (4.4) in Chapter 1, the number in the second phase has variance $\theta_i(1+f)/2 + (\theta_i(1+f)/2)^2$ and is independent of the number in the first phase so

$$\mathrm{var}\,(D_i) = ED_i + (\theta_i(1+f)/2)^2$$

There are $L + 2$ parameters. These can be estimated by solving the following $L + 2$ equations:

$$\sum_{i=1}^{L} S_i^A = C(n_A)\sum_{i=1}^{L} \hat{\theta}_i$$

$$\sum_{i=1}^{L} S_i^B = C(n_B)\hat{f}\sum_{i=1}^{L} \hat{\theta}_i$$

$$\sum_{i=1}^{L} D_i = (\hat{T} + (1+\hat{f})/2)\sum_{i=1}^{L} \hat{\theta}_i$$

and for $1 \leq i \leq L - 1$

$$S_i^A + S_i^B + D_i = \hat{\theta}_i \left\{ \hat{T} + (1 + \hat{f})/2 + C(n_A) + C(n_B) \right\}$$

These equations may look complicated but they are simple to solve. The first can be used to compute $\sum_{i=1}^{L} \hat{\theta}_i$, the second can then be used to find $\hat{f}$, the third to compute $\hat{T}$, and then the individual $\hat{\theta}_i$ can be computed from the remaining $L - 1$. We do not need the equation with $i = L$ since we have already computed the sum of the $\hat{\theta}_i$.

To measure the goodness of fit of these parameters, we can use

$$
\begin{aligned}
X^2 \;=\; & \sum_{i=1}^{L} (S_i^A - \hat{E}(S_i^A))^2 / \widehat{\mathrm{var}}(S_i^A) \\
& + \sum_{i=1}^{L} (S_i^B - \hat{E}(S_i^B))^2 / \widehat{\mathrm{var}}(S_i^B) \\
& + \sum_{i=1}^{L} (D_i - \hat{E}(D_i))^2 / \widehat{\mathrm{var}}(D_i)
\end{aligned}
$$

If the quantities S_i^A, S_i^B, D_i were stochastically independent of each other and normally distributed, then the statistic X^2 should be approximately χ^2 with $3L - (L+2) = 2L - 2$ degrees of freedom. For n_A, n_B, and T sufficiently large, all of these quantities are approximately normally distributed. Since the loci are unlinked, S_i^A is independent of S_j^A and S_j^B when $j \neq i$. Also, S_i^A is independent of S_i^B as long as T is large enough so that there are no shared polymorphisms. However, a small positive correlation is expected between S_i^A and D_i, and between S_i^B and D_i, because a positive fraction of the mutations that contribute to polymorphism also contribute to differences between species. The last observation and the fact that the normality is only asymptotic forces the test to be carried out by doing simulations with the estimated parameters.

Example 3.1. Adh. The first application of the HKA test was to the alcohol dehydrogenase locus in *Drosophila melanogaster*. The polymorphism data came from a four-cutter restriction enzyme survey of 81 isochromosomal lines of *D. melanogaster* studied by Kreitman and Aguadé (1986ab). Nine polymorphic restriction sites were identified in the flanking region and eight in the *Adh* locus. They estimated the effective number of sites to be 414 in the flanking region and 79 in the *Adh* locus. Their interspecific data were based on a sequence comparison of one *D. melanogaster* sequence and one *D. sechelia* sequence. This comparison revealed 210 differences in 4052 bp of flanking sequence and 18 differences in 324 bp in the *Adh* locus. The next table summarizes the data:

	within *D. melanogaster*			between species		
	sites	variable	%	sites	variable	%
flanking region	414	9	0.022	4052	210	0.052
Adh locus	79	8	0.101	324	18	0.056

Note that the divergence between species is almost the same in the two regions but there is a considerably higher rate of polymorphism in the *Adh* locus compared to the flanking sequence.

We have no data on the variability within *D. simulans* so we will suppose that the ancestral population size is the same as the current population size, that is, $f = 1$. To take account of the differing number of sites in the comparisons within ($w_1 = 414$, $w_2 = 79$) and between ($b_1 = 4052$, $b_2 = 324$) species and to prepare for the fact that in the next example the two sample sizes will be different (here $n_1 = n_2 = 81$), we let μ_i be the per nucleotide mutation rate at the ith locus, let $\pi_i = 4N\mu_i$, and note that

$$
\begin{aligned}
ES_1^A &= C(n_1) \cdot w_1 \pi_1 \\
ES_2^A &= C(n_2) \cdot w_2 \pi_2 \\
ED_1 &= b_1 \pi_1 (T+1) \\
ED_2 &= b_2 \pi_2 (T+1)
\end{aligned}
$$

Adding the equations as before, we arrive at

$$
\begin{aligned}
S_1^A + S_2^A &= C(n_1) \cdot w_1 \hat{\pi}_1 + C(n_2) \cdot w_2 \hat{\pi}_2 \\
D_1 + D_2 &= (b_1 \hat{\pi}_1 + b_2 \hat{\pi}_2)(\hat{T}+1) \\
S_1^A + D_1 &= C(n_1) \cdot w_1 \hat{\pi}_1 + b_1 \hat{\pi}_1 (\hat{T}+1)
\end{aligned}
$$

These equations are not as easy to solve as the previous ones. Letting $x = \hat{\pi}_1$, $y = \hat{\pi}_2$, and $z = \hat{T}+1$, they have the form

$$
\begin{aligned}
c &= ax + by \\
f &= dxz + eyz \\
i &= gx + hxz
\end{aligned}
$$

The three equations can be written as

$$
z = \frac{f}{dx + ey} \qquad y = \frac{c - ax}{b} \qquad (1 - gx)\frac{f}{z} = fhx
$$

Using the first two in the third equation leads to $\alpha x^2 + \beta x + \gamma = 0$, where

$$
\begin{aligned}
\alpha &= g\left(d - \frac{ea}{b}\right) \\
\beta &= \frac{gec}{b} + hf - i\left(d - \frac{ea}{b}\right) \\
\gamma &= \frac{-iec}{b}
\end{aligned}
$$

At this point, there are two cases to consider. If $n_1 = n_2$, $b_1 = w_1$, and $b_2 = w_2$, then

$$d - \frac{ea}{b} = b_1 - \frac{b_2 C(n_1) w_1}{C(n_2) w_2} = 0$$

In this case, $\alpha = 0$ so we solve the linear equation to get $x = -\gamma/\beta$. When $\alpha \neq 0$, the root of the quadratic equation that we want is

$$x = \frac{-\beta + \sqrt{\beta^2 - 4\alpha\gamma}}{2\alpha}$$

In either case, once x is found, we can compute y and z.

Carrying out the arithmetic in this example gives

$$\hat{\pi}_1 = 6.558 \times 10^{-3}, \quad \hat{\pi}_2 = 8.971 \times 10^{-3}, \quad \hat{T} = 6.734$$

Using the relationships

$$
\begin{aligned}
\text{var}\,(S_i^A) &= E S_i^A + (w_i \pi_i)^2 C_2(n_i) \\
\text{var}\,(D_i) &= E D_i + (b_i \pi_i)^2
\end{aligned}
$$

we can compute $X^2 = 6.09$. Monte Carlo simulations with the parameters set equal to these estimates show that the probability of $X^2 > 6.09$ is approximately 0.016. As the reader may have noticed, the flanking sequence is not far enough from the gene region to make it reasonable to assume that the two are unlinked. However, the positive correlation that results from interlocus linkage will shift the distribution of X^2 toward smaller values and make rejections based on the model conservative. Likewise, the intralocus recombination we are ignoring will reduce the variance of the quantities estimated and tend to decrease the value of X^2.

Having identified a significant departure from neutrality, the next step is to seek an explanation. The fact that there is more polymorphism in the coding region than in the adjacent flanking sequence suggests that something is acting there to make the genealogies larger than they would be under the neutral model. In Section 3.3, we argued that one explanation for this was balancing selection acting on the fast/slow polymorphism.

Example 3.2. Drosophila fourth chromosome.

Berry, Ajioka, and Kreitman (1991) studied a 1.1kb fragment of the *cubitus interruptus Dominant* (ci^D) locus on the small nonrecombining fourth chromosome for ten lines of *Drosophila melanogaster* and nine of *Drosophila simulans*. They found no polymorphism within *Drosophila melanogaster* and a single polymorphism within *Drosophila simulans*. To perform the HKA test they used data on the 5' region of *Adh* from 11 sequences of Kreitman and Hudson (1991) as their comparison neutral locus. This yielded the following data

	ci^D	$5'\,Adh$
nucleotides	1106	3326
polymorphism	0	30
divergence	54	78

Calculating as in the previous example we find

$$\hat{\pi}_1 = 3.136 \times 10^{-3} \quad \hat{\pi}_2 = 2.072 \times 10^{-2} \quad \hat{T} = 11.74$$

and $X^2 = 6.85$. Using the result of Hudson, Kreitman, and Aguadé (1987) that in this case the statistic has approximately a chi-square distribution with 1 degree of freedom, Berry, Ajioka, and Kreitman (1991) concluded that the probability of an X^2 value this large is < 0.01. (Note that the value of 1 here contrasts with the $2L - 2 = 2$ degrees of freedom that the statistic would have if S_i^A and D_i were independent.)

One explanation for these data is purifying selection: original population sizes in both species were small, permitting effectively neutral drift of mildly deleterious alleles and causing the accumulation of fixed differences between the two species. Subsequent population expansion has increased the efficacy of selection against such mildly deleterious mutations, and what we see, within species, is the wholesale removal of variation by purifying selection. While this explanation is possible, it seems unlikely. Given the lack of variation at both silent and replacement sites, a slightly deleterious allele model would require that selection coefficients against both silent and replacement sites would fall between $1/2N_2$ and $1/2N_1$, where N_1 and N_2 are the pre- and post-expansion population sizes. It is unlikely that these two types of mutations, which have entirely different functional consequences, would have similar selection coefficients.

A second explanation is that a selective sweep eliminated variation in this region for both species. In order to estimate the time of occurrence of such a sweep we note that if T_{tot} is the total time in the genealogy of our sample, μ is the mutation rate per nucleotide per generation, and k is the number of silent sites, then the expected number of segregating sites

$$ES = T_{tot}\mu k$$

To simplify calculations, we will suppose that the sweep was recent enough so that the resulting genealogy is star-shaped. In this case $T_{tot} = nt$, where n is the sample size and t is the time of the sweep. For the *Drosophila melanogaster* sample, $S = 0$ so we are left with an estimate of $t = 0$. For *D. simulans* substituting 1 for ES, and taking $n = 9$, $k = 331$, and $\mu = 1 \times 10^{-9}$ we arrive at

$$t = \frac{ES}{nk\mu} = \frac{1}{9 \cdot 331 \cdot 10^{-9}} = 3.35 \times 10^5 \text{ generations ago}$$

Assuming 10 generations per year, this translates into 33,500 years.

Having assumed a star-shaped phylogeny and calculated a time, we should go back and check to see if our assumption is justified. The probability of no coalescence in a sample of size n during t generations in a population of size N is

$$\approx \exp\left(-\binom{n}{2}\frac{t}{2N}\right)$$

If we take $2N = 5 \times 10^6$, $n = 9$, and $t = 3.35 \times 10^5$ then the above

$$= \exp\left(-36\frac{3.35}{50}\right) = e^{-2.412} = 0.0896$$

i.e., it is very likely that there has been at least one coalescence. Once one abandons the assumption of a star-shaped phylogeny, calculations become difficult and it is natural to turn to simulation. Using $4N\mu = 3$ for $D.$ *simulans*, Berry, Ajioka, and Kreitman (1991) computed that there was a 50% probability of sweep in the last $0.36N$ generations, or 72,000 years.

Example 3.3. yellow-achaete. The *yellow-achaete (y-ac), phosphoglu- conte dehydrogenase (Pgd), and period (per)* loci are three gene regions of varying distance from the telomere of the X chromosome and range from very low to moderate rates of recombination in $D.$ *simulans*. Begun and Aquadro (1991) used the HKA test to compare these gene regions to each other and to the *rosy* locus which is located on the right arm of chromosome 3 and was studied by Aquadro, Lado, and Noon (1988).

Since females have two X chromosomes but males have only one, the effective population size of an X linked gene is only $3N/4$. When testing two X-linked genes, the HKA test can be applied as for two autosomal genes. However, when comparing autosomal and X-linked genes, the equations must be modified to take into account the difference in population sizes. Let locus 1 be autosomal with neutral mutation rate μ_1 and locus 2 be X-linked with neutral mutation rate μ_2. If the sample sizes are n_A and $n_B = 1$, then the equations must be modified as follows:

$$ES_2^A = C(n_A) \cdot \frac{3\theta_2}{4} \qquad \text{var}\,(S_2^A) = E(S_2^A) + C_2(n_A) \cdot \left(\frac{3\theta_2}{4}\right)^2$$

$$ED_2 = \theta_2(T + 3/4) \qquad \text{var}\,(D_2) = ED_2 + (3\theta_2/4)^2$$

Adding the equations as before, we arrive at

$$\begin{aligned}
S_1^A + S_2^A &= C(n_A) \cdot \hat{\theta}_1 + C(n_A) \cdot \hat{\theta}_2 \\
D_1 + D_2 &= \theta_1(\hat{T} + 1) + \theta_2(\hat{T} + 3/4) \\
S_1^A + D_1 &= C(n_A) \cdot \hat{\theta}_1 + \hat{\theta}_1(\hat{T} + 1)
\end{aligned}$$

Using the HKA to compare these four genes, Begun and Aquadro (1991) found

Region	y-ac	Pgd	per	rosy
y-ac	—	3.42	4.71*	9.23**
Pgd		—	0.09	1.80
per			—	1.64

* $p < 0.05$, ** $p < 0.005$

To interpret these data, Begun and Aquadro argued that the 5.4% divergence at y-ac is similar to estimates from other regions, which range from about 3% for hsp70 and Pgd to 5% for per and rosy. In contrast the levels of variation are very low: 0.0001 for y-ac versus 0.0011 for Pgd, 0.0070 for per, and 0.0190 for rosy. The fact that the two significant departures from neutrality involved y-ac suggests that there has been a reduction in variation at y-ac consistent with a selective sweep.

4.4 MacDonald-Kreitman

To describe the test of MacDonald and Kreitman (1991), we need some notation. Of M possible mutations in a coding region, let M_r be the number of possible neutral replacement mutations (i.e., ones that change the amino acid but not the effectiveness of the protein) and let M_s be the number of possible neutral synonymous mutations. By definition all of the $M - M_r - M_s$ remaining mutations are deleterious. Let μ be the mutation rate per nucleotide, so that the mutation rate for any one of the three possible changes at a site is $\mu/3$. Under the neutral theory, the expected number of fixed replacement substitutions in a set of alleles is $T_b(\mu/3)M_r$, where T_b is the total time on between-species branches. The expected number of fixed synonymous substitutions in a set of alleles is $T_b(\mu/3)M_s$. For a particular phylogeny and mutation rate, the number of replacement substitutions is independent of the number of synonymous substitutions. Therefore the ratio of the expected replacement to expected synonymous fixed mutations is

$$\frac{T_b(\mu/3)M_r}{T_b(\mu/3)M_s} = \frac{M_r}{M_s}$$

If T_w is the total time on within species branches then the ratio of expected replacement to expected synonymous polymorphic mutations is

$$\frac{T_w(\mu/3)M_r}{T_w(\mu/3)M_s} = \frac{M_r}{M_s}$$

Thus, if protein evolution occurs by neutral processes, the two ratios are the same and we can use standard statistical tests for 2×2 contingency tables to test this null hypothesis. Under the alternative model of adaptive protein evolution, there should be relatively more replacement substitution between species than replacement polymorphism within a species, so a deviation in this direction is interpreted as evidence for positive selection.

Example 4.1. To explain the workings of the test, we will begin with the original data set of MacDonald and Kreitman (1991). They compared DNA sequences of the *Adh* locus in *Drosophila melanogaster*, *D. simulans*, and *D. yakuba*. The DNA sequence data can be found on page 653 of their paper. To carry out the test, the following summary is sufficient:

	Fixed	Polymorphic
Replacement	7	2
Synonymous	17	42

To analyze the table, we first compute the number of observations we expect to find in each cell (given in parentheses in the next table):

	Fixed	Polymorphic	Total
Replacement	7 (3.176)	2 (5.824)	9
Synonymous	17 (20.824)	42 (38.176)	59
Total	24	44	68

Then we compute the χ^2 statistic

$$\frac{(7-3.176)^2}{3.176} + \frac{(2-5.824)^2}{5.824} + \frac{(17-20.824)^2}{20.824} + \frac{(42-38.176)^2}{38.176} = 8.198$$

The number of degrees of freedom in this case is 1, so the χ^2 distribution is just the square of a standard normal, χ, and we can use a table of the standard normal to conclude that the probability of a deviation this large by chance is $2P(\chi > \sqrt{8.198}) = 0.0042$. MacDonald and Kreitman analyzed the contingency table with a G test of independence (with the Williams correction for continuity) finding $G = 7.43$ and $p = 0.006$.

Geneticists have embraced the MacDonald-Kreitman test as a useful tool for looking for positive selection. However, the initial paper did not get such a warm reception. Graur and Li, and Whittam and Nei, each wrote letters that appeared in the November 14, 1991 issue of *Nature* suggesting that the test had serious problems. Both pairs of authors objected to some of the bookkeeping involved in the three-species comparison. For example, at position 1590 all the alleles in *D. melanogaster* have T and all of the alleles in *D. yakuba* have C, while in *D. simulans* half the alleles have T, and the other half have C. MacDonald and Kreitman count this as one polymorphic site, whereas two mutations, one within *D. simulans* and one between two of the species, are needed to produce the observed pattern.

This first point is a legitimate concern but is moot if, as in most applications, one only compares two species. Li and Graur go on to make two further points about MacDonald and Kreitman's paper. "Second, they fail to consider the fact that a polymorphism in a species does not necessarily imply that the polymorphism arose with the species." "Third, their decision as to whether or not a site is polymorphic is highly sensitive to the number (n) of sequences sampled and n is only 6 for *D. simulans*." To counter these objections, one has only to look back at the assumptions. We assume there is no recombination so that the entire locus has the same genealogy and that in this genealogy all of the lineages within each species coalesce before coalescing with a lineage from the other species. In this picture mutations that occur on the edges connecting the two most recent common ancestors of the individuals in the two species are fixed differences between the two samples, while the other mutations produce polymorphisms in one of the two samples. That is, in the test, the terms "fixed difference" and "polymorphism" are defined with respect to the samples and not with respect to the populations, so no problem arises if some site is polymorphic in the population but not in the sample.

In view of the concerns about the bookkeeping in the three-way comparison and in order to show the reader what the data look like, we will now consider only the data for $D.$ $melanogaster$ and $D.$ $simulans$, given on the next two pages. The contingency table is now much different, with the 24 fixed differences having been reduced to just 4.

	Fixed	Polymorphic	Total
Replacement	2	2	4
Synonymous	2	26	28
Total	4	28	32

Since the cell counts are small, we analyze the results with $Fisher's$ $exact$ $test$. To derive this test, we note that if we condition on the number of replacement substitutions n_r, then the number of fixed replacements, n_{fr} is binomial(n_r,p), where $p = T_b/(T_w + T_b)$. Likewise, if we condition on the number of synonymous substitutions n_r then the number of fixed synonymous substitutions, n_{fs}, is binomial(n_s,p). Let n_f and n_p be the number of fixed and polymorphic substitutions. The probability of a given table conditioned on the marginal values n_r, n_s, n_f, n_p is

$$\frac{n_r!}{n_{fr}!n_{pr}!}p^{n_{fr}}(1-p)^{n_{pr}} \cdot \frac{n_s!}{n_{fs}!n_{ps}!}p^{n_{fs}}(1-p)^{n_{ps}} = \frac{C}{n_{fr}!n_{pr}!n_{fs}!n_{ps}!}$$

where C is a constant independent of $(n_{fr}, n_{pr}, n_{fs}, n_{ps})$.

There are only five 2×2 tables with the indicated row and column sums: n_{fr} can be 0, 1, 2, 3, or 4 and this determines the rest of the entries. Of these, the ones with $n_{fr} = 2,3,4$ are more extreme than the indicated table. Using the preceding formula, it is easy to compute the conditional probability that $n_{fr} = k$ given the row and column sums

k	0	1	2	3	4
prob.	0.569383	0.364405	0.063070	0.003115	0.000028

From this we see that the probability of a table this extreme is $0.066212 > 0.05$.

D. melanogaster

pos.	con.	a	b	c	d	e	f	g	h	i	j	k	l
781	G	T	T	T	T	T	T	T	T	T	T	T	T
816	G	T	T	T	T	.	.	.	.	.	.	.	T
834	T	.	.	.	.	.	.	.	.	.	.	.	.
870	C	T	T	T	T	T	T	T	T	T	T	T	T
950	G	.	.	.	.	.	.	.	.	.	.	.	.
974	G	.	.	.	.	.	.	.	.	.	.	.	.
1068	C	T	T	.	.	.	.	.	.	.	.	.	.
1089	C	.	.	.	.	.	.	.	.	.	.	.	.
1199	C	.	T	.	.	.	.	.	.	.	.	.	.
1203	C	.	.	.	.	.	.	.	.	.	.	.	.
1229	T	.	.	C	C	C	C	C	C	C	C	C	C
1235	C	.	.	.	.	.	.	.	.	.	.	A	.
1271	A	.	.	.	.	.	.	.	.	.	.	.	.
1283	C	A	A	.	.	.	.	.	.	.	.	.	.
1304	C	.	.	.	.	.	.	.	.	.	.	.	.
1316	C	.	.	.	.	.	.	.	.	.	.	.	.
1425	C	A	A	.	.	.	.	.	.	.	.	.	.
1431	T	C	C	.	.	.	.	.	.	.	.	.	.
1443	T	.	.	.	.	.	.	G	G	G	G	G	G
1452	C	.	.	.	.	.	T	T	T	T	T	T	T
1490	A	.	.	.	.	.	.	C	C	C	C	C	C
1504	C	T	T	T	T	T	T	T	T	T	T	T	T
1518	C	.	.	.	.	.	T	T	T	T	T	T	T
1527	C	T	T	T	T	T	T	.	.	.	.	.	.
1551	C	.	.	.	.	.	.	.	.	.	.	.	.
1555	C	.	.	.	.	.	.	.	.	.	.	.	T
1557	C	A	A	A	A	A	.	.	.	.	.	.	.
1560	G	.	.	.	.	.	.	.	.	.	.	.	.
1590	C	T	T	T	T	T	T	T	T	T	T	T	T
1596	G	.	.	A	A	.	A	.	.	.	.	.	A
1614	C	.	.	.	.	.	.	.	.	.	.	.	.

In contrast, if we compare *D. simulans* with *D. yakuba* using the data in MacDonald and Kreitman (1991)

	Fixed	Polymorphic	Total
Replacement	6	0	6
Synonymous	17	29	46
Total	23	29	52

then Fisher's exact test gives that the probability $n_{fr} = 6$ given the row and column sums is 0.00493, so there is a clear departure from neutral evolution.

D. simulans

pos.	con.	a	b	c	d	e	f		
781	G	.	.	.	.	.	.	Rep	Fixed
816	G	T	T	T	T	T	T	Syn	Poly
834	T	C	C	.	.	.	C	Syn	Poly
870	C	.	.	.	.	.	.	Syn	Fixed
950	G	.	A	.	.	.	.	Syn	Poly
974	G	T	.	T	T	T	T	Syn	Poly
1068	C	.	.	.	.	.	.	Syn	Poly
1089	C	A	A	A	A	A	A	Rep	Fixed
1199	C	.	.	.	.	.	.	Syn	Poly
1203	C	.	.	T	.	.	.	Syn	Poly
1229	T	.	.	.	.	.	.	Syn	Poly
1235	C	.	.	.	.	.	.	Syn	Poly
1271	A	.	T	.	T	.	.	Syn	Poly
1283	C	.	.	.	.	.	.	Syn	Poly
1304	C	.	.	.	.	T	.	Syn	Poly
1316	C	.	.	T	T	.	.	Syn	Poly
1425	C	.	.	.	.	.	.	Syn	Poly
1431	T	.	.	.	.	.	.	Syn	Poly
1443	T	.	.	.	.	.	.	Syn	Poly
1452	C	.	.	.	.	.	.	Syn	Poly
1490	A	.	.	.	.	.	.	Rep	Poly
1504	C	.	.	.	.	.	.	Syn	Fixed
1518	C	.	.	.	.	.	.	Syn	Poly
1527	C	.	.	.	.	.	.	Syn	Poly
1551	C	.	.	.	T	.	.	Syn	Poly
1555	C	.	.	.	.	.	.	Rep	Poly
1557	C	.	.	.	.	.	.	Syn	Poly
1560	G	.	.	.	A	.	.	Syn	Poly
1590	C	T	T	T	.	.	.	Syn	Poly
1596	G	.	.	.	.	.	.	Syn	Poly
1614	C	.	G	.	.	.	.	Syn	Poly

Example 4.2. Eanes, Kirchner, and Yoon (1993) sequenced 32 and 12 copies of the glucose-6-phosphate dehydrogenase gene (*G6pd*) in *Drosophila melanogaster* and *D. simulans* respectively. This revealed the following results (the number of observations we expect to find in each cell is given in parentheses):

	Fixed	Polymorphic	Total
Replacement	21 (12.718)	2 (10.282)	23
Synonymous	26 (34.282)	36 (27.717)	62
Total	47	38	85

The χ^2 statistic is 16.541. The probability of a χ^2 value this large by chance is < 0.0001. Thus, there is a very strong signal of departure from neutral evolution. The most likely explanation is that replacement substitutions are not neutral but have been periodically selected through the populations of one or both species as advantageous amino acid mutations.

Example 4.3. Accessory gland proteins are specialized proteins in the seminal fluid of *Drosophila*. They have been suggested to be involved in egg-laying stimulation, remating inhibition, and sperm competition, so there is reason to suspect that they are under positive selection. Tsaur, Ting, and Wu (1998) studied the evolution of *Acp26Aa*. They sequenced 39 *D. melanogaster* chromosomes, which they combined with 10 published *D. melanogaster* sequences and 1 *D. simulans* sequence in Aguade, Miyashita, and Langley (1992). The reader's first reaction to the sample size of 1 for *D. simulans* may be that this makes it impossible to determine whether sites are polymorphic in *D. simulans*. This does not ruin the test, however. It just reduces T_w to the total time in the genealogy for the *D. melanogaster* sample.

The next table gives the data as well as the number of observations we expect to find in each cell (given in parentheses):

	Fixed	Polymorphic	Total
Replacement	75 (69.493)	22 (27.507)	97
Synonymous	21 (26.507)	16 (10.492)	37
Total	96	38	134

The χ^2 statistic is 5.574. The probability of a χ^2 value this large by chance is $2P(\chi \geq \sqrt{5.574}) = 0.0181$. It is interesting to note that while the MacDonald-Kreitman test leads to a rejection of the neutral model, Tajima's D, which is -0.875, and Fu and Li's D, which is -0.118, do not come close to rejection.

Example 4.4. The phenomenon of rapid evolution of male reproductive proteins also occurs in humans. Mammalian sperm DNA is the most densely packed form of eukaryotic DNA. This highly condensed form is thought to be achieved by packaging of DNA molecules in side-by-side linear arrays, brought about through the action of protamines. There are two types of protamines in mammals: Protamine P1, consisting of 50–53 amino acids, is the major sperm protamine while Protamine P2, a larger molecule with 99–102 amino acids, is expressed only in primates and rodents. Wykcoff, Wang, and Wu (2000) studied the corresponding genes. They sequenced 600 bp of *Prm-1* from 26 humans, 4 chimpanzees, 1 bonobo, and 2 gorillas and 930 bp of *Prm-2* from 16 humans, 1 chimpanzee, 1 bonobo, and 1 gorilla finding the following results:

Prm-1	Fixed	Polymorphic
Replacement	9	0
Synonymous	9	6

Prm-2	Fixed	Polymorphic
Replacement	7	0
Synonymous	11	9

Using Fisher's exact test, they computed p values of 0.037 and 0.035, respectively. For a different approach to the study of protamine evolution, see Rooney and Zhang (1999).

Example 4.5. The first four examples have all shown a larger ratio of replacement to silent changes between species. Mitochondrial DNA shows the opposite pattern. Nachman (1998) describes the results of 25 comparisons involving a wide variety of organisms. Seventeen of the contingency tables deviate from the neutral expectation, and most of the deviations (15 of 17) are in the direction of greater ratio of replacement to silent variation within species. A typical example is the comparison of the ATPase gene 6 from *Drosophila melanogaster* and *D. simulans* from Kaneko, Satta, Matsura, and Chigusa (1993). As before, the number of observations we expect to find in each cell is given in parentheses:

	Fixed	Polymorphic	Total
Replacement	4 (1.482)	4 (6.518)	8
Synonymous	1 (3.518)	18 (15.482)	19
Total	5	22	27

The χ^2 statistic is 7.467. The probability of a χ^2 value this large by chance is $2P(\chi \geq \sqrt{7.467}) = 0.0064$. One explanation for a larger ratio of replacement to silent changes within populations is that many of the replacement polymorphisms are mildly deleterious.

5
Genome Rearrangement

Up to this point, we have only considered the effect of small-scale processes: nucleotide substitutions, insertions, and deletions. In this chapter, we will consider a variety of large-scale processes as well as the possibility of genome duplication.

5.1 Chromosome Size

In this section, we will begin our consideration of the evolution of genomes due to reciprocal translocation, the exchange of genetic material between nonhomologous chromosomes. Here we will consider only the sizes of the chromosomes and not their gene content or order. Sankoff and Ferretti (1996) were the first to introduce a stochastic model for the evolution of the sizes of k chromosomes. On each step, two of the chromosomes are chosen "at random" and each is broken at a place that is uniformly distributed along the length. They then pair the left half of one with the right half of the other as illustrated in the following picture:

$$xxxxxxxx|xxxx \qquad xxxxxxxx|oooooo$$
$$ooooooo|oooooo \qquad ooooooo|xxxx$$

Sankoff and Ferretti explored two different meanings for the phrase "at random": (i) all chromosomes are equally likely to be chosen (the *uniform model*), and (ii) each chromosome is chosen with a probability proportional to its length (the *proportional model*).

If there are only two chromosomes, the two schemes are identical since in either case both chromosomes are always chosen. Sankoff and Ferretti were able to show that if the chromosome lengths are normalized to sum to 1, then in equilibrium the longer chromosome has length Y, where Y has probability density function

(1.1) $$P(Y = y) = 12y(1 - y) \qquad \text{for } y \in [1/2, 1]$$

We will prove this result in (1.7) below. From (1.1) and calculus, it follows that the expected value $EY = 11/16$. In other words, on average, the longer chromosome will be about 70% of the entire genome.

Sankoff and Ferretti also considered in some detail the case of three chromosomes. Unfortunately, they defined the state of the system to be the lengths in decreasing order $\ell_1 > \ell_2 > \ell_3$. With this scheme, a translocation may change the rank of the lengths of any number of the chromosomes, so the equation for the stationary distribution became very complicated, and they were not able to find a simple formula for the stationary distribution. Without a simple formula, Sankoff and Ferretti were forced to "compute" the stationary distribution by simulation.

Sankoff and Ferretti restricted their attention to the autosomes (nonsex chromosomes) since the X and Y chromosomes do not undergo reciprocal translocations with the autosomes (Ohno 1967). Comparing their results to data from *Muntlacus muntjak* (barking deer) with $k = 3$ autosomes, the pea with $k = 7$, *Zea mays* (corn) with $k = 10$, *Oriza sativa* (rice) with $k = 12$, wheat with $k = 21$, and humans with $k = 22$, they found in all cases that the shortest chromosomes produced by their model were too short compared to those observed and the longest ones in the model were too long. Faced with this problem, Sankoff and Ferretti modified the model to impose a lower bound on the size of chromosomes that could be created. This modification resulted in a good fit for four of their examples, but for humans and wheat the long chromosomes were still too long.

Here we will take a slightly different approach to modeling chromosome lengths. Consider k chromosomes with centromeres. Letting ℓ_{2j-1} and ℓ_{2j} be the lengths of the two arms of the jth chromosome, we arrive at a model with $2k$ chromosome arms. To keep the Markov chain theory simple, we will suppose that the length of the ith chromosome arm is a positive integer ℓ_i. More sophisticated readers can work directly with the corresponding chain with state space the set of vectors $(x_1, \ldots, x_{2k})$ of nonnegative real numbers that add up to 1. However, since reality corresponds to a discrete model with total genome size T in the millions or billions of nucleotides, we will first develop a theory that works for any fixed finite genome length T and then investigate the simplifications in the solution that occur when $T \to \infty$.

The set of possible states of our model will be those length vectors $(\ell_1, \ldots \ell_{2k})$ with $\ell_1 + \cdots + \ell_{2k} = T$, where T is the total genome size. In contrast to Sankoff and Ferretti, we will not write the lengths in order.

To be picturesque, we will consider the ith chromosome as being made up of LEGO bricks. On any given move, we may take from 1 to ℓ_i bricks from the ith stack. Each chromosome thus has ℓ_i "cut points" and the genome has a total of T "cut points." On each transition, we will pick two of these T possible cut points at random. We then pair the left half of one with the right half of the other. This procedure may pick the same chromosome arm twice and hence not make a perceptible difference in chromosome length. In addition, our two cut points may be on different arms of the same chromosome. When this occurs, the total length of the chromosome does not change but the centromere may move. Biologists call this event a *pericentric inversion*.

Following Sankoff and Ferretti, we will first examine the case of two chromosome arms. That is, we have only one chromosome and all that is at stake is the position of the centromere on that chromosome. Specializing further, we will consider the case of two chromosome arms with a total of $T = 9$ LEGO bricks. Since our rules guarantee that each arm always has at least one brick, the state space is $(8,1), (7,2), \ldots (1,8)$. By considering the $\binom{9}{2} = 36$ possible choices of two distinct breakpoints one can easily compute that 36 times the transition probability for our chain is:

	(8,1)	(7,2)	(6,3)	(5,4)	(4,5)	(3,6)	(2,7)	(1,8)
(8,1)	28+1	1	1	1	1	1	1	1
(7,2)	1	22+2	2	2	2	2	2	1
(6,3)	1	2	18+3	3	3	3	2	1
(5,4)	1	2	3	16+4	4	3	2	1
(4,5)	1	2	3	4	16+4	3	2	1
(3,6)	1	2	3	3	3	18+3	2	1
(2,7)	1	2	2	2	2	2	22+2	1
(1,8)	1	1	1	1	1	1	1	28+1

Here the diagonal elements are written as a sum of the number of choices that pick the same arm twice and the number that pick different arms and make no change in order to make the patterns in the entries more apparent.

This transition probability is symmetric:

$$(1.2) \qquad\qquad p(u, v) = p(v, u)$$

From (1.2) it follows that in the special case of nine bricks and two chromosome arms, the stationary distribution is the uniform distribution $\pi(u) = 1/8$ for each of the 8 states. It is easy to see that the j arm model has the same symmetry property. On a given step, we will either (a) choose the same arm twice and nothing will happen or (b) choose two different arms. In the second case, we can assume without loss of generality that the two arms chosen are the first and the second. This having been done, the third to jth arms play no role, so we are reduced to the case of two chromosome arms.

Theorem 1.1. *The stationary distribution for the j arm model with total genome size T is uniform over the set of all $(\ell_1, \ldots \ell_j)$ with $\ell_1 + \cdots + \ell_j = T$.*

The human genome corresponds to the case $T = 3 \times 10^9$ nucleotides, so it is sensible to consider the rescaled lengths $x_i = \ell_i/T$ and let $T \to \infty$ to get a process with state space the set of all $(x_1, \ldots x_j)$ with $x_i \geq 0$ and $x_1 + \cdots + x_j = 1$. Let $P(X_i = x)$ be the probability density function for the length of the ith chromosome arm. Symmetry implies that $P(X_i = x) = P(X_1 = x)$. It follows from Theorem 1.1 that

$$(1.3) \quad P(X_1 = x) = C \operatorname{vol}(x_1 = x, x_2 + \cdots + x_{j-1} \leq 1 - x) = C'(1 - x)^{j-2}$$

by scaling since we are taking the volume of a $j-2$ dimensional set. In order for (1.3) to define a probability distribution, we must have $C' = (j - 1)$. A little calculus shows that each chromosome arm has average size $1/j$, which must be true by symmetry.

To connect our results for the LEGO brick chain with a discrete version of the proportional model of Sankoff and Ferretti, let $h(u)$ be the probability that in our scheme we pick the same arm twice when the collection of lengths is $u = (\ell_1, \ldots, \ell_j)$. If we follow the rules of Sankoff and Ferretti and pick two different arms with probabilities proportional to their lengths, we arrive at a Markov chain with transition probability

$$(1.4) \qquad s(u, v) = \begin{cases} \frac{p(u,v)}{1-h(u)} & \text{if } u \neq v \\ \frac{p(u,v)-h(u)}{1-h(u)} & \text{if } u = v \end{cases}$$

When $T = 9$, the transition probability matrix is

	(8,1)	(7,2)	(6,3)	(5,4)	(4,5)	(3,6)	(2,7)	(1,8)
(8,1)	1/8	1/8	1/8	1/8	1/8	1/8	1/8	1/8
(7,2)	1/14	2/14	2/14	2/14	2/14	2/14	2/14	1/14
(6,3)	1/18	2/18	3/18	3/18	3/18	3/18	2/18	1/18
(5,4)	1/20	2/20	3/20	4/20	4/20	3/20	2/20	1/20
(4,5)	1/20	2/20	3/20	4/20	4/20	3/20	2/20	1/20
(3,6)	1/18	2/18	3/18	3/18	3/18	3/18	2/18	1/18
(2,7)	1/14	2/14	2/14	2/14	2/14	2/14	2/14	1/14
(1,8)	1/8	1/8	1/8	1/8	1/8	1/8	1/8	1/8

This matrix is not symmetric about the diagonal, owing to the different normalizations of the rows, so it is harder to guess the stationary distribution. However, from the definition of s given in (1.4) it is easy to see that if $u \neq v$ then

$$(1.5) \qquad \{1 - h(u)\} s(u, v) = p(u, v) = p(v, u) = \{1 - h(v)\} s(v, u)$$

Summing equation (1.5) over u and using $\sum_u s(v, u) = 1$ gives

$$\sum_u \{1 - h(u)\} s(u, v) = 1 - h(v)$$

so the transition probability $s(u, v)$ has stationary distribution $\sigma(u) = C_T(1 - h(u))$, where C_T is a constant that depends on the total genome size T, and is chosen to make the sum of the $\sigma(u)$ equal to one.

Considering scaled chromosome arm lengths $x_i = \ell_i/T$ and letting $T \to \infty$, we see that for Sankoff and Ferretti's proportional model $h(x) = x_1^2 + \cdots + x_j^2$, so the stationary distribution is

$$(1.6) \qquad C(1 - x_1^2 - x_2^2 \cdots - x_j^2) \quad \text{when } x_i \geq 0 \text{ and } \sum_i x_i = 1$$

In the case of two chromosomes, if we let $x_1 = x$ and $x_2 = 1 - x$, then the length of the first chromosome has density

$$(1.7) \qquad P(X_1 = x) = C'x(1 - x) \quad \text{for } 0 < x < 1$$

In order for (1.7) to be a probability density, we must have $C' = 6$. To make the connection with Sankoff and Ferretti's result note that if $X^1 = \max\{X_1, X_2\}$ is the length of the longer chromosome then $P(X^1 = x) = 2P(X_1 = x)$ for $x \in [1/2, 1]$, in agreement with (1.1).

The calculations above show that Sankoff and Ferretti's proportional model is a time change of ours. In other words, if we ignore the transitions in our model that choose the same arm twice, then the result is the model of Sankoff and Ferretti. To understand the differences between the stationary distributions, we turn to simulation. With the human genome in mind, we choose $k = 22$. The figure on the next page shows the sizes of the 22 human chromosomes as dots. The curves give the average chromosome lengths in the Sankoff and Ferretti proportional model (line with tick marks) and in our model with 44 chromosome arms (smooth lines). In both cases, the chromosomes that the models produce have been sorted in order of increasing size and normalized so that their total length is 1. The curve gives the average of 100 simulations.

The line with tick marks that starts lower on the left and ends higher on the right is the result of the Sankoff and Ferretti model. The smooth line, which is somewhat closer to the data, is from our model. The reason for the difference between the models becomes clear if one simulates a random breakage model in which the unit interval is fractured into 22 pieces that are sorted in order of increasing size. The average of 100 simulations in this case is almost indistinguishable from the averages for the Sankoff and Ferretti model. Since our stationary distribution results from breaking the unit interval into 44 pieces and then adding randomly chosen pairs, chromosome sizes will be more uniform.

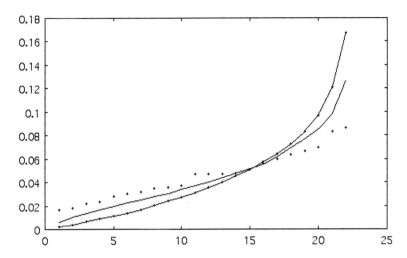

As the figure shows, the stationary distribution of our new model is more uniform than that of Sankoff and Ferretti, but still has short chromosomes that are too short and long chromosomes that are too long. As mentioned above, Sankoff and Ferretti fixed this problem by imposing an absolute lower limit on chromosome sizes. Here we will start with a softer version of their constraint by introducing a fitness function $\phi(u)$ that describes the relative fitness of an individual with chromosome arm lengths $u = (\ell_1, \ldots, \ell_j)$.

To develop a concrete formula for $\phi(u)$, we will take as inspiration the fact that recombination is an important mechanism for pairing homologous chromosomes during meiosis. Since the rate of crossing over per base pair is not constant we now switch over to writing chromosome lengths in terms of centiMorgans (cM), a measure of chromosomal distance that corresponds to a 1% probability of recombination per generation. With lengths written in Morgans (= 100 cM) crossovers are a rate one Poisson process. We define our fitness $\phi(u)$ to be the probability that each pair of homologous chromosome arms experiences at least one recombination event:

$$(1.8) \qquad \phi(u) = \prod_{i=1}^{j} (1 - e^{-\ell_i})$$

Having decided on a form for our fitness function, the next step is to decide on how to modify the dynamics. Inspired by the well-known Metropolis algorithm, which can be used to look for the maximum of a function ϕ, we introduce the modified chain with transition probability:

$$(1.9) \qquad q(u,v) = \begin{cases} p(u,v) & \text{if } \phi(v) \geq \phi(u) \\ p(u,v) \cdot \frac{\phi(v)}{\phi(u)} & \text{if } \phi(v) \leq \phi(u) \end{cases}$$

In words, if the new state proposed by the transition probability has greater fitness, we always accept the proposed move. Otherwise, we accept the transition with probability $\phi(v)/\phi(u)$.

We will refer to this new Markov chain as the model with recombination fitness. The next result describes its stationary distribution.

Theorem 1.2. *The transition probability defined in (1.8) and (1.9) has*

$$(1.10) \qquad\qquad \phi(u)q(u,v) = \phi(v)q(v,u)$$

Consequently, $q(u,v)$ has stationary distribution $C_T\phi(u)$, where C_T is a constant chosen to make the sum of the probabilities equal to 1.

Proof. We can suppose without loss of generality that $\phi(v) \geq \phi(u)$ so $q(u,v) = p(u,v)$ and $q(v,u) = p(v,u)\phi(u)/\phi(v)$. Using the last two equalities we have

$$\phi(u)q(u,v) = \phi(u)p(u,v) = \phi(v) \cdot \frac{\phi(u)}{\phi(v)}p(v,u) = \phi(v)q(v,u)$$

where the second equality follows from the fact that $p(u,v) = p(v,u)$. Having checked (1.10), the second conclusion follows immediately; see page 61 of Durrett (1999). ◻

To test the model, we first found data on the world wide web on chromosome lengths measured in centiMorgans for several different species. We then compared the predicted chromosome lengths from our model with recombination fitness to the observed data. The figures on the next pages show four fits. On each graph the line gives the observed sizes of chromosomes sorted in increasing order. The bars give 90% confidence intervals for the sizes of chromosomes in our stochastic model. For humans and rats, the data stay between the 90% confidence intervals.

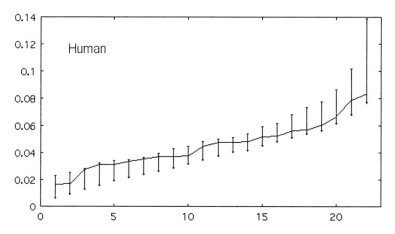

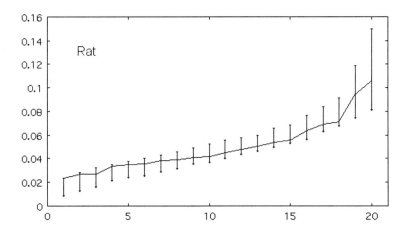

In the case of sheep the line of observed chromosome sizes are too small for chromosomes 19–23 and then suddenly too high on chromosomes 24 and 25. One possible explanation for the long chromosomes is that fusions have recently occurred and the system has not returned to its stationary distribution. In the case of wheat, the observed chromosome arm lengths are more uniform than predicted by our model. One possible explanation for this is the fact that since its divergence from rice, the wheat genome has undergone hexaploidization, which increased its haploid chromosome number from 7 to 21, see e.g., page 1973 of Gale and Devos (1998). After events like this one, it takes some time for chromosome sizes to return to equilibrium.

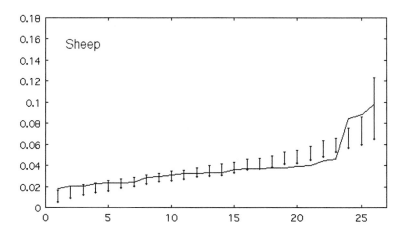

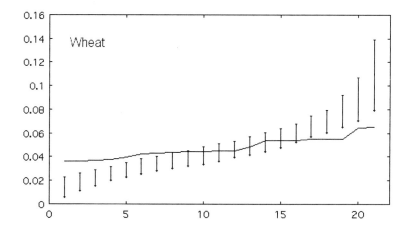

To improve the fit in the bad cases, we can make another change in the model. Sankoff and Ferretti modified their model by forbidding chromosomes that are too short. Here we will forbid chromosomes that are too long. In the notation of definition (1.9), we will use a fitness function that is

$$(1.11) \qquad \phi(u) = \prod_{i=1}^{j}(1 - e^{-\ell_i}) \cdot 1_{(l_i \leq b)}$$

Here $1_{(l_i \leq b)}$ is 1 if $l_i \leq b$, is 0 otherwise, and b represents the bound on the maximum length of a chromosome arm, which is adjusted for fitting purposes. We will call the Markov chain that results from using our new ϕ in (1.9) the truncated model.

In support of this fitness function, we can cite Schubert and Oud (1997), whose experiments with the bean *Vicia fabia* suggested that "for the normal development of an organism, the longest chromosome arm must not exceed half of the spindle axis at telophase." In simpler language, if the end of a chromosome is in the wrong half of the cell while division occurs, then it becomes entangled with the cell wall, with disastrous consequences for the genetic material. See page 518 of Schubert and Oud for some pictures of this disaster. Results presented in Table 1 on page 517 of Schubert and Oud (1997) show that when the longest chromosome arm is at most 21.3% of the whole genome, plants are normal, but when the longest arm is 21.7% or more, the offspring are mostly sterile. We take this as evidence that the sharp cutoff imposed in (1.11) is a reasonable approximation.

As in the case of our first model with fitness (see Theorem 1.2), the new model has stationary distribution $C'_T \phi(u)$, where C'_T is a new constant chosen to make the sum of the probabilities one. The figures below show the new truncated model fit to our two bad cases. The truncation makes the fit for sheep worse for the three largest chromosomes and now has chromosomes 16 to 23 too small.

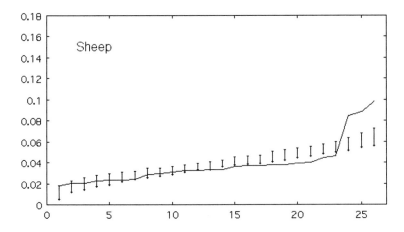

The fit for wheat is improved since the data were more uniform than the previous prediction, and the new selection forces chromosome sizes to be more uniform.

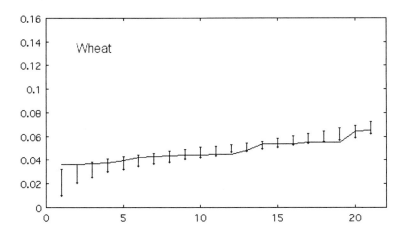

Of course, the mere fact that the new model fits better does not mean that selection against chromosomes that are too long is acting to make chromosome size distributions more uniform. In wheat, for example, the hexaploidization mentioned above is another explanation for the departure from the model's equilibrium distribution. However, comparison of observed chromosome lengths with that of a model of random translocations suggests that some form of selection is causing the distribution of lengths to be more uniform.

5.2   Inversions

Palmer and Herbon (1988) discovered that while the genes in the mitochondrial genomes of cabbage (*Brassica oleracea*) and turnip (*Brassica
campestris*) are 99% identical, the gene order is quite different. If the order
of the segments is 1, 2, 3, 4, 5 in turnip then the order in cabbage is 1,
−5, 4, −3, 2, where the negative numbers indicate that the segment in
cabbage is reversed relative to turnip. A little experimentation reveals that
it is possible to turn cabbage into turnip with three inversions.

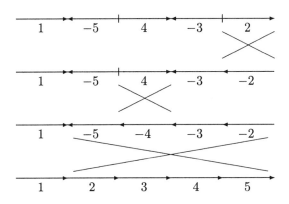

In this simple example it is not hard to see that three inversions are
necessary, but to handle more complicated examples such as the comparison
between cytomegalovirus (CMV) 1, 2, 3, 4, 5, 6, 7 and Epstein-Barr Virus
(EBV) 1, −2, −3, −6, −5, 7, −4 studied by Hannenhalli et al. (1995), we
will need to develop some theory. Our first step is to define the *breakpoint
graph*. To do this we first replace k by $2k − 1 : 2k$, $−k$ by $2k : 2k − 1$, and
then add 0, at the beginning and ,15 at the end to generate two strings

$$\begin{aligned} CMV \quad & 0,1{:}2,3{:}4,5{:}6,7{:}8,9{:}10,11{:}12,13{:}14,15 \\ EBV \quad & 0,1{:}2,4{:}3,6{:}5,12{:}11,10{:}9,13{:}14,8{:}7,15 \end{aligned}$$

The vertices separated by commas in EBV are connected by "black edges,"
the thick lines in the picture below. Those separated by commas in CMV
are connected by "gray edges," the thin lines.

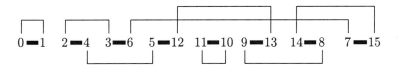

Each vertex in the breakpoint graph has degree 2 and is an endpoint of one black edge and one gray edge. Starting with a black edge and following the alternating sequence of black and gray edges, we can see that this graph has three cycles: 0-1-0, 2-4-5-12-13-9-8-14-15-7-6-3-2, 11-10-11. When EBV has been rearranged to match CMV there will be eight cycles.

$$0 \blacksquare 1 \quad 2 \blacksquare 3 \quad 4 \blacksquare 5 \quad 6 \blacksquare 7 \quad 8 \blacksquare 9 \quad 10 \blacksquare 11 \quad 12 \blacksquare 13 \quad 14 \blacksquare 15$$

A move corresponds to cutting two black edges and reversing the segment in between. Since the best thing that can happen is that one cycle can be cut into two, this can at most increase the number of cycles by 1. Therefore if we let $d(\pi)$ denote the minimum number of reversals to make the signed permutation π into the identity and let $c(\pi)$ be the number of cycles in the breakpoint graph, then we have

$$(2.1) \qquad\qquad d(\pi) \geq n + 1 - c(\pi)$$

where n is the number of segments. In the current example, $n = 7$ and $c(\pi) = 3$, so this says that $d(\pi) \geq 5$.

Another consequence of (2.1) is that if at each stage we can increase the number of cycles by 1, then we can find a path of length 5. A reversal is called *proper* if it increases the number of cycles by 1. A little thought shows this holds if and only if when the two black edges are eliminated, then the left end of one black edge is connected to the left edge of the other black edge by the edges that remain. An example of a proper reversal above is the one involving the black edges 2-4 and 3-6. The result is

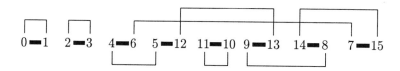

$$0 \blacksquare 1 \quad 2 \blacksquare 3 \quad 4 \blacksquare 6 \quad 5 \blacksquare 12 \quad 11 \blacksquare 10 \quad 9 \blacksquare 13 \quad 14 \blacksquare 8 \quad 7 \blacksquare 15$$

Using black edges 4-6 and 5-12 now leads to

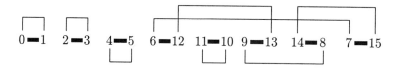

$$0 \blacksquare 1 \quad 2 \blacksquare 3 \quad 4 \blacksquare 5 \quad 6 \blacksquare 12 \quad 11 \blacksquare 10 \quad 9 \blacksquare 13 \quad 14 \blacksquare 8 \quad 7 \blacksquare 15$$

At this point, if we tried the black edges 9-13 and 14-8, then the number of cycles would not change. This happens whenever the left end of one black edge is connected to the right end of the other. 6-12 and 7-15 is a proper reversal and leads to

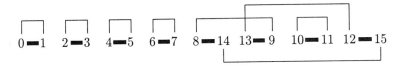

Using 8-14 and 12-15 now leads to

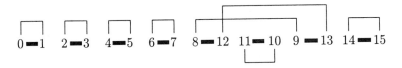

A fifth and final move using 8-12 and 9-13 puts all of the numbers in order. The construction shows $d(\pi) \leq 5$ so with (2.1) we can conclude that the distance to the identity is indeed equal to 5.

Comparison / Source	Segments n	Postulated Distance	Actual Distance
B. oleracea vs. *B. campestris* Palmer and Herbon 1988	5	3	3
B. rapus vs. *B. campestris* Palmer and Herbon 1988	5	3	3
B. nigra vs. *B. campestris* Palmer and Herbon 1988	12	11	9
R. sativa vs. *B. campestris* Palmer and Herbon 1988	15	14	13
B. hirta vs. *B. campestris* Palmer and Herbon 1987	12	10	10
Ogura vs. normal radish Makarov and Palmer 1988	12	10	8
Tobacco vs. *Lobelia fervens* Knox et al 1993	7	5	5
Anemone vs. Clematis Hoot and Palmer 1994	6	6	6
Subclover vs. alfalfa Milligan et al 1989	10	8	8
Pea vs. soybean Palmer et al. 1988	13	8	8

The method above has been applied by Bafna and Pevzner (1995, 1996) to a number of examples in the biology literature. In a few cases, the distance they found was smaller than the most parsimonious path biologists found by hand. The latter is not surprising. When the number of segments is 12, the number of permutations is $12! = 479{,}001{,}600$ and the number of possible reversals at each stage is $\binom{13}{2} = 78$.

In each case here, and indeed in all biological examples that we know of, the lower bound in (2.1) gives the distance. The next example, which is the breakpoint graph for the permutation 3, 2, 1, shows that this is not always true.

(⋆)

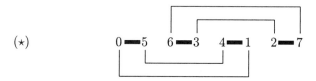

There are two cycles 0-5-4-1-0 and 6-3-2-7-6. However, since in each case the left end of one black edge is connected to the right end of the other, there is no proper reversal. The reversal involving 0-5 and 4-1 does not decrease the number of cycles. However, after this is done, the situation becomes

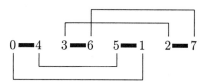

At this point, the reversal involving 3-6 and 2-7 has become proper. Performing it leads to

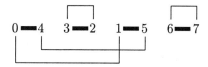

Now the reversal involving 0-4 and 1-5 is proper. Doing it puts the numbers in order. Since there are three segments in this example and two cycles in the breakpoint graph, the bound that (2.1) gives is $d(\pi) \geq 4 - 2$. However, on our first move we could not increase the number of cycles so we ended up with $d(\pi) = 3$.

To explain the obstruction we encountered here requires some terminology. Let π be the current permutation. At the beginning of the example above, i.e., in $(\star)$, we have

$$\pi_0 = 0, \ \pi_1 = 5, \ \pi_2 = 6, \ \pi_3 = 3, \ \pi_4 = 4, \ \pi_5 = 1, \ \pi_6 = 2, \ \pi_7 = 7$$

We say that a reversal $\rho(i, j)$ acts on black edges (π_{i-1}, π_i) and (π_{j-1}, π_j). Here i and j will always be odd numbers. A gray edge is said to be *oriented* if the reversal acting on the two black edges incident to it is proper, and *unoriented* otherwise. In $(\star)$ all gray edges are unoriented. A cycle is said to be *oriented* if it contains an oriented gray edge. Otherwise it is *unoriented*. In $(\star)$ both cycles are unoriented.

Gray edges (π_i, π_j) and $\pi_k, \pi_\ell)$ are interleaving if the intervals $[i, j]$ and $[k, \ell]$ overlap but neither contains the other. In $(\star)$, $(0,1)$ and $(6,7)$ are interleaving but $(0,1)$ and $(5,4)$ are not. Two cycles, C_1 and C_2, are said to be *interleaving* if there are gray edges $g_i \in C_i$ so that g_1 and g_2 are interleaving. In $(\star)$, the two cycles are interleaving. Let $\mathcal{C}_\pi$ be the set of cycles in the breakpoint graph of a permutation π. Define the interleaving graph H_π to have vertices $\mathcal{C}_\pi$ and edges connecting any two interleaving cycles. In $(\star)$ the graph consists of two vertices connected by one edge.

A connected component of H_π is said to be *oriented* if it contains an oriented cycle and is unoriented otherwise. In $(\star)$, there is only one unoriented cycle in the interleaving graph, so it is a *hurdle*. Hannenhalli and Pevzner (1995a) have shown that if $h(\pi)$ is the number of hurdles, then

$$(2.2) \qquad\qquad d(\pi) \geq n + 1 - c(\pi) + h(\pi)$$

In $(\star)$, $n = 3$, $c(\pi) = 2$ and $h(\pi) = 1$, so this new lower bound $4 - 2 + 1 = 3$ gives the right answer.

To see the reason for distinguishing oriented from unoriented cycles we need a more complicated example. Consider the permutation $3, -5, 8, -6, 4, -7, 9, 2, 1$, which has the following breakpoint graph.

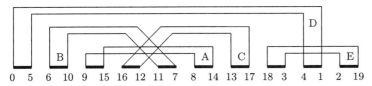

This time there are five cycles, as indicated in the figure. A is oriented but the other four are not. Cycle A is interleaving with B and C but not with D and E. Cycles B and C, and D and E, are interleaving, but the other pairs we have not mentioned are not.

The interleaving graph consists of two components: a triangle ABC that is oriented and an edge DE that is not. Again, there is only one unoriented component, so the number of hurdles is 1. Since $n = 9$ and $c(\pi) = 5$, the lower bound from (2.2) is $10 - 5 + 1 = 6$. To see that this can be achieved, note that if we start with the reversal that cuts the black edges 9-15 and 8-14, then we increase the number of cycles by 1 and the result is

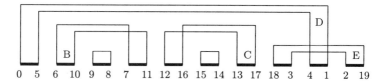

The cycles B and C are now oriented. Reversals using 6-10 and 7-11 then 12-16 and 13-17 put the numbers 6 to 17 in order. The pair DE is equivalent to $(\star)$ so it can be sorted in 3 moves for a total distance of 6.

To understand the final complexities in the general definition of hurdles we need another more complicated example. Consider 5, 7, 6, 8, 1, 3, 2, 4, for which the breakpoint graph is

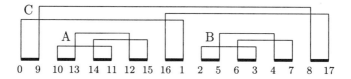

This time there are three cycles, as indicated in the figure. All three are unoriented and no two of them are interleaving, so the interleaving graph H_π consists of three connected components that are isolated points, all of which are unoriented. For a connected component U of H_π, define the leftmost and rightmost positions in U by

$$U_{min} = \min_{\pi_i \in C \in U} i \quad \text{and} \quad U_{max} = \max_{\pi_i \in C \in U} i$$

Here $A_{min} = 2$, $A_{max} = 7$, $B_{min} = 10$, $B_{max} = 15$, $C_{min} = 0$, and $C_{max} = 17$. Consider the set of unoriented components, and define the *containment partial order* $U \prec V$ if $[U_{min}, U_{max}] \subset [V_{min}, V_{max}]$. An unoriented component that is minimal with respect to this order is a *minimal hurdle*.

There are also potential hurdles at the top of the partial order. We say that a component U separates V and W if there is a gray edge (π_i, π_j) in U so that $[V_{min}, V_{max}] \subset [i, j]$ but $[W_{min}, W_{max}] \not\subset [i, j]$. In our most recent example C separates A and B by virtue of the edge $(0,1)$. If U is a maximal oriented component with respect to $\prec$ and it does not separate any two hurdles, then U is called a *maximal hurdle*. This example has two minimal hurdles and no maximal hurdle, so $h(\pi) = 2$. Since $n = 8$ and $c(\pi) = 3$, the lower bound that results from (2.2) is $9 - 3 + 2 = 8$.

To see the reason for the no separation condition in the definition of maximal hurdle, we apply the reversal that involves black edges 12-15 and 2-5:

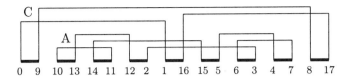

$$0 \quad 9 \quad 10 \quad 13 \quad 14 \quad 11 \quad 12 \quad 2 \quad 1 \quad 16 \quad 15 \quad 5 \quad 6 \quad 3 \quad 4 \quad 7 \quad 8 \quad 17$$

The gray edges $(0,1)$ and $(16,17)$ in cycle C are now oriented. The cycles A and B have merged into 1, but the gray edges $(14,15)$ and $(2,3)$ are now oriented. The number of cycles is now 2 but both hurdles have been destroyed so the lower bound from (2.2) is now $9 - 2 + 0 = 7$. With both cycles oriented we can compute as before to find seven moves that bring this permutation to the identity.

The bound in (2.2) is very close to the right answer. Hannenhalli and Pevzner (1995a) showed that

$$(2.3) \qquad\qquad d(\pi) = n + 1 - c(\pi) + h(\pi) + f(\pi)$$

where $f(\pi) = 1$ if the permutation is a fortress and 0 otherwise. The details of the definition of a fortress are somewhat complicated, so we refer the reader to Chapter 10 of Pevzner (2000) for it and the proofs of (2.2) and (2.3). All of the steps in the proof of (2.3) are constructive, so it leads to an algorithm for computing the reversal distance in $O(n^4)$ time, where n is the number of segments. The n^4 makes this method somewhat painful for large n. However, it is remarkable that there is a polynomial time algorithm. Caprara (1997) has shown that the corresponding problem for unoriented permutations is NP-hard. Much earlier, Even and Goldreich (1981) had shown that the general problem of computing the distance to the identity for a given set of generators of the permutation group is NP-hard.

Example 2.1. All of the examples considered above have been mitochondrial, chloroplast, or viral genomes, where there is a single chromosome. As we will see in Section 5.3, the situation is much more complicated for multichromosome genomes, where nonhomologous chromosomes exchange genetic material by a process called reciprocal translocation. The sex chromosomes do not participate in this process, so the change in their gene order is due only to reversals. Taking the order of conserved blocks in mice to be 1, 2, 3, 4, 5, 6, 7, 8, the order in humans is -4, -6, 1, 7, -2, -3, 5, 8. Ignoring block 8, the breakpoint graph is as follows

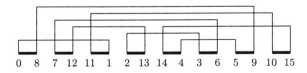

$$0 \quad 8 \quad 7 \quad 12 \quad 11 \quad 1 \quad 2 \quad 13 \quad 14 \quad 4 \quad 3 \quad 6 \quad 5 \quad 9 \quad 10 \quad 15$$

There are two cycles here: 0-8-9-5-4-14-15-10-11-1-0 and 7-12-13-2-3-6-7, so $d(\pi) \geq 8 - 2 = 6$. The following sequence shows that 6 moves suffice. Here we have reinstated the final segment 8, and for reasons that will become clear in a moment have introduced a 0 at the beginning. Parentheses mark the segments that are reversed in going to the next line.

$$
\begin{array}{ccccccccc}
0 & (-4 & -6 & 1 & 7 & -2 & -3) & 5 & 8 \\
0 & (3 & 2 & -7 & -1) & 6 & 4 & 5 & 8 \\
0 & 1 & (7 & -2) & 3 & 6 & 4 & 5 & 8 \\
0 & 1 & 2 & -7 & (3 & 6) & 4 & 5 & 8 \\
0 & 1 & 2 & (-7 & -6 & 3 & 4 & 5) & 8 \\
0 & 1 & 2 & (-5 & -4 & -3) & 6 & 7 & 8 \\
0 & 1 & 2 & 3 & 4 & 5 & 6 & 7 & 8
\end{array}
$$

As is the case in most biological examples, the situation is much simpler than the general case. However, it is somewhat surprising that things aren't even simpler. To explain this, we note that if we model the chromosome as the unit interval and generate breakpoints uniformly distributed on $(0,1)$, then each reversal introduces two new *breakpoints*, i.e., consecutive blocks that are neither $i, (i + 1)$ nor $-(i + 1), -i$. In the original permutation there are eight breakpoints. This suggests that four inversions would suffice. However six are needed, since in four cases the inversion reduces the number of breakpoints by only one. A second remarkable aspect of the reversal distance problem is the lack of uniqueness of the minimal path. Bafna and Pevzner (1995) have computed that there are 1872 scenarios that transform the human into the mouse X chromosome with six reversals.

Example 2.2. Our final topic is to use the methods described above to investigate the evolutionary relationship between three species. Hannenhalli et al. (1995) considered 10 Herpes virus genomes. Here we will restrict our attention to three: Herpes Simplex Virus (HSV), Epstein Barr Virus (EBV), and Cytomegalovirus (CMV). Comparing the gene orders in these viruses leads to the following segments:

$$
\begin{array}{ll}
HSV & 1, 2, 3, 4, 5, 6, 7 \\
EBV & 1, 2, 3, -5, 4, 6, -7 \\
CMV & 1, -2, -3, 7, -4, 5, 6
\end{array}
$$

Constructing the breakpoint graph for the NSV-EBV comparison

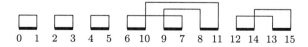

$$
\begin{array}{cccccccccccccc}
0 & 1 & 2 & 3 & 4 & 5 & 6 & 10 & 9 & 7 & 8 & 11 & 12 & 14 & 13 & 15
\end{array}
$$

and using (2.1), we have $d(HSV, EBV) \geq 8-5 = 3$. For the other direction, we note that performing the reversal involving the black edges 6-10 and 8-11 leaves a situation where two more reversals will put the numbers in order.

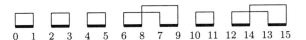

0 1 2 3 4 5 6 8 7 9 10 11 12 14 13 15

At the beginning of the section, we showed that $d(EBV, CMV) = 5$. The breakpoint graph for the HSV-CMV comparison is

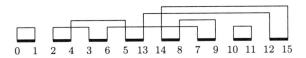

0 1 2 4 3 6 5 13 14 8 7 9 10 11 12 15

(2.1) implies that $d(HSV, CMV) \geq 8 - 3 = 5$. We leave it to the reader to show that $d(HSV, CMV) = 8 - 3 = 5$.

If we connect HSV, EBV, and CMV in an unoriented tree, then there will be one intermediate genome X.

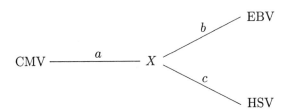

If we let a, b, and c be the number of changes on the indicated edges, then

$$a + b \geq 5 \qquad a + c \geq 5 \qquad b + c \geq 3$$

Adding the three inequalities, we have $2(a + b + c) \geq 13$, so $a + b + c \geq 7$. There are three triples (a, b, c) with sum 7 that satisfy these inequalities: $(4, 2, 1)$, $(4, 1, 2)$, and $(3, 2, 2)$. To check this note that $b + c$ can only be 3 or 4. In the first case, $a = 4$, $b \geq 1$, and $c \geq 1$, while in the second $a = 3$, $b \geq 2$, and $c \geq 2$.

For a given triple, say $(4, 2, 1)$, Hannenhalli et al. (1995) used a computer to generate all permutations that were distance 4 from CMV, distance 2 from EBV, and distance 1 from HSV. There is one that is in all three sets $1, 2, 3, -4, 5, 6, 7$, so it represents one possibility for genome X. Considering $(4, 1, 2)$ leads to another possibility: $1, 2, 3, -4, 5, 6, -7$. The third $(3, 2, 2)$

does not lead to any scenario with seven inversions, so we have only two most parsimonious scenarios.

The considerations above become increasingly more difficult as the number of species increases. Sankoff and Blanchette (1998ab) have attacked this problem by replacing the reversal distance by the more simply computed breakpoint distance, i.e., the number of breakpoints/2.

5.3   Translocations

As mentioned earlier, genomes evolve by inversions within chromosomes and reciprocal translocation of genetic material between autosomes, i.e., the nonsex chromosomes. This section is devoted to a study of the latter mechanism. We begin with an account of a remarkable paper of Nadeau and Taylor (1984). At that point, there was very little genetic data compared to what exists today. However, there were 54 loci in humans whose chromosomal locations were also known in mice. These data gave rise to 13 conserved segments where the genes were adjacent in both species. The genes involved, the length of the segment in centiMorgans, and the chromosome locations in mice and humans are given in the next table. The p's and q's in the human column refer to the chromosome arms on which the genes are located.

Genes	length	Mouse	Human
B2m, Sdh-1	1	2	15q
Galt, Aco-1	5	4	9p
Pgm-2, Pgd, Gpd-1	24	4	1p
Pgm-1, Pep-7, Alb-1	12	5	4q
Gus, Mor-1	11	5	7q
Got-2, Prt-2	4	7	19
Ups, Es-17	10	8	16q
Mpi, Pk-3	6	9	15q
Pgm-3, Mod-1	3	9	6q
Acy-1, Trf, Bgl	10	9	3p
Igh, Pi	12	12	14q
Glo-1, H-2, C-4, Upg-1	9	17	6p

The lengths in the table above are the distances between the genes at the end of the segment. The actual conserved segment will be larger than this measurement. To estimate how much larger, we note that if n genes are put randomly in a segment of length m, then the expected distance r between the leftmost and rightmost gene is

(3.1) $$r = m(n-1)/(n+1)$$

Here and in what, follows we use the notation of Nadeau and Taylor (1984), even though in some cases it will look strange to probabilists. To explain (3.1) we will draw a picture:

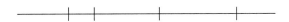

Here the $n = 4$ genes define $n + 1 = 5$ segments. Symmetry implies that the segments have the same average length so the average distance between the leftmost and rightmost gene is $(n - 1)/(n + 1)$ times the total length m. For the reader who does not like the appeal to symmetry in the last argument, we give the following

Proof. We can suppose without loss of generality that $m = 1$. The probability that none of the genes fall in $[0, x]$ is $(1 - x)^n$. Differentiating, we find that the location of the leftmost gene Y_1 has density function $P(Y_1 = x) = n(1 - x)^{n-1}$. Integrating by parts, we have

$$EY_1 = \int_0^1 x \cdot n(1 - x)^{n-1}\, dx = \int_0^1 (1 - x)^n\, dx = -\frac{(1 - x)^{n+1}}{n + 1}\bigg|_0^1 = \frac{1}{n + 1}$$

Reflection symmetry implies that if Y_n is the location of the rightmost gene, then $E(1 - Y_n) = 1/(n + 1)$. Combining these two facts, we have

$$E(Y_n - Y_1) = 1 - E(1 - Y_n) - EY_1 = \frac{n - 1}{n + 1} \qquad \square$$

Inverting the relationship in (3.1), we have

$$\hat{m} = r\frac{(n + 1)}{n - 1}$$

In words, the estimated length is the observed range multiplied by $(n + 1)/(n - 1)$. In the data above, segments with 2, 3, and 4 genes have their lengths multiplied by 3, 2, and 5/3. A little arithmetic then shows that the average length of conserved segments observed is 20.9 cM.

Because conserved segments were identified by the presence of two or more linked homologous markers, segments lacking identifiable markers and segments with a single identifiable marker were necessarily excluded in estimates of conserved segment length. As a result, the estimate of the mean length of conserved segments is biased toward long segments. To account for this bias, let T be the total number of mapped homologous markers, G be the genome size in centiMorgans, and $D = T/G$ be the density of markers. If we let L be the mean length of conserved segments, and we assume that these breakpoints are distributed "at random," then their locations will follow a Poisson process and the lengths will have an exponential distribution with mean L:

$$f(x) = \frac{1}{L}e^{-x/L}$$

We assume that markers are also distributed "at random," so the probability that a segment of length x will have at least two markers is

$$1 - e^{-Dx} - Dxe^{-Dx}$$

and the relative frequency of segments of length x in the sample is

$$S(x) = [1 - e^{-Dx} - Dxe^{-Dx}] f(x)$$

Normalizing this relative frequency to integrate to 1, we see that the expected value of observed lengths is

$$Ex' = \frac{\int_0^\infty xS(x)\,dx}{\int_0^\infty S(x)\,dx}$$

Recalling $\int_0^\infty e^{-\lambda x}\,dx = 1/\lambda$, $\int_0^\infty xe^{-\lambda x}\,dx = 1/\lambda^2$, and $\int_0^\infty x^2 e^{-\lambda x}\,dx = 2/\lambda^3$, we have

$$\int_0^\infty S(x)\,dx = 1 - \frac{1}{L(D+L^{-1})} - \frac{D}{L(D+L^{-1})^2}$$

$$\int_0^\infty xS(x)\,dx = L - \frac{1}{L(D+L^{-1})^2} - \frac{2D}{L(D+L^{-1})^3}$$

Combining the last three formulas, we have

$$Ex' = \frac{[L^2(D+L^{-1})^3 - (D+L^{-1}) - 2D]/(D+L^{-1})^3}{[L(D+L^{-1})^2 - (D+L^{-1}) - D]/(D+L^{-1})^2}$$

Expanding out the cube in the numerator and the square in the denominator, a lot of cancelation occurs, leaving us with

$$Ex' = \frac{L^2[D^3 + 3D^2L^{-1}]}{LD^2 \cdot (D+L^{-1})} = L \cdot \frac{LD+3}{LD+1}$$

In the case under consideration, the total number of markers $T = 54$ and the genome size of mouse is $G = 1600$ centiMorgans, so $D = 0.338$ markers/cM. Setting

$$20.9 = \frac{L^2 D + 3L}{LD+1}$$

and solving, we have $0.338L^2 + (3 - 20.9 \cdot 0.338)L - 20.9 = 0$, which gives $L = 8.1$. To calculate the number of segments, we divide $1600/8.1 = 197.53$. However, 18 of the breakpoints are caused by the ends of the 19 mouse chromosomes, so our estimate of the number of breakpoints caused by translocations is 179.53.

The final step in Nadeau and Taylor's (1984) analysis is to assign an uncertainty to the estimate. If the uncertainty in the estimation of x' were small, then the relationship between L and x' could be approximated by a linear function with slope dL/dx'. Using $\text{var}(cx') = c^2\,\text{var}(x')$, then we have

$$\text{var}(L) \approx \text{var}(x') \cdot \left(\frac{dL}{dx'}\right)^2$$

The standard deviation of the transformed lengths of the 13 conserved segments in our sample is 12.8 cM. This leads to an estimate of $(12.8)^2/13 = 12.6$ for $\text{var}(x')$. To evaluate the second term, we use calculus to conclude that

$$\frac{dx'}{dL} = \frac{(2DL+3)(LD+1) - D(L^2D + 3L)}{(LD+1)^2}$$

and $dL/dx' = 1/(dx'/dL)$. Substituting the numerical values of L, D, and $V(x')$, we estimate the standard deviation of our estimate of L to be 1.6 cM. Dividing this leads to an estimate of 178 ± 39 breakpoints or 89 ± 20 reciprocal translocations between the genomes of man and mouse.

Over time the number of markers in the comparative map between mouse and man has grown but the estimates of the average length of conserved segments (in centiMorgans) based on the theory in Nadeau and Taylor (1984) have remained roughly constant.

source	markers	segments	estimate
Nadeau and Taylor (1984)	54	13	8.1
Nadeau (1989)	157	27	10.1
Copeland et al. (1993)	917	101	8.8
Debry and Seldin (1996)	1416	181	7.7

As gene mapping efforts have proceeded, however, the gene orders in some previously defined segments have been found to be different. As Nadeau and Sankoff (1998) discuss, there are two types of problems. *Disrupted synteny* occurs when a small chromosome segment is missing from a larger chromosome segment on one chromosome and is instead located on another chromosome. An example is *Xpg* on mouse chromosome 1, whose homolog in humans is located on chromosome segment 13q32.2-33. Most of the genes that flank *Xpg* in humans have homologs on mouse chromosome 14. The genetic length of the anomalous segment marked by *Xpg* is about 1.6 cM.

The second type of problem is *disrupted linkage but not synteny*, where rearranged segments are embedded within larger conserved segments as though a small inversion occurred within a long conserved segment. For example, Koizumi et al. (1992) found that in the Huntington disease region of chromosome segment 4p16.3 in humans, most markers are in the same order as in a corresponding part of chromosome 5 in mice, but *Idua* is not in its expected location. A second example of this form is provided by 11 genes in the region of human chromosome 22q11 associated with DiGeorge syndrome. When Botta et al. (1997) compared them with the corresponding region of mouse chromosome 16, they found that the gene order of the last four genes was inverted, *DGCR6* was first in humans but 6th in mice, and *CLTCL* has no homologue in mice. For more examples of these types of problems, see Nadeau and Sankoff (1998).

Having discovered problems on a small scale, it is natural to ask if the large-scale structure of the comparative map is compatible with our uniform breakage model. One way of investigating this question is to look at the distribution of the number of genes per conserved segment. If breakpoints were a Poisson process with rate n and genes were a Poisson process with rate m, then the number of genes in a segment would have a shifted geometric distribution with success probability $n/(m+n)$. That is the probability of r genes would be

$$(3.2) \qquad \left(\frac{m}{m+n}\right)^r \cdot \frac{n}{m+n} \qquad \text{for } r = 0, 1, 2, \ldots$$

Taking a different approach to this question, Sankoff and Nadeau (1996) have shown:

Consider a linear interval of length 1, with $n > 0$ uniformly distributed breakpoints that partition the interval into $n+1$ segments. Suppose that there are m genes also uniformly distributed on the interval between 0 and 1, and independently of the breakpoints. For an arbitrary segment, the probability that it contains r genes, $0 \le r \le m$, is

$$(3.3) \qquad P(r) = \frac{nm!(n+m-r-1)!}{(n+m)!(m-r)!}$$

To make the connection with (3.2) we can write (3.3) as

$$\frac{m}{n+m} \cdot \frac{m-1}{n+m-1} \cdots \frac{m-r+1}{n+m-r+1} \cdot \frac{n}{n+m-r}$$

Proof. The segment length between two adjacent breakpoints has probability density $f(x) = n(1-x)^{n-1}$. For a segment of length x, the probability that it has r genes is given by the binomial distribution. Thus

$$P(r) = \int_0^1 n(1-x)^{n-1} \binom{m}{r} x^r (1-x)^{m-r} \, dx$$

Repeated integration by parts shows that

$$\int_0^1 x^a (1-x)^{b-a} \, dx = \frac{b-a}{a+1} \int_0^1 x^{a+1}(1-x)^{b-a-1} \, dx$$

$$= \frac{(b-a) \cdot (b-a-1) \cdots 1}{(a+1) \cdot (a+2) \cdots b} \int_0^1 x^b \, dx = \frac{(b-a)!a!}{(b+1)!}$$

Using this result with $a = r$ and $b = n + m - 1$ shows

$$P(r) = n \cdot \frac{m!}{r!(m-r)!} \cdot \frac{(n+m-r-1)!r!}{(n+m)!}$$

which is the indicated result.   □

Sankoff, Parent, Marchand, and Ferretti (1997) applied this result to the human/mouse map that was available at the time their paper was written. Since one cannot observe n_0 the number of segments having no genes, they had to compare $f(r) = n_r / \sum_{k>0} n_k$ with $Q(r) = P(r)/(1 - P(0))$. They found that the fit was generally pretty good, but $f(1)$ was much larger than $Q(1)$.

As in the case of reversals, one can ask how many translocations, fissions, and fusions are needed to transform the autosomes of the mouse genome into those of the human genome. Kececioglu and Ravi (1995) were the first to consider this problem. They gave an approximate algorithm for computing the *translocation distance*; that is, the minimum number of translocations needed to convert one genome into another, which computes the correct answer within a factor of 2. Hannenhalli (1995) followed up this work by giving a polynomial algorithm for computing the exact distance. The first step in the solution is the same as for reversal distance. One introduces the cycle graph with black and gray edges and shows that if there are n segments, N chromosomes, and c_A components in the cycle graph, then the distance for an arrangement A satisfies

$$d(A) \geq n - N - c_A$$

As in the case of reversals, there are additional parameters associated with the genome that are important in computing the translocation distance. This time the hurdles that must be overcome are subpermutations (SPs): a set of genes close together within a chromosome in both genomes but not in the same order. The definition of subpermutation and the ensuing analysis are somewhat complicated, so we refer the reader to Hannenhalli's paper for the proof of the following result.

(3.4) If s_A is the number of subpermutations, then

$$d(A) = n - N - c_A + s_A + \begin{cases} 2 & \text{if } A \text{ has even isolation} \\ 1 & \text{if } A \text{ has an odd number of minimal SPs} \\ 0 & \text{otherwise} \end{cases}$$

Hannenhalli and Pevzner (1995b) extended Hannenhalli's analysis of the translocation distance to compute the *genomic distance*, that is, the minimal number of reversals, translocations, fissions, and fusions needed to transform one genome into another one. The answer is in terms of seven parameters capturing different combinatorial properties of the sets of strings so we will not go into the details here. Using the comparative map information available at that time Hannenhalli and Pevzner computed that the human/mouse genomic distance was 131.

5.4   Genome Duplication

In this section, we will consider three examples where DNA sequence data indicate that the whole genome has undergone duplication: yeast (*Saccharomyces cerevisiae*), maize, and *Arabidopsis thalia*. Smith (1987) was the first to suggest that the yeast genome had undergone duplication based on the fact that the core histone genes occur as duplicate pairs. A few years later, Lalo et al. (1993) showed that there was a large duplication between chromosomes III and XIV covering the centromeric regions of these two chromosomes. The completion of the sequencing of the yeast genome in 1997 made it possible for Wolfe and Shields (1997) to study this question in more detail.

To look for duplicated blocks, they used the BLASTP to compare the amino acid sequences of all genes in the yeast genome. A BLASTP score of ≥ 200 (which will occur randomly with probability $p = 10^{-18}$ or less) was taken as evidence that two genes are homologues. The process of looking for duplicated blocks is complicated by the fact that after genes are duplicated, it is often the case that one member of the pair loses function and similarity is erased by the accumulation of mutations. For this reason, Wolfe and Shields defined a duplicate region when there were (a) at least three pairs of homologues with intergenic distances of at most 50 kb, and (b) conservation of gene order and orientation (with allowance for small inversions within some blocks). With these criteria they found 55 duplicate regions containing 376 pairs of homologous genes. The duplicated regions were an average of 55 kb long and together they span about 50% of the yeast genome.

How did these 55 duplicated regions arise? They were formed either by many successive independent duplications (each involving dozens of kilobases) or simultaneously by a single duplication of the entire genome (tetraploidy) followed by reciprocal translocation between chromosomes to produce a mosaic of duplicated blocks. In support of the tetraploidy and translocation model, one can observe that for 50 of the 55 blocks, the orientation of the entire block with respect to the centromere is the same in the two copies. Block orientation is expected to be conserved if the blocks were formed by reciprocal translocation between chromosomes, whereas if each block was made by an independent duplication event, the orientation should be random. Since 50 heads or 50 tails in 55 tosses of a fair coin is extremely unlikely, this is evidence for the tetraploidy explanation.

To obtain more evidence for duplication and to estimate the age of the event, Wolfe and Shields (1987) compared 12 *S. cerevisiae* duplicate pairs with homologues in *Kluveromyces* and an outgroup. In 9 of these pairs, there was strong bootstrap support ($\geq 89\%$) for a branching order that places the two *S. cerevisiae* sequences together; in the others there was no strong support for any order. They then estimated the ages of the duplications in *S. cerevisiae* compared with the divergence from *Kluveromyces*. Three of the gene pairs yield very young ages, indicating that they have been involved in recent gene duplications. Of the five pairs for which there were sufficient data to calculate a confidence interval based on bootstrapping, the mean relative age of duplication is 0.74 (with a standard deviation of 0.12). Since the divergence of *Kluveromyces* and *S. cerevisiae* has been estimated at 1.5×10^8 years ago, this places the genome duplication in yeast at roughly 10^8 years ago. For more on the comparison of gene order in *Kluveromyces* and *S. cerevisiae*, see Keogh, Seoighe, and Wolfe (1998).

Seoighe and Wolfe (1998, 1999) followed up on this work by using simulation and analytical methods of Nadeau and Taylor (1984) to investigate the extent of genome rearrangement after duplication in yeast. To simplify things they took the distance between two genes to be the number of genes between them rather than the distance in kilobases. In their simulations, an original genome with eight chromosomes was duplicated and genes were deleted at random until something resembling present-day yeast remained: 5790 genes on 16 chromosomes. Reciprocal translocations were then made between randomly chosen points in the genome, and blocks of duplicated genes were identified by using criteria similar to those in Wolfe and Shields (1997): three homologues with a maximum distance of 45 genes between them. Of all of the parameter combinations they considered, a probability of 8% for retaining a duplicate pair and 75 reciprocal translocations produced the best fit to what was observed. It produced 62 duplicate blocks spanning 54% of the genome and containing 350 duplicate pairs. This was the only case in which all three statistics were within two standard deviations of their means.

To explain Seoighe and Wolfe's use of results of Nadeau and Taylor (1984), we need to distinguish between chromosomal regions demarcated by reciprocal translocations, called *segments*, and the number of duplicate regions that could be identified, called *blocks*. If we let L be the mean length of segments, then, as in Section 5.3, segment lengths have an exponential distribution:

$$\frac{1}{L}e^{-x/L}$$

The reader should not be too hasty to accept this generalization of the previous results since segment lengths are now numbers of genes rather than kb. However, our estimate of L will turn out to be 16.45, so we probably do not make much of an error approximating the geometric here by the exponential and the binomial in the next step by the Poisson distribution.

Having pointed out this slight inaccuracy, we now return to performing the computation as Seoighe and Wolfe (1998) have done and using their notation. The probability that a segment of length x contains three or more homologues is

$$1 - e^{-Dx} - Dxe^{-Dx} - \frac{(Dx)^2}{2}e^{-Dx}$$

where D is the density of homologous pairs in the whole genome. Thus the fraction of the genome covered by segments has expected value

$$F = N \int_0^\infty (1 - e^{-Dx} - Dxe^{-Dx} - \frac{(Dx)^2}{2}e^{-Dx})\frac{1}{L}xe^{-x/L}\,dx$$

where N is the number of segments. Replacing N by $5790/L$ and recalling

(4.1)
$$\int_0^\infty x^k e^{-\lambda x}\,dx = k!/\lambda^{k+1}$$

where $0! = 1$, we have

(4.2) $$F = \frac{5790}{L}\left(L - \frac{1}{L(D+L^{-1})^2} - \frac{2D}{L(D+L^{-1})^3} - \frac{3D^2}{L(D+L^{-1})^4}\right)$$

As in Nadeau and Taylor (1984), if m is the expected length of a segment that contains n paralogues separated by a total distance r then

$$m = r(n+1)/(n-1)$$

Using this, the fraction of the genome covered by blocks, 0.496, translates into a fraction 0.686 of the genome in identified segments. Using this in (4.1) we have $L = 5790/16.45 = 352$ segments organized as 176 pairs. Eight of these breakpoints are chromosome ends, yielding an estimate of 84 reciprocal translocations.

As a further check on the predictions of the calculations above we can observe that the probability that a segment of length x contains y homologues is $e^{-Dx}(Dx)^y/y!$, so the expected number of segments of length x with y homologues is

(4.3) $$N \int_0^\infty e^{-Dx}\frac{(Dx)^y}{y!} \cdot \frac{1}{L}e^{-x/L}\,dx = \frac{ND^y}{L(D+L^{-1})^{y+1}}$$

where we have used (4.1) to evaluate the integral. Comparing the expected values from (4.1) with the data gives the result in the following table. Here simulation refers to a model with 446 pairs of retained duplicates and 84 reciprocal translocations, and the intervals in this column are the mean $\pm$ 2 standard deviations. Since the simulation parameters are closely related to the parameters used in evaluating (4.3), it should come as no surprise that (4.3) agrees well with the simulation. The agreement between the data and simulation is not so good. In six cases (3, 5, 8, 10, 12, 13) the data lie outside the approximate 95% confidence interval based on the simulation.

Since blocks are defined by the occurrence of 3 or more homologues, there are no data for 0, 1, or 2. The additional number of two-member blocks found in the real data is 34. This is larger than the theoretical prediction, but might reflect the fact that there have been some small-scale duplications since the whole genome duplication event.

y	data	(4.3)	simulation
0		49.6	49.4
1		35.6	35.9 ± 5.9
2		25.6	26.2 ± 5.2
3	10	18.4	18.5 ± 4.3
4	10	13.2	13.2 ± 3.5
5	6	9.5	9.6 ± 3.1
6	4	6.8	6.8 ± 2.5
7	6	4.9	4.8 ± 2.1
8	6	3.5	3.3 ± 1.7
9	1	2.5	2.4 ± 1.4
10	4	1.8	1.8 ± 1.2
11	2	1.3	1.3 ± 1.1
12	1	0.9	0.9 ± 1.0
13	4	0.7	0.6 ± 0.7
14	0	0.5	0.4 ± 0.6
15	0	0.3	0.3 ± 0.6
16–20	1	0.8	0.6 ± 2.6
21–25	0	0.1	0.0

Having estimated the number of reciprocal translocations since genome duplication, it is natural to inquire about the minimum number of translocations needed to rearrange the duplicated genes on the 16 chromosomes so that the yeast genome consists of two sets of 8 chromosomes with identical gene order. Seoighe and Wolfe found that after three initial inversions were performed to correct the orientation of the five blocks whose orientation relative to the centromere is opposite to their copies, this could be done in 41 steps. This is considerably smaller than the estimate of 84 given above. However, the reader should note that this only requires that the conserved blocks be brought into a symmetrical arrangement, while simulations in Seoighe and Wolfe (1998) show that the number of moves required to do this can be much smaller than the number performed to scramble the genome. El-Marbrouk, Bryant, and Sankoff (1999) attacked this problem using Hannenhalli's breakpoint graph. They did not use any inversions and found that a duplication followed by 45 translocations is necessary and sufficient to produce the current order of duplicated genes. For more on genome halving problems, see El-Marbrouk, Nadeau, and Sankoff (1999).

Recently, Friedman and Hughes (2000) have taken another look at duplicated genes in yeast. They used a cutoff score of $p = 10^{-50}$ to define homologous genes. By comparing the number of matches in windows of fixed size for the yeast genome with that of a randomly scrambled version, they determined that for their fixed window size 4 matches disregarding order were needed to define a block. With this criterion, they identified 39 blocks. To test the hypothesis of a single genome duplication they looked at the distribution of the fraction of synonymous substitutions, p_s. They found that the distribution of p_s was distinctly bimodal, indicating that some duplications were recent but a subset of 28 duplications occurred in the distant past. For the more ancient duplications they estimated an age of 200–300 million years in contrast to Wolfe and Shield's estimate of 100 million years.

Maize

Ahn and Tanksley (1993) constructed genetic linkage maps for rice and maize. They found that in some instances entire chromosomes or chromosome arms were nearly identical with respect to gene content and gene order. Their analysis also revealed that most ($> 72\%$) of the single-copy loci in rice were duplicated in maize, suggesting the presence of a polyploidization event. This pattern extends to many other cereals. Moore et al. (1995) showed that the genomes of rice, wheat, maize, foxtail millet, sugar cane, and sorghum could be aligned by dissecting the individual chromosomes into segments and rearranging the linkage blocks into similar structures. Further work by Devos and Gale (1997) and Gale and Devos (1998) has brought more detail to the picture. However, their circular comparative maps are hard for us to interpret so we will stick with the simple linear picture in Moore et al. (1995). Using numbers and letters to indicate segments of rice chromosomes, the maize genome can be written as follows

$$
\begin{array}{rclcccccc}
M3 & = & 12a & 1a & 1b \\
M6 & = & \underline{6a} & \underline{6b} & \underline{5a} & \underline{5b} \\
M1 & = & \underline{3c} & 8 & 10 & 3b & 3a \\
M4 & = & 11a & 2 \\
M2 & = & \underline{4a} & \underline{4b} & 9 & 7 \\
\\
M8 & = & 1a & \underline{5a} & \underline{5b} & 1b \\
M9 & = & \underline{6a} & \underline{6b} & 8 & \underline{3c} \\
M5 & = & 2 & 10 & 3b & 3a \\
M7 & = & 11a & \underline{9 \;\; 7} \\
M10 & = & \underline{4a} & \underline{4b} & 12a \\
\end{array}
$$

The underlined groups are conserved between the two sets of chromosomes, so we will call them segments. Making choices about the orientation of the segments of length one that will minimize the distance leads to the following:

$$
M3 \;\; = \;\; +1 \;\; +2 \;\; +3
$$

$$
\begin{aligned}
M6 &= +4 \quad +5 \\
M1 &= +6 \quad +7 \\
M4 &= +8 \quad +9 \\
M2 &= +10 \quad +11 \\
M8 &= -2 \quad +5 \quad +3 \\
M9 &= +4 \quad -6 \\
M5 &= -9 \quad +7 \\
M7 &= +8 \quad +11 \\
M10 &= +10 \quad -1
\end{aligned}
$$

If we invert $-2, 5$ in $M8$, then $M8 = -5 + 2 + 3$ and the resulting genomes are cotailed in the terminology of Hannenhalli. That is, the same blocks appear on the ends. The reader may notice that $+6$ is on the front end of $M1$ while -6 is on the back end of $M9$. However, this is exactly what we want. If we flip $M9$, then it has $+6$ on the front.

To construct the breakpoint graph, we follow the procedure in Section 5.1, but now we use 0's for the chromosome ends:

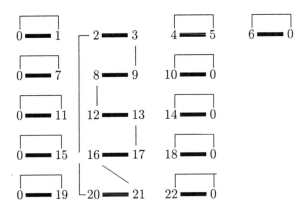

When M8, M9, M5, M7, and M10 are rearranged to match the order in the other five chromosomes, there will be 16 cycles. Now there are 12, so a minimum of 4 translocations is needed. It is easy to see that this is sufficient. We first make $M8$ match $M3$, then make $M9$ match $M6$, etc., and we are done in four moves.

The solution to undoubling the maize genome is elegant and parsimonious. Unfortunately, it is also wrong. The absence of duplicated blocks in millets, sorghum, and sugarcane locates the duplication at the indicated place in the phylogeny. Comparing with the haploid chromosome number x of closely related species makes it appear unlikely that the progenitor maize genome had five chromosomes. Wilson et al. (1999) have suggested that the progenitor maize genome had eight chromosomes, even though this requires six fusions after duplication to reduce the number to the current ten. Their suggestion for the makeup of the predoubling genome can be found in Figure 4 of their paper. It requires in addition six inversions and one insertion to produce the current maize genome.

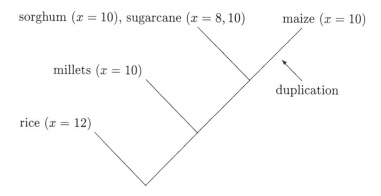

sorghum ($x = 10$), sugarcane ($x = 8, 10$)   maize ($x = 10$)

millets ($x = 10$)

duplication

rice ($x = 12$)

The tetraploid event in the evolution of maize could be an autotetraploid event (the doubling of one genome) or an allotetraploid event (the hybridization of two closely related species). Hexaploid bread wheat (*Triticum aestivum*) is an allopolyploid with genome construction AABBCC, formed through hybridization of *T. uratu* with a B genome of unknown origin, and subsequent hybridization only about 8000 years ago with C genome diploid, *T. tauschii*. In order to distinguish between these two scenarios, Gaut and Doebley (1997) examined the ages of 14 duplicate genes in maize.

loci	distance
orp1, orp2	0.298(1.44)
ant1, ant2	0.277(1.32)
ohp1, ohp2	0.254(1.19)
r, b	0.241(0.83)
cpna, cpnb	0.186(0.55)
cdc2a, cdc2b	0.177(1.04)
whp1, c2	0.169(0.66)
fer1, fer2	0.168(1.44)
cI, plI	0.159(1.05)
ibp1, ibp2	0.150(0.36)
tbp1, tbp2	0.147(1.20)
vpl4a, vpl4b	0.121(0.29)
obf1, obf2	0.104(0.48)
pgpa1, pgpa2	0.102(0.39)

In an autotetraploid, the divergence of the gene copies will all start at the time the species returns to being a diploid. In an allotetraploid, during the time of tetrasomic inheritance, genetic drift (or selection) could bring the alleles of one parent species to fixation. These genes would begin to diverge at the time of the shift to disomic inheritance, while loci that retain alleles from both parents would date to the time of the divergence of the two species that combined to make the allotetraploid. Thus the presence of two distinct age classes would be evidence for allotetraploidy. The next table gives the synonymous distance between the duplicated loci with the variance time 1000 in parentheses. A χ^2 test soundly rejects ($p < 0.0001$) the hypothesis that all of these random variables have the same mean. The group above the line (group A) and the group below the line (group B) have 95% confidence intervals that don't overlap. A χ^2 homogeneity test was not significant for either group (group A, $p = 0.65$, and group B, $p = 0.08$).

Having demonstrated the existence of two groups of duplicated sequence pairs, Gaut and Doebley's next step was to explore how the duplication events are related to the divergence of maize and sorghum. To do this we first need an estimate of the rate of nucleotide substitutions. Gaut et al. (1996) estimated the synonymous substitution rate between the *Adh1* and *Adh2* loci of grasses at 6.5×10^{-9} substitutions per synonymous site per year. Given this rate, sequences in group A diverged roughly

$$\frac{0.267}{2 \cdot 6.5 \times 10^{-9}} = 20,500,000 \quad \text{years ago}$$

and pairs of duplicated sequences in group B diverged approximately 11.4 million years ago. Quite remarkably the average divergence between maize and sorghum falls between the group A distance and the group B distances, suggesting that the sorghum genome is more closely related to one of the maize sub genomes than to the other one. For more on this topic, see Gaut et al. (2000).

Arabidopsis thaliana

was chosen as a model diploid plant species because of its compact genome size. Thus it was surprising when a 105 kilobase bacterial artificial chromosome clone from tomato sequenced by Ku et al. (2000) showed conservation of gene order and content with four different segments in chromosomes 2–5 of *Arabidopsis*. This pattern suggests that these four segments were derived from a common ancestral segment through two or more rounds of large scale genome duplication events, or by polyploidy. Comparison of the divergence of the gene copies suggested that one of the duplication events is ancient and may predate the divergence of *Arabidopsis* and tomato approximately 112 million years ago, while the other is more recent.

When the complete sequence of *Arabidopsis* was later published (see Nature **408**, 796–815), dot-matrix plots of genic similarities showed (see also Paterson et al. 2000) that much of the genome fell into pairs. These plots provide compelling evidence in support for one polyploidy event, which the authors of *Arabidopsis* Genome Initiative took to be the more recent event proposed by Ku et al. (2000). A significantly different conclusion was made by Vision, Brown, and Tanksley (2000), who analyzed the duplications in the completed genome sequenced. Their results suggest that there were three rounds of duplications where 25, 36, and 23 blocks were duplicated 100, 140, and 170 years ago. An independent analysis of the duplicated genes by Lynch and Conrey (2000) suggested that there was one whole genome duplication 65 million years ago.

References

Aguadé, M., Miyashita, N., and Langley, C.H. (1989) Reduced variation in the *yellow-achete-scute* region in natural populations of *Drosophila melaongaster*. *Genetics*. **122**, 607–615

Aguadé, M., Miyashita, N., and Langley, C.H. (1992) Polymorphism and divergence in *Mst26A* male accessory gland gene region in *Drosophila*. *Genetics*. **132**, 755–770

Ahn, S., and Tanksley, S.D. (1993) Comparative linkage maps of the rice and maize genomes. *Proc. Natl. Acad. Sci. USA*. **90**, 7980–7984

Aldous, D.J. (1985) Exchangeability and related topics. Pages 1–198 in Lecture Notes in Math. **1117**, Springer-Verlag, New York

Anderson, S. et al. (1981) Sequence and organization of the human mitochondrial genome. *Nature*. **290**, 457–465

Aquadro, C.F. (1991) Molecular population genetics of *Drosophila*. In *Molecular Approaches in Pure and Applied Entomology*. Edited by J. Oakeshott and M. Whitten. Springer-Verlag, New York

Aquadro, C.F., Begun, D.J., and Kindahl, E.C. (1994) Pages 46–56 in *Non-neutral Evolution: Theories and Molecular Data*. Edited by B. Golding. Chapman and Hall, New York.

Aquadro, C.F., and Greenberg, B.D. (1983) Human mitochondrial DNA variation and evolution: Analysis of nucleotide sequences from seven individuals. *Genetics*. **103**, 287–312

Aquadro, C.F., Lado, K.M., and Noon, W.A. (1988) The *rosy* region of *Drosophila melanogaster* and *Drosophila simulans*. I. Contrasting levels of naturally occurring DNA restriction map variation and divergence. *Genetics.* **119**, 875–888

Arratia, R., Barbour, A.D., and Tavaré, S. (1992) Poisson process approximations for the Ewens sampling formula. *Ann. Appl. Prob.* **2**, 519–535

Athreya, K.B., and Ney, P.E. (1972) *Branching Processes.* Springer, New York

Bafna, V., and Pevzner, P. (1995) Sorting by reversals: Genome rearrangements in plant organelles and the evolutionary history of *X* chromosome. *Mol. Biol. Evol.* **12**, 239–246

Bafna, V., and Pevzner, P. (1996) Genome rearrangements and sorting by reversals. *SIAM J. Computing.* **25**, 272–289

Begun, D.J., and Aquadro, C.F. (1991) Molecular population genetics of the distal portion of the *X* chromosome in *Drosophila*: Evidence for genetic hitchhiking of the *yellow-achaete* region. *Genetics.* **129**, 1147–1158

Berry, A.J., Ajioka, J.W., and Kreitman, M. (1991) Lack of polymorphism on the *Drosophila* fourth chromosome resulting from selection. *Genetics.* **129**, 1111–1117

Birky, C.W., and Walsh, J.B. (1988) Effects of linkage on rates of molecular evolution. *Proc. Natl. Acad. Sci. USA.* **85**, 6414–6418

Botta, A., et al. (1997) Comparative mapping of the DiGeorge syndrome region in mouse shows inconsistent gene order and differential degree of gene conservation. *Mammalian Genome.* **8**, 890–895

Braverman, J.M., Hudson, R.R., Kaplan, N.L., Langley, C.H., and Stephan, W. (1995) The hitchhiking effect on the site frequency spectrum of DNA polymorphisms. *Genetics.* **140**, 783–796

Brown, A.H.D., Feldman, M.W., and Nevo, E. (1980) Multilocus structure of natural populations of *Hordeum spontaneum. Genetics* **96**, 523–536

Brown, W.M., George, Jr., M., and Wilson, A.C. (1979) Rapid evolution of mitochondrial DNA. *Proc. Natl. Acad. Sci. USA.* **76**, 1967–1971

Cann, R.L., Stoneking, M., and Wilson, A.C. (1987) Mitochondrial DNA and human evolution. *Nature.* **325**, 31–36

Cannings, C. (1974) The latent roots of certain Markov chains arising in genetics: A new approach. I. Haploid models. *Adv. Appl. Prob.* **6**, 260–290

Caprara, A. (1997) Sorting by reversals is difficult. Pages 75–83 in the proceedings of RECOMB 97, ACM, New York

Charlesworth, B., Morgan, M.T., and Charlesworth, D. (1993) The effects of deleterious mutations on neutral molecular variation. *Genetics.* **134**, 1289–1303

Charlesworth, D., Charlesworth, B., and Morgan, M.T. (1995) The pattern of neutral molecular variation under the background selection model. *Genetics.* **141**, 1619–1632

Chovnick, A., Gelbart, W., and McCarron, M. (1977) Organization of the *rosy* locus in *Drosophila melanogaster. Cell.* **11**, 1–10

Clark, A.G., et al. (1998) Haplotype structure and population genetic inferences from nucleotide sequence variation in human lipoprotein lipase. *Am. J. Hum. Genetics.* **63**, 595–612

Clifford, P., and Sudbury, A. (1973) A model of spatial conflict. *Biometrika.* **60**, 581–588

Copeland, N.G., et al. (1993) A genetic linkage map of mouse: Current applications and future prospects. *Science.* **262**, 57–66

Cox, J.T. (1989) Coalescing random walks and voter model consensus times on the torus in $\mathbf{Z}^d$. *Ann. Prob.* **17**, 1333–1366

Cox, J.T., and Durrett, R. (2002) The stepping stone model: New formulas expose old myths. *Ann. Appl. Prob.*, to appear

Cox, J.T., and Greven, A. (1991) On the long term behavior of finite particle systems: A critical dimension example. Pages 203–213 in *Random Walks, Brownian Motion and Interacting Particle Systems*. Edited by R. Durrett and H. Kesten. Birkhauser, Boston

Cox, J.T., and Griffeath, D. (1986) Diffusive clustering in the two dimensional voter model. *Ann. Prob.* **14**, 347–370

Coyne, J.A. (1976) Lack of genic similarity between two sibling species of *Drosophila* as revealed by varied techniques. *Genetics.* **84**, 593–607

Crow, J.F., and Aoki, K. (1984) Group selection for a polygenic trait: Estimating the degree of population subdivision. *Proc. Natl. Acad. Sci. USA.* **81**, 6073–6077

Crow, J.F., and Simmons, M.J. (1983) The mutation load in *Drosophila*. Pages 1–35 in *The Genetics and Biology of Drosophila*. Edited by M. Ashburner, H.L. Carson, and J.N. Thompson. Academic Press, London

DeBry, R.W., and Seldin, M.F. (1996) Human/mouse homology relationships. *Genomics.* **33**, 337–351

Devos, K.M., and Gale, M.D. (1997) Comparative genetics in the grasses. *Plant Molecular Biology.* **35**, 3–15

DiRienzo, A., et al. (1994) Mutational processes of simple sequence repeat loci in human populations. *Proc. Natl. Acad. Sci. USA* **91**, 3166–3170

Donnelly, P., Kurtz, T.G., and Tavaré, S. (1991) On the functional central limit theorem for the Ewens sampling formula. *Ann. Appl. Prob.* **1**, 539–545

Donnelly, P., and Tavaré, S. (1986) The ages of alleles and a coalescent. *Adv. Appl. Prob.* **18**, 1–19

Donnelly, P., and Tavaré, S. (1997) *Progress in Population Genetics and Human Evolution*. IMA Volumes in Mathematics and Its Applications, **87**. Springer, New York

Drake, J.W., Charlesworth, B., Charlesworth, D., and Crow, J.F. (1998) Rates of spontaneous mutation. *Genetics*. **148**, 1667–1686

Durrett, R. (1995) *Probability: Theory and Examples, 2nd Ed.* Duxbury Press, Pacific Grove, CA

Durrett, R. (1996) *Stochastic Calculus: A Practical Introduction*. CRC Press, Boca Raton, FL

Durrett, R. (1999) *Essentials of Stochastic Processes*. Springer-Verlag, New York

Eanes, W.F., Kirchner, M., and Yoon, J. (1993) Evidence for adaptive evolution of the *G6pd* in the *Drosophila melanogaster* and *Drosophila simulans* lineages. *Proc. Natl. Acad. Sci. USA*. **90**, 7475–7479

El-Mabrouk, N., Bryant, D., and Sankoff, D. (1999) Reconstructing the pre-doubling genome. Pages 154–163 in the Proceedings of RECOMB 99. ACM, New York

El-Mabrouk, N., Nadeau, J.H., and Sankoff, D. (1999) Genome halving. Pages 235–250 in *Proceedings of the 9th Annual Symposium on Combinatorial Pattern Matching*. Lecture Notes in Computer Science **1448**, Springer, New York

Even, S. and Goldreich, O. (1981) The minimum-length generator sequence problem is NP-hard. *J. of Algorithms*. **2**, 311–313

Ewens, W.J. (1972) The sampling theory of selectively neutral alleles. *Theor. Popul. Biol.* **3**, 87–112

Ewens, W.J. (1979) *Mathematical Population Genetics*. Springer-Verlag, Berlin

Felsenstein, J. (1981) Evolutionary trees from DNA sequences: A maximum likelihood approach. *J. Mol. Evol.* **17**, 368–376

Fitch, W.M. (1977) On the problem of discovering the most parsimonious tree. *Am. Nat.* **44**, 223–257

Friedman, R., and Hughes, A.L. (2000) Gene duplication and the structure of eukaryotic genomes. *Genome Research*. **11**, 373–381

Fu, Y.X. (1996) New statistical tests of neutrality for DNA samples from a population. *Genetics*. **143**, 557–570

Fu, Y.X. (1997) Statistical tests of neutrality of mutations against population growth, hitchhiking and background selection. *Genetics*. **147**, 915–925

Fu, Y.X. and Li, W.H. (1993) Statistical tests of neutrality of mutations. *Genetics*. **133**, 693–709

Gale, M.D., and Devos, K.M. (1998) Comparative genetics in the grasses. *Proc. Natl. Acad. Sci. USA* **95**, 1971–1974

Gaut, B.S., and Doebley, J.F. (1997) DNA sequence evidence for the segmental allotetraploid origin of maize. *Proc. Natl. Acad. Sci. USA.* **94**, 6809–6814

Gaut, B.S., Le Thierry d'Ennequin, M., Peek, A.S., and Sawkins, M.C. (2000) Maize as a model for the evolution of plant nuclear genomes. *Proc. Natl. Acad. Sci. USA* **97**, 7008–7015

Gaut, B.S., Morton, B.R., McCaig, B.M., and Clegg, M.T. (1996) *Proc. Natl. Acad. Sci. USA.* **93**, 10274–10279

Gojobori, T., Ishii, K., and Nei, M. (1982) Estimation of average number of nucleotide substitutions when the rate of substitution varies with nucleotide. *J. Mol. Evol.* **18**, 414–423

Gonick, L., and Wheelis, M. (1991) *The Cartoon Guide to Genetics.* Harper-Collins, New York

Griffiths, R.C., and Marjoram, P. (1996) Ancestral inference from samples of DNA sequences with recombination. *J. Comp. Biol.* **3**, 479–502

Griffiths, R.C., and Marjoram, P. (1997) An ancestral recombination graph. Pages 257–270 in Donnelly and Tavaré (1997).

Griffiths, R.C., and Tavaré, S. (1994a) Ancestral inference in population genetics. *Stat. Sci.* **9**, 307–319

Griffiths, R.C., and Tavaré, S. (1994b) Sampling theory for neutral alleles in a varying environment. *Philos. Trans. R. Soc. London B.* **344**, 403–410

Hamblin, M.T., and Aquadro, C.F. (1996) High nucleotide sequence variation in a region of low recombination in *Drosophila simulans* is consistent with the background selection model. *Mol. Biol. Evol.* **13**, 1133–1140

Hamblin, M.T., and Veuille, M. (1999) Population structure among African and derived populations of *Drosophila simulans*; evidence for ancient subdivision and recent admixture. *Genetics.* **153**, 305–317

Hannenhalli, S. (1995) Polynomial algorithm for computing translocation distance between genomes. Pages 162–176 in *Sixth Annual Symposium on Combinatorial Pattern Matching.* Springer Lecture Notes in Computer Science **937**, Springer, Berlin

Hannenhalli, S., and Pevzner, P.A. (1995a) Transforming cabbage into turnip (polynomial algorithm for sorting signed permutations by reversals). Pages 178–189 in *Proceedings of the 27th Annual ACM Symposium on the Theory of Computing.* Full version in the *Journal of the ACM.* **46**, 1–27

Hannenhalli, S., and Pevzner, P. (1995b) Transforming men into mice (polynomial algorithm for the genomic distance problem. Pages 581–592 in *Proceedings of the 36th Annual IEEE Symposium on Foundations of Computer Science.* IEEE, New York

Hannenhalli, S., Chappey, C., Koonin, E.V., and Pevzner, P.A. (1995) Genome sequence comparisons and scenarios for gene rearrangements: A test case. *Genomics.* **30**, 299–311

Hansen, J.C. (1990) A functional central limit theorem for the Ewens sampling formula. *J. Appl. Prob.* **27**, 28–43

Harding, R.M., Fullerton, S.M., Griffiths, R.C., Bond, J., Cox, M.J., Schneider, J.A., Moulin, D.S., and Clegg, J.B. (1997) Archaic African and Asian lineages in the genetic ancestry of modern humans. *Am. J. Hum. Genet.* **60**, 772–789

Hasegawa, M., Kishino, H., and Yano, T. (1985) Dating of the human-ape splitting by a moecular clock of mitochondrial DNA. *J. Mol. Evol.* **22**, 160–174

Hey, J. (1991) A multi-dimensional coalescent process applied to multiallelic selection models and migration models. *Theor. Popul. Biol.* **39**, 30–48

Hey, J. (1997) Mitochondrial and nuclear genes present conflicting portraits of human origins. *Mol. Biol. Evol.* **14**, 166–172

Hey, J., and Wakeley, J. (1997) A coalescent estimator of the population recombination rate. *Genetics.* **145**, 833–846

Holley, R.A., and Liggett, T.M. (1975) Ergodic theorems for weakly interacting systems and the voter model. *Ann. Prob.* **3**, 643–663

Hoot, S.B., and Palmer, J.D. (1994) Structural rearrangments, including parallel inversions, within the chloroplast genome of *Anemone* and related genera. *J. Mol. Evol.* **38**, 274–281

Hoppe, F. (1984) Polya-like urns and the Ewens' sampling formula. *J. Math. Biol.* **20**, 91–94

Horai, S., and Hayasaka, K. (1990) Intraspecific nucleotide sequence differences in the major noncoding region of human mitochondrial DNA. *Am. J. Hum. Genet.* **46**, 828–842

Hudson, R.R. (1983) Properties of a neutral allele model with intragenic recombination. *Theor. Popul. Biol.* **23**, 183–201

Hudson, R.R. (1987) Estimating the recombination parameter of a finite population model without selection. *Genet. Res.* **50**, 245–250

Hudson, R.R. (1991) Gene genealogies and the coalescent process. Pages 1–44 in *Oxford Surveys in Evolutionary Biology.* Edited by D. Futuyama and J. Antonovics. Oxford University Press

Hudson, R.R., Boos, D.D., and Kaplan, N.L. (1992) A statistical test for detecting geographic subdivision. *Mol. Biol. Evol.* **9**, 138–151

Hudson, R.R., and Kaplan, N. (1985) Statistical properties of the number of recombination events in the history of a sample of DNA sequences. *Genetics.* **111**, 147–164

Hudson, R.R., and Kaplan, N.L. (1988) The coalescent process in models with selection and recombination. *Genetics.* **120**, 831–840

Hudson, R.R., and Kaplan, N.L. (1994) Gene trees with background selection. Pages 140–153 in *Nonneutral Evolution: Theories and Molecular Data.* Edited by G.B. Golding. Chapman and Hall, New York

Hudson, R.R., and Kaplan, N.L. (1995) Deleterious background selection with recombination. *Genetics.* **126**, 1605–1617

Hudson, R.R., and Kaplan, N.L. (1996) The coalescent process and background selection. Pages 57–65 in *New Uses for New Phylogenies.* Edited by P. Harvey et al. Oxford University Press

Hudson, R.R., Kreitman, M., and Aguadé (1987) A test of neutral evolution based on nucleotide data. *Genetics.* **116**, 153–159

Hudson, R.R., Slatkin, M., and Maddison, W.P. (1992) Estimation of levels of gene flow from DNA seqeunce data. *Genetics.* **132**, 583–589

Johnson, N.L., and Kotz, S. (1973) *Distributions in Statistics: Discrete Distributions.* Houghton-Mifflin, Boston

Joyce, P., and Tavaré, S. (1987) Cycles, permutations and the structure of the Yule process with immigration. *Stoch. Proc. Appl.* **25**, 309–314

Jukes, T.H., and Cantor, C.R. (1969) Evolution of protein molecules. In *Mammalian Protein Metabolism, II.* Edited by H.N. Munro. Academic Press, New York

Kaessmann, H., Heissig, F., von Haeseler, A., and Pääbo, S. (1999) *Nature Genetics.* **22**, 78–81

Kaessmann, H., Wiebe, V., and Pääbo, S. (1999) Extensive nuclear DNA diversity among chimpanzees. *Science.* **286**, 1159–1162

Kaessmann, H., Wiebe, V., Weiss, G., and Pääbo, S. (2001) Great ape DNA sequences reveal a reduced diversity and an expansion in humans. *Nature Genetics.* **27**, 155–156

Kaneko, M., Satta, Y., Matsura, E.T., and Chigusa, S. (1993) Evolution of the mitochondrial ATPase 6 gene in *Drosophila*: Unusually high level of polymorphism in *D. melanogaster. Genet. Res.* **61**, 195–204

Kaplan, N.L., Darden, T., and Hudson, R.R. (1988) The coalescent in models with selection. *Genetics.* **120**, 819–829

Kaplan, N.L., and Hudson, R.R. (1985) The use of sample genealogies for studying a selectively neutral *m*-locus model with recombination. *Theor. Popul. Biol.* **28**, 382–396

Kaplan, N.L., Hudson, R.R., and Langley, C.H. (1989) The "hitchhiking effect" revisited. *Genetics.* **123**, 887–899

Kececioglu, J., and Ravi, R. (1995) Of mice and men: Evolutionary distance between genomes under translocation. Pages 604–613 in *Proceedings of* the 6th Annual ACM-SIAM Symposium on Discrete Algorithms. ACM, New York

Keightley, P.D. (1994) The distribution of mutation effects on viability in Drosophila melanogaster. Genetics. **138**, 1315–1322

Keogh, R.S., Seoighe, C., and Wolfe, K.H. (1998) Evolution of gene order and chromosome number in Saccharomyces, Kluyveromyces, and related fungi. Yeast. **14**, 443–457

Kimura, M. (1953) "Stepping stone" model of population. Ann. Rep. Natl. Inst. Genetics Japan. **3**, 62–63

Kimura, M. (1962) On the probability of fixation of mutant genes in a population. Genetics. **47**, 713–719

Kimura, M. (1968) Evolutionary rate at the molecular level. Nature. **217**, 624–626

Kimura, M. (1969) The number of heterozygous nucleotide sites maintained in a finite population due to a steady flux of mutations. Genetics. **61**, 893–903

Kimura, M. (1971) Theoretical foundations of population genetics at the molecular level. Theor. Popul. Biol. **2**, 174–208

Kimura, M. (1980) A simple method for estimating evolutionary rates of base substitutions through comparative studies of nucleotide sequences. J. Mol. Evol. **16**, 111–120

Kimura, M. (1981) Estimation of evolutionary distances between homologous nucleotide sequences. Proc. Natl. Acad. Sci. USA. **78**, 454–458

Kimura, M., and Crow, J.F. (1964) The number of alleles that can be maintained in a finite population. Genetics. **49**, 725–738

Kimura, M., and Maruyama, T. (1966) The mutational load with epistatic gene interactions in fitness. Genetics. **54**, 1337–1351

Kimura, M., and Maruyama, T. (1971) Patterns of neutral polymorphism in a geographically structured population. Genet. Res. **18**, 125–131

Kimura, M., and Ohta, T. (1969) The average number of generations until the fixation of a mutant gene in a finite population. Genetics. **61**, 763–771

Kimura, M., and Weiss, G.H. (1964) The stepping stone model of population structure and the decrease of genetic correlation with distance. Genetics. **49**, 561–576

Kingman, J.F.C. (1982a) The coalescent. Stoch. Proc. Appl. **13**, 235–248

Kingman, J.F.C. (1982b) Exchangeability and the evolution of large populations. Pages 97–112 in Exchangeability in Probability and Statistics. Edited by G. Koch and F. Spizzichino. North-Holland, Amsterdam

Knox, E.B., Downie, S.R., and Palmer, J.D. (1993) Chloroplast genome rearrangements and the evolution of giant lobelias from herbaceous ancestors. Mol. Biol. Evol. **10**, 414–430

Kocher, T.D., and Wilson, A.C. (1991) Sequence evolution of mitochondrial DNA in human and cchimpanzee control region and a protein-coding region. Pages 391–413 in *Evolution of Life: Fossils, Molecules, and Cultures.* Edited by S. Osawa and T. Honjo. Springer, Tokyo

Koizumi, T., et al. (1992) Linkage but not gene order, of homologous loci, including α-L-iduronidase (*Idua*), is conserved in the Huntington disease region of the mouse and human genomes. *Mammalian Genome.* **3**, 23–27

Kreitman, M. (1983) Nucleotide polymorphism at the alcohol dehydrogenase locus of *Drosophila melanogaster. Nature.* **304**, 412–417

Kreitman, M., and Aguadé, M. (1986a) Genetic uniformity in two populations of *Drosophila melanogaster* as revealed by filter hybridization of four-nucleotide-recognizing restriction enzyme digests. *Proc. Natl. Acad. Sci. USA* **83**, 3562–3566

Kreitman, M., and Aguadé, M. (1986b) Excess polymorphism at the *Adh* locus in *Drosophila melanogaster. Genetics.* **114**, 93–110

Kreitman, M., and Hudson, R.R. (1991) Inferring the evolutionary histories of the *Adh* and *Adh-dup* loci in *Drosophila melanogaster* from patterns of polymorphism and divergence. *Genetics.* **127**, 565–582

Krone, S.M., and Neuhauser, C. (1997) The genealogy of samples in models with selection. *Genetics.* **145**, 519–534

Kruglyak, L. (1999) Prospects for whole-genome linkage disequilibrium mapping of common disease genes. *Nature Genetics.* **22**, 139–144

Kruglyak, L., and Nickerson, D.A. (2001) Variation is the spice of life. *Nature Genetics.* **27**, 234–236

Ku, H.M., Vision, T., Liu, J., and Tanksley, S.D. (2000) Comparing sequenced segments of the tomato and *Arabidopsis* genomes: Large scale duplication followed by selective gene loss creates a network of synteny. *Proc. Natl. Acad. Sci. USA* **97**, 9121–9126

Lalo, D., Stettler, S., Mariotte, S., Slominski, P.P., and Thuriaux, P. (1993) Two yeast chromosomes are related by a fossil duplication of their centromeric regions. *C.R. Acad. Sci. III.* **316**, 367–373

Li, W.H. (1977) Distribution of nucleotide differences between two randomly chosen cistrons in a finite population. *Genetics.* **85**, 331–337

Li, W.H. (1997) *Molecular Evolution.* Sinauer, Sunderland, MA

Li, W.H., and Sadler, L.A. (1991) Low nucleotide diversity in man. *Genetics.* **129**, 513–523

Lynch, M., and Conrey, J.S. (2000) The evolutionary fate and consequences of duplicated genes. *Science.* **290**, 1151–1159

Lynch, M., and Crease, T.J. (1990) The analysis of population survey data on DNA sequence variation. *Mol. Biol. Evol.* **7**, 377–394

MacDonald, J.H., and Kreitman, M. (1991) Adaptive protein evolution at the *Adh* locus in *Drosophila*. *Nature*. **351**, 652–654

Makarov, C.A., and Palmer, J.D. (1988) Mitochondrial DNA rearrangements and transcriptional alterations in the male-sterile cytoplasm and ogura radish. *Molecular and Cell Biology*. **8**, 1474–1480

Malécot, G. (1967) Identical loci and relationship. *Proceedings of the 5th Berkeley Symp*. **4**, 317-332, U. of California Press

Malécot, G. (1969) *The Mathematics of Heredity*. Freeman, San Francisco

Martial, J.A., Hallewell, R.A., Baxter, J.D., and Goodman, H.M. (1979) Human growth hormone: complimentarity and expression in bacteria. *Science*. **205**, 602–607

Maruyama, T. (1970) Effective number of alleles in a subdivided population. *Theor. Popul. Biol.* **1**, 273–306

Maruyama, T. (1971) Analysis of population structure. II. Two dimensional stepping stone models of finite length and other geographically structured populations. *Ann. Hum. Genet. London* **35**, 179–196

Maynard Smith, J. and Haigh, J. (1974) The hitchhiking effect of a favorable gene. *Genet. Res.* **23**, 23–35

Milligan, B.G., Hampton, J.N., and Palmer, J.D. (1989) Dispersed repeats and structural reorganization in subclover chloroplast DNA. *Mol. Biol. Evol.* **6**, 355–368

Miyata, T., Hayashida, H., Kikuno, R., Hasegawa, M., Kobyashi, M., and Koike, K. (1982) Molecular clock of silent substitution: At least a six-fold preponderance of silent changes in mitochondrial genes over those in nuclear genes. *J. Mol. Evol.* **19**, 28–35

Moore, G., Devos, K.M., Wang, Z., and Dale, M.D. (1995) Grasses, line up and form a circle. *Current Biology*. **5**, 737–739

Moran, P.A.P. (1958) Random processes in genetics. *Proc. Cambridge. Philos. Soc.* **54**, 60–71

Nachman, M.W. (1998) Deleterious mutations in animal mitochondrial DNA. *Genetica*. **102/103**, 61–69

Nachman, M.W., and Crowell, S.L. (2000) Contrasting evolutionary histories of two introns of the Duchene muscular dystrophy gene, *Dmd*, in humans. *Genetics*. **155**, 1855–1864

Nachman, M.W., Bauer, V.L., Crowell, S.L., and Aquadro, C.F. (1998) DNA variability and recombination rates at X-linked loci in humans. *Genetics*. **150**, 1133–1141

Nadeau, J.H. (1989) Maps of linkage and synteny homologies between mouse and man. *Trends in Genetics*. **5**, 82–86

Nadeau, J.H., and Sankoff, D. (1998) The lengths of undiscovered conserved segments in comparative maps. *Mammalian Genome*. **9**, 491–495

Nadeau, J.H., and Taylor, B.A. (1984) Lengths of chromosomal segments conserved since divergence of man and mouse. *Proc. Natl. Acad. Sci. USA.* **81**, 814–818

Nagylaki, T. (1974) The decay of genetic variability in geographically structured populations. *Proc. Natl. Acad. Sci. USA* **71**, 2932–2936

Nei, M. (1975) *Molecular Population Genetics and Evolution.* American Elsevier, North-Holland, Amsterdam

Nei, M., Maruyama, T., and Chakraborty, R. (1975) The bottleneck effect and genetic variability in populations. *Evolution.* **29**, 1–10

Nei, M., and Takahata, N. (1993) Effective population size, genetic diversity, and coalescence time in subdivided populations. *J. Mol. Evol.* **37**, 240–244

Neuhauser, C., and Krone, S.M. (1997) Ancestral processes with selection. *Theor. Popul. Biol.* **51**, 210–237

Nickerson, D.A., et al. (1998) DNA sequence diversity in a 9.7kb segment of the human lipoprotein lipase gene. *Nature Genetics.* **19**, 233–240

Nordborg, M., Charlesworth, B., and Charlesworth, D. (1996) The effect of recombination on background selection. *Genet. Res.* **67**, 159–174

Oakeshott, J.G., et al. (1982) Alcohol dehydrogenase and glycerol-3-phosphate dehydrogenase clines in *Drosophila melanogaster* on different continents. *Evolution.* **36**, 86–92

Ohno, S. (1967) *Sex Chromosomes and Sex-linked Genes.* Springer-Verlag, New York

Ohta, T. and Kimura, M. (1975) The effect of selected linked lcous on the heterozygosity of neutral alleles (the hitch-hiking effect). *Genet. Res.* **25**, 313–326

Palmer, J.D., and Herbon, L.A. (1987) Unicircular structure of the *Brassica hirta* mitochondrial genome. *Current Genetics.* **11**, 565–570

Palmer, J.D., and Herbon, L.A. (1988) Plant mitochondrial DNA evolves rapidly in structure but slowly in sequence. *J. Mol. Evol.* **28**, 87–97

Palmer, J.D., Osorio, B., and Thompson, W.F. (1988) Evolutionary significance of inversions in legume chloroplast DNAs. *Current Genetics.* **14**, 65–74

Paterson, A.H., et al. (2000) Comparative genomics of plant chromosomes. *Plant Cell.* **12**, 1523–1540

Pevzner, P. (2000) *Computational Molecular Biology: An Algorithmic Approach.* MIT Press, Cambridge, MA

Przeworski, M., Hudson, R.R., and DiRienzo, A. (2000) Adjusting the focus on human variation. *Trends in Genetics.* **16**, 296–302

Rogers, A.R., and Harpending, H. (1992) Population growth makes waves in the distribution of pairwise genetic differences. *Mol. Biol. Evol.* **9**, 552–569

Rooney, A.P., and Zhang, J. (1999) Rapid evolution of a primate sperm protein: Relaxation of function constraint or positive Darwinian selection. *Mol. Biol. Evol.* **16**, 706–710

Sankoff, D., and Blanchette, M. (1998a) Multiple genome rearrangement and breakpoint phylogeny. *J. Comp. Biol.* **5**, 555-570

Sankoff, D., and Blanchette, M. (1998b) Breakpoint phylogenies. Pages 243–247 in the proceedings of RECOMB 98, ACM, New York

Sankoff, D., and Ferretti, V. (1996) Karyotype distributions in a stochastic model of reciprocal translocation. *Genome Research.* **6**, 1–9

Sankoff, D., and Nadeau, J.H. (1996) Conserved synteny as a measure of genomic distance. *Discrete Appl. Math.* **71**, 247–257

Sankoff, D., Parent, M.N., Marchand, I., Ferretti, V. (1997) On the Nadeau-Taylor theory of conserved chromosome segments. Pages 262–274 in *Combinatorial Pattern Matching, Eighth Annual Symposium.* Edited by A. Apostolico and J. Hein. Lecture Notes in Computer Science **1264** Springer, Berlin

Schaeffer, S.W., and Miller, E.L. (1993) Estimation of linkage disequilibrium and the recombination parameter determined from the alcohol dehydrogenase region of *Drosophila pseudoobscura. Genetics.* **135**, 541–552

Schubert, I., and Oud, J.L. (1997) There is an upper limit of chromosome size for normal development of an organism. *Cell.* **88**, 515–520

Seeburg, P.H., Shine, J., Martial, J.A., Baxter, J.D., and Goodman, H.M. (1977) Nucleotide sequence and amplification in bacteria of structural gene for rat grwoth hormone. *Nature.* **270**, 486–494

Seielstad, M.T., Minch, E., and Cavalli-Sforza, L.L. (1998) Genetic evidence for a higher migration rate in humans. *Nature Genetics.* **20**, 278–280

Seoighe, C., and Wolfe, K.H. (1998) Extent of genome rearrangement after genome duplication in yeast. *Proc. Natl. Acad. Sci. USA.* **95**, 4447–4452

Seoighe, C., and Wolfe, K.H. (1999) Updated map of duplicated regions in the yeast genome. *Gene.* **238**, 253–261

Simonsen, K.L., Churchill, G.A., and Aquadro, C.F. (1995) Properties of statistical tests of neutrality for DNA polymorphism data. *Genetics.* **141**, 413–429

Singh, R.S., Lewontin, R.C., and Felton, A.A. (1976) Genetic heterogeneity within electrophoretic "alleles" of xanthine dehydrogenase in *Drosophila pseudoobscura. Genetics.* **84**, 609–629

Slade, P.F. (2000a) Simulation of selected genealogies. *Theor. Popul. Biol.* **57**, 35–49

Slade, P.F. (2000b) Most recent common ancestor probability distributions in gene genealogies under selection. *Theor. Popul. Biol.* **58**, 291–305

Slatkin, M. (1987) The average number of sites separating DNA sequences drawn from a subdivided population. *Theor. Popul. Biol.* **32**, 42–49

Slatkin, M. (1991) Inbreeding coefficients and coalescent times. *Genet. Res. camb.* **58**, 167–175

Slatkin, M. (1993) Isolation by distance in equilibrium and non-equilibrium populations. *Evolution.* **47**, 264–279

Slatkin, M., and Barton, N.H. (1989) A comparison of three indirect methods of estimating average levels of gene flow. *Evolution.* **43**, 1349–1368

Slatkin, M., and Hudson, H. (1991) Pairwise comparison of mitochondrial DNA sequences in stable and exponentially growing populations. *Genetics.* **129**, 555–562

Smith, M.M. (1987) Molecular evolution of *Saccharomyces cerevisiae* histone gene loci. *J. Mol. Evol.* **24**, 252–259

Stephan, W., Wiehe, T., and Lenz, M.W. (1992) The effect of strongly selected substitutions on neutral polymorphism: Analytical results based on diffusion theory. *Theor. Popul. Biol.* **41**, 237–254

Stoneking, M., Bhatia, K., and Wilson, A.C. (1986) Rates of sequence divergence estimated from restriction maps of mitochondrial DNAs from Papua New Guinea. *Cold Spring Harbor Symposia on Quantitative Biology.* **51**, 433–439

Strobeck, C. (1987) Average number of nucleotide differences in a sample from a single subpopulation: A test for population subdivision. *Genetics.* **117**, 149–153

Tajima, F. (1983) Evolutionary relationship of DNA sequences in finite populations. *Genetics.* **105**, 437–460

Tajima, F. (1989) Statistical method for testing the neutral mutation hypothesis by DNA polymorphism. *Genetics.* **123**, 585–595

Tajima, F., and Nei, M. (1982) Biases of the estimates of DNA divergence obtained by the restriction enzyme technique, *J. Mol. Evol.* **18**, 115–120

Tajima, F., and Nei, M. (1984) Estimation of evolutionary distance between nucleotide sequences. *Mol. Biol. Evol.* **1**, 269–285

Takahata, N. (1983) Gene identity and genetic differentiation of populations in the finite island model. *Genetics.* **104**, 497–512

Takahata, N. (1995) A genetic perspective on the origins and history of humans. *Annu. Rev. Ecol. Syst.* **26**, 343–372

Takahata, N., and Nei, M. (1984) F_{ST} and G_{ST} statistics in the finite island model. *Genetics.* **107**, 501–504

Tamura, K., and Nei, M. (1993) Estimation of the number of nucleotide substitutions in the control region of mitochondrial DNA in human and chimpanzees. *Mol. Biol. Evol.* **10**, 512–526

Tavaré, S. (1984) Line of descent and genealogical processes, and their applications in population genetics models. *Theor. Popul. Biol.* **26**, 119–164

Tavaré, S. (1987) The birth process with immigration, and the genealogical structure of large populations. *J. Math. Biol.* **25**, 161–168

Tsaur, S.C., Ting, C.T., and Wu, C.I. (1998) Positive selection driving the evolution of a gene of male reproduction, *Acp26Aa*, of *Drosophila*: II. Divergence versus polymorphism. *Mol. Biol. Evol.* **15**, 1040–1046

Vigilant, L., Pennington, R., Harpending, H., Kocher, T.D., and Wilson, A.C. (1989) Mitochondrial DNA sequences in single hairs from a southern African population. *Proc. Natl. Acad. Sci. USA.* **86**, 9350–9354

Vision, T.J., Brown, D.G., and Tanksley, S.D. (2000) The origin of genomic duplications in *Arabidopsis. Science.* **290**, 2114–2117

Wakeley, J. (1993) Sustitution rate variation among sites in hypervariable region 1 of human mitochondrial DNA. *J. Mol. Evol.* **37**, 613–623

Wakeley, J. (1997) Using the variance of pairwise differences to estimate the recombination rate. *Genet. Res.* **69**, 45–48

Wall, J.D. (2000) A comparison of estimators of the population recombination rate. *Mol. Biol. Evol.* **17**, 156–163

Wall, J.D., and Przeworski, M. (2000) When did the human population size start increasing? *Genetics.* **155**, 1865–1874

Ward, R.H., Frazier, B.L., Dew-Jager, K., and Pääbo, S. (1991) Extensive mitochondrial diversity within a single Amerindian tribe. *Proc. Natl. Acad. Sci. USA.* **88**, 8720–8724

Watson, G.N. (1966) *A Treatise on the Theory of Bessel Functions.* Cambridge University Press

Watson, J.D., and Crick, F.H.C. (1953a) A structure for deoxyribonucleic acids. *Nature.* **171**, 737–738

Watson, J.D., and Crick, F.H.C. (1953b) The structure of DNA. *Cold Spring Harbor Symp. Quant. Biol.* **18**, 123–131

Watterson, G.A. (1975) On the number of segregating sites in genetical models without recombination. *Theor. Popul. Biol.* **7**, 256–276

Watterson, G.A. (1977) Heterosis or neutrality? *Genetics.* **85**, 789–814

Watterson, G.A. (1978) An analysis of multi-allelic data. *Genetics.* **88**, 171–179

Weir, B.S. and Cockerham, C.C. (1984) Estimating *F*-statistics for the analysis of population structure. *Evolution.* **38**, 1358–1370

Weiss, G.H., and Kimura, M. (1965) A mathematical analysis of the stepping stone model of genetic correlation. *J. Appl. Prob.* **2**, 129–149

Weiss, G., and von Haeseler, A. (1998) Inference of population history using a likelihood approach. *Genetics.* **149**, 1539–1546

Wiehe, T., and Stephan, W. (1993) Analysis of genetic hitchhiking model and its application to DNA polymorphism data from *Drosophila melanogaster. Mol. Biol. Evol.* **10**, 842–854

Wilson, W.A., Harrington, S.E., Woodman, W.L., Lee, M., Sorrells, M.E., and McCouch, S.R. (1999) Inferences on the genome structure of progenitor maize through comparative analysis of rice, maize, and the domesticated panicoids. *Genetics.* **153**, 453–473

Wolfe, K.H., and Shields, D.C. (1997) Molecular evidence for an ancient duplication of the entire yeast genome. *Nature.* **387**, 708–713

Wright, S. (1943) Isolation by distance. *Genetics* **28**, 114–156

Wright, S. (1951) The genetical structure of populations. *Ann. Eugen.* **15**, 323–354

Wyckoff, G.J., Wang, W., and Wu, C.I. (2000) Rapid evolution of male reproductive genes in the descent of man. *Nature.* **403**, 304–308

Yang, Z. (1996) Among-site rate variation and its impact on phylogenetic analyses. *Trends. Ecol. Evol.* **11**, 367–372

Zharkikh, A. (1994) Estimation of evolutionary distances between nucleotide sequences. *J. Mol. Evol.* **39**, 315–329

Index

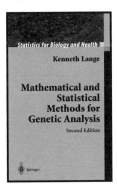
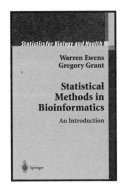
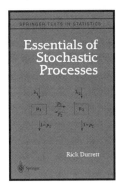
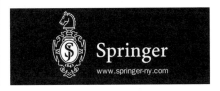